The Heart Attack Germ

The Heart Attack Germ

◆

Prevent Strokes, Heart Attacks and the Symptoms of Alzheimer's by Protecting Yourself from the Infections and Inflammation of Cardiovascular Disease

*Louis A. Dvonch, M.D. and
Russell Dvonch*

Writer's Showcase
New York Lincoln Shanghai

The Heart Attack Germ
Prevent Strokes, Heart Attacks and the Symptoms of Alzheimer's by Protecting Yourself from the Infections and Inflammation of Cardiovascular Disease

All Rights Reserved © 2003 by Louis A. Dvonch, M.D. and Russell Dvonch

No part of this book may be reproduced or transmitted in any form or by any means, graphic, electronic, or mechanical, including photocopying, recording, taping, or by any information storage retrieval system, without the written permission of the publisher.

Writer's Showcase
an imprint of iUniverse, Inc.

For information address:
iUniverse, Inc.
2021 Pine Lake Road, Suite 100
Lincoln, NE 68512
www.iuniverse.com

ISBN: 0-595-26220-1

Printed in the United States of America

In memory of Julie

Contents

Introduction 1

PART 1: How Infection and Inflammation Create Strokes, Heart Attacks and the Symptoms of Alzheimer's Disease

Chapter 1	The Heart Attack Germ 7
Chapter 2	The Chlamydia Story 26
Chapter 3	A Refresher Course in Strokes and Heart Attacks 35
Chapter 4	The Response to Injury 57
Chapter 5	Chronic Inflammation 67
Chapter 6	Inflammatory Atherosclerosis 76
Chapter 7	Vulnerable Plaque and Blood Clots 96
Chapter 8	The Triggers of Strokes and Heart Attacks 108
Chapter 9	Risk Factors—Old and New 127
Chapter 10	Bugs in the System: The Link between Infection, Inflammation and Cardiovascular Disease 152
Chapter 11	The Germs of Strokes and Heart Attacks 160
Chapter 12	The Arguments for Chlamydia Pneumoniae as a Cause of Strokes and Heart Attacks 184

CHAPTER 13	Antibiotics and the Prevention of Cardiovascular Disease	200
CHAPTER 14	Cardiovascular Germs and the Symptoms of Alzheimer's Disease	214

PART 2: Preventing Strokes, Heart Attacks and the Symptoms of Alzheimer's Disease with WIN/WIN Therapy

CHAPTER 1	A Philosophy of Healing	227
CHAPTER 2	The Five Steps of WIN/WIN Therapy	235
CHAPTER 3	An Added Advantage of WIN/WIN Therapy	326
CHAPTER 4	The Future of WIN/WIN Therapy and the Heart Attack Germ	329
CHAPTER 5	The Heart Attack Germ on the Web at www.theheartattackgerm.com	333

About the Authors 335
Endnotes 337

Acknowledgment

The authors wish to thank Barbara Hogenson, Jeffrey Couchman, Douglas Borton and the family of Dr. Dvonch for their help and encouragement in the preparation of this book.

NOTE:

A key principle of *The Heart Attack Germ* is that treating atherosclerosis and cardiovascular disease always requires the care of a physician. Always consult your physician before starting or changing any medical treatment.

Visit *The Heart Attack Germ* on the web at
www.theheartattackgerm.com
for announcements and the latest news on the cause and cure of strokes, heart attacks and the symptoms of Alzheimer's disease.

Introduction

Question: What's the most important "risk factor" for strokes and heart attacks?

Answer: Not reading this book!

It's true. *The Heart Attack Germ* is the first book written for the general public that reveals the amazing story of *Chlamydia pneumoniae*—The Heart Attack Germ. This tiny bacterium has sparked a gigantic revolution in the understanding and treatment of strokes and heart attacks. Only *The Heart Attack Germ* explains how you can benefit from this revolution, right now.

Let me give you two quick examples of the groundbreaking medical discoveries revealed in *The Heart Attack Germ* that may prevent a stroke or heart attack in your future.

First, the latest scientific studies by hospitals and universities have found that strokes, heart attacks and the symptoms of Alzheimer's disease begin with inflammation in the arteries of the heart and brain. This inflammation can be caused by bacterial and viral infections. The germs that cause these infections are so common that, at some point in our lives, nearly all of us will get infected by at least one of them.

The contagious germs of cardiovascular disease are easily passed from person to person, which means you can "catch" a stroke or heart attack in much the same way as you catch the flu or a cold. Up until a few years ago, this fact was completely unknown by just about everybody, including your doctor. And because it was unknown, all previous attempts to prevent strokes and heart attacks were largely ineffective.

It is only in the past few years that medical journals from around the world began reporting on cardiovascular inflammation and the germs of cardiovascular disease. Now, you can read for yourself the full story of this remarkable breakthrough that explains the mystery behind the number one killer in America. If you're suffering from atherosclerosis, angina, stroke, heart attack or the symptoms of Alzheimer's, you won't know what's making you sick unless you read *The Heart Attack Germ*.

Now, here is a second recent medical discovery: cardiovascular infections and their inflammation can be treated cheaply, painlessly and effectively with familiar antibiotic, antiviral and anti-inflammatory drugs, thus preventing the onset of strokes and heart attacks and reducing the need for dangerous surgery, such as angioplasty or bypass operations.

These two discoveries alone make *The Heart Attack Germ* unlike any other cardiovascular book you have ever read. Current books do not address infection and inflammation as the twin evils of cardiovascular trouble. Instead, they focus on secondary or contributing factors, such as diet, exercise, cholesterol levels and so on. Therefore, even if you follow the advice in these books, *you are still at risk for a stroke or heart attack* because infection and inflammation have not been treated.

Contrary to popular belief, it doesn't matter how much you exercise or how little cholesterol you eat—if you have infection or inflammation of the heart or brain arteries, you are at risk for stroke, heart attack and the symptoms of Alzheimer's. Only *The Heart Attack Germ* explains this vital information and outlines the steps necessary to insure your maximum protection against cardiovascular disease.

The Heart Attack Germ is not a rehash of old news. You won't find endless charts detailing the sodium content of fast food, pep-talks on how to stop smoking, or pages of low-fat recipes like *Grilled Chicken Breasts with Honey Mustard Glaze* to pad out the last half of the book. The ideas presented in *The Heart Attack Germ* are based on revolutionary breakthroughs in knowledge and technology, backed up by rigorous scientific study and my own experiences during 50 years in private practice. Almost everything you read in this book will be new to you, and will forever change your ideas about the cause and cure of cardiovascular disease.

As a doctor, my goal is to prevent strokes and heart attacks in my patients. As a writer, my goal is to do the same for my readers. With the knowledge contained in *The Heart Attack Germ*, I believe that you, in partnership with your physician, will have the best chance ever of preventing strokes, heart attacks and the symptoms of Alzheimer's disease.

That's pretty much all I have to say by way of an Introduction. As promised, it was quick. But was it convincing?

Are strokes and heart attacks really caused by infections and inflammation? Can you catch a heart attack the same way you catch a cold? Is it possible to prevent a heart attack by taking antibiotic drugs?

Obviously, it will take more than an Introduction to convince you that it's all true. So my advice is…keep reading!

See you in Chapter One!

PART 1:
How Infection and Inflammation Create Strokes, Heart Attacks and the Symptoms of Alzheimer's Disease

1

The Heart Attack Germ

At this very moment, you may be located in the cardiovascular health section of your favorite bookstore, skimming through *The Heart Attack Germ* to judge whether it's worth buying. You'd much rather be paging through the latest John Grisham novel, but right now you've got some serious questions on your mind.

That's because, most likely, you or someone you love is standing in the shadows of cardiovascular disease. So you've decided to scour the bookshelves for authoritative information and sound advice on how to prevent strokes and heart attacks.

In many respects, the news you've found sounds promising. You've read that the rate of strokes and heart attacks has dropped in the past few decades. Many hospitals routinely offer advanced surgical procedures such as coronary bypass and angioplasty for their patients with heart disease. And the shelves are packed with books offering advice on the latest diets and cardiovascular exercises, all designed to reduce your risk of a stroke or heart attack.

And yet...

You have the uneasy feeling that—despite all the words, charts and diagrams you've studied—nobody seems to really understand cardiovascular disease. Least of all, you.

It appears to be a disease without any specific cause...only "risk factors" such as cholesterol levels and a lack of physical exercise. And, as you've no doubt discovered, simply reducing your risk factors is no guarantee that you won't suffer a stroke or heart attack. After all, *nearly half of all patients with cardiovascular disease have no known risk factors.*

And what if you're already suffering from advanced cardiovascular disease? The treatments before you are a gloomy mix of major surgical procedures you'd rather avoid, arduous rehabilitation and radical changes in lifestyle—with no assurance that any of it will do you much good. After all, *cardiovascular disease remains the number one killer in America.*

And so—without much hope that you'll find anything new or encouraging—you picked up a book with the title *The Heart Attack Germ: Prevent Strokes, Heart Attacks and the Symptoms of Alzheimer's by Protecting Yourself from the Infections and Inflammation of Cardiovascular Disease*—which seems an unlikely name. What does a germ have to do with heart attacks? Or inflammation, for that matter. The words "infections" and "inflammation" weren't mentioned in all those other books you'd read. And if there *is* such a thing as a "heart attack germ," then why haven't you heard about it before now?

Welcome to something new and encouraging.

First, the "something new" part. A common bacterium named *Chlamydia pneumoniae* has been identified by scientists and researchers the world over as the Heart Attack Germ. People infected with the germ are at a significantly increased risk for stroke, heart attack and other cardiovascular problems, including the symptoms of Alzheimer's disease. Several other common bacteria and viruses have also been associated with an increased risk of stroke and heart attack. All of these germs are contagious and easily transmitted from person to person. In fact, the odds are that you've *already* been infected by one or more of the germs of cardiovascular disease.

If the news that you might already be infected with the Heart Attack Germ or one of its cardiovascular cousins makes you feel uneasy, take a deep breath and relax because here comes the "encouraging" part.

The recent advances in knowledge and technology that led to the discovery of the Heart Attack Germ have created a radical rethinking about cardiovascular disease. This new understanding has produced improved treatments that—for the first time—attack the underlying cause of strokes, heart attacks and the symptoms of Alzheimer's. These treatments dramatically reduce the risk of many cardiovascular troubles—safely, painlessly, inexpensively and without surgery.

As surprising as it sounds, the fact that science has finally linked strokes, heart attacks and the symptoms of Alzheimer's with infectious germs is very good news! Your doctor has many effective treatments against the Heart Attack Germ and the other germs associated with cardiovascular disease, and more treatments are on the way. After decades of false starts and half-measures, the medical world is finally on the right track toward a cure for cardiovascular disease.

But you don't have to wait for the future. Many of these treatments are available right now, and this book will show you how to start benefiting from them immediately, significantly reducing your risk of stroke, heart attack and the symptoms of Alzheimer's. And that really *is* encouraging news.

As an example of how completely different *The Heart Attack Germ* is from anything else you may have heard about, let's first consider…

The Cause and Prevention of Strokes and Heart Attacks

Despite all you've read, there *is* a particular cause—and a new, preventive therapy—for cardiovascular disease. Thanks to the latest work by hundreds of researchers the world over, the story behind strokes and heart attacks can be summed up in a few short paragraphs…and here they are, with key concepts in bold type:

> Most strokes and heart attacks begin with **inflammation**, often as the result of **germs** that infect the **arteries of the heart and brain**. Although several cardiovascular germs

have been identified, most of the research has centered on the **Heart Attack Germ,** *Chlamydia pneumoniae*—a type of bacteria that is the chief suspect behind many strokes and heart attacks.

Chlamydia pneumoniae, and the other cardiovascular germs, establish **long-lasting, hidden infections** that damage the walls of the artery, producing inflammation. **Constant, long-lasting inflammation creates cholesterol plaque**, which clings to the damaged artery wall.

Over time, mounds of cholesterol plaque build up inside the artery, reducing the flow of blood. This disease process is called **atherosclerosis**. Additional factors—such as **high blood pressure, diabetes and smoking**—contribute to the damage of the artery, which further increases inflammation and the risk of stroke or heart attack.

It usually takes more than the presence of plaque, however, to provoke a stroke or heart attack. Most often, it takes **the sudden appearance of a blood clot** inside the artery. Blood clots appear when "soft cholesterol," which is normally contained within cholesterol plaque, **suddenly leaks out into the bloodstream**. As long as the mounds of cholesterol plaque hold together, and soft cholesterol doesn't leak out, the risk for a stroke or heart attack is low. But **constant inflammation weakens plaque, making it vulnerable to rupture**, allowing soft cholesterol to escape and mix with the bloodstream.

There are certain times when the risk of plaque rupture increases dramatically. Periods of **physical or mental stress** can cause an artery to go into violent contractions called **spasm**. The crushing force of spasm will literally crack open a mound of cholesterol plaque, letting soft cholesterol spurt into the bloodstream. The **soft cholesterol creates an instant blood clot**, which completely shuts down the flow of blood through the artery, **triggering a stroke or heart attack.**

With this new understanding of **the infectious/inflammatory cause of atherosclerosis**, new and more effective treatments become obvious. The best way to prevent strokes and heart attacks is a **preventive cure**—treat infection and inflammation of the arteries as soon as they appear, before the build-up of plaque can even begin. **By preventing infection and inflammation, you can prevent strokes and heart attacks. If a patient is already suffering from cardiovascular disease, treating infection and inflammation will dramatically reduce the risk of further events.**

One of the easiest, safest and surest ways of preventing infection and inflammation is the use of **antibiotic and antiviral drugs**, which are effective in killing or suppressing the germs linked to cardiovascular disease.

Combining anti-infective and anti-inflammatory treatments with the truly helpful, more traditional therapies offers you the greatest protection against cardiovascular disease. It also prevents the unnecessary damage done by **risky surgical procedures** such as bypass surgery and angioplasty. Thanks to the new concepts of infection and inflammation, scientists are already working on **vaccines** that may someday eradicate most strokes and heart attacks.

How THE HEART ATTACK GERM creates strokes and heart attacks

1. The Heart Attack Germ *Chlamydia pneumoniae* enters the body through the mouth and nose, infecting the lungs and causing respiratory diseases such as bronchitis and pneumonia.

2. To cure the infection, the body uses immune cells in the lungs, which surround the germs, swallow them whole, and kill them. But the Heart Attack Germ is difficult to kill and may actually live and multiply inside immune cells.

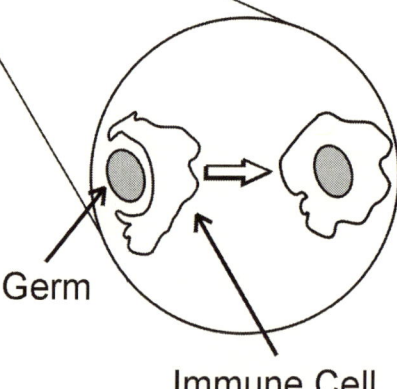

Germ

Immune Cell

How THE HEART ATTACK GERM creates strokes and heart attacks

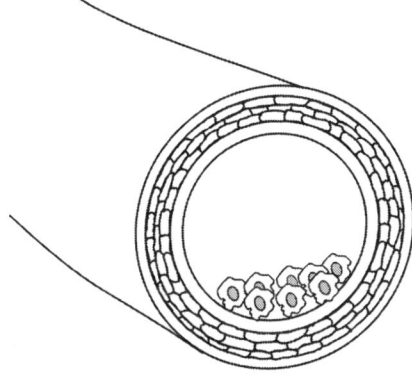

3. Immune cells exit the lungs, carrying the living germs through the bloodstream and into the arteries of the heart and brain. Once inside an artery, the germs multiply, damaging the artery wall and creating long-term infection and inflammation.

4. Long-term infection and inflammation continually draws cholesterol into the artery. Over time, mounds of cholesterol plaque clog the artery, shutting down circulation and setting the stage for a stroke or heart attack.

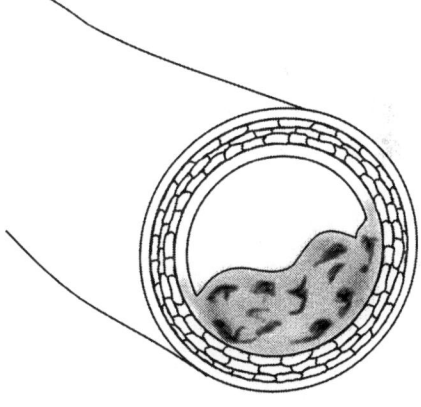

And there you have it.

This—condensed to a few, short paragraphs—is what *The Heart Attack Germ* is all about. During the course of the book, I will explain in detail exactly how infection and inflammation lead to cardiovascular disease and how to use this information—*right now*—to dramatically reduce your risk of strokes and heart attacks.

Even in bite-sized paragraphs, however, all that information may be a little difficult to digest. So let me break it down even further so you'll really understand what lies ahead—and why *The Heart Attack Germ* is unlike any book you've ever read before.

The Heart Attack Germ has two main sections: "Part I: How Infection and Inflammation Create Strokes, Heart Attacks and the Symptoms of Alzheimer's Disease" and "Part II: Preventing Strokes, Heart Attacks and the Symptoms of Alzheimer's Disease with WIN/WIN Therapy." Let's start with…

Part I: How Infection and Inflammation Create Strokes, Heart Attacks and the Symptoms of Alzheimer's Disease

Without question, the most surprising news about strokes and heart attacks is that they can arise from an infectious, contagious disease—so contagious, that nearly every person in America will become infected by *Chlamydia pneumoniae*—the Heart Attack Germ—during the course of a lifetime. And because this germ is easily passed from person to person, you can "catch" a stroke or heart attack the same way you catch the flu or the common cold.

In addition to *Chlamydia pneumoniae*, other germs that infect the cardiovascular system have also been linked to strokes and heart attacks. Like *Chlamydia*, these germs are contagious and will infect the majority of people by the time of late adulthood.

If the news that germs can lead to cardiovascular disease sounds astonishing to you, be assured that the researchers who made the discovery were no less astonished. Yet, study after study has confirmed the news. Only now is this information emerging from the scientific medical journals and appearing in the popular media. Here, in outline, is a closer look at how infective germs can lead to strokes and heart attacks:

Strokes and heart attacks begin with inflammation in the arteries of the heart and brain.

Inflammation is the body's response to injury. It's a protective mechanism that the body uses to heal itself. During inflammation, the body responds to injury with a complex collection of cells and chemicals that work together to kill infective germs, and repair and restore damaged cells and tissues. Most of the time, inflammation is good news—it means that your body has discovered an injury and is functioning properly to heal the damage.

Germs can infect the arteries of the heart and brain, creating inflammation.

Research has now demonstrated that, just like any other part of the body, arteries can become infected by bacteria and viruses such as *Chlamydia pneumoniae*, the Heart Attack Germ. Nearly everyone, at some point in his life, becomes infected by the germs of cardiovascular disease. But because these infections produce no obvious symptoms, they remain hidden from view. Despite being hidden, this infection damages the lining of the arteries, which provokes the healing inflammatory response.

Cholesterol plaque begins as the body attempts to heal itself through inflammation.

As surprising as it sounds, cholesterol plaque begins, *not* as a disease, but as a normal, healthy response by the body. Cholesterol plaque contains many of the inflammatory elements that are designed to destroy infectious germs and repair damaged tissue. These elements are drawn to injured and infected arteries as part of the healing process. That's why—at least, in the beginning—cholesterol plaque is not an abnormal disorder, but a natural part of your body's defense system against disease.

Infection and inflammation in the arteries can last for years or decades.

Although inflammation is the body's way of killing germs, the germs that infect arteries can be very difficult for the body to eliminate completely. Small pockets of bacteria and viruses can linger for a lifetime, slowly spreading disease throughout the artery. Because infections tend to hang on year after year, the artery continues to be inflamed, year after year.

This is where the real trouble begins. Inflammation is designed to be helpful only for the short-term; long-term episodes of inflammation can do great damage to the body.

Long-term infection and inflammation create atherosclerosis, which clogs the artery with cholesterol plaque.

The build-up of plaque within an artery is called atherosclerosis and it's the direct result of long-term inflammation. Since plaque is naturally drawn to the site of inflammation, long-term infection and inflammation continually draws cholesterol plaque to the artery over an extended period of time. As the years pass by—and infection and inflammation secretly simmer away inside their unsuspecting victims—layer after layer of plaque is deposited inside the artery. These layers build into mounds of cholesterol that reduce the flow of blood through the artery, eventually causing many of the symptoms of cardiovascular disease. Even more dangerous, however, is when atherosclerosis creates *no* early symptoms and the first sign of trouble is a sudden stroke or heart attack that seems to appear from out of the blue.

Additional factors—such as high blood pressure, diabetes and smoking—contribute to inflammation, which increases the risk for stroke and heart attack.

For many years, doctors knew that certain medical conditions (such as high blood pressure and diabetes) and certain health habits (such as smoking and obesity) contributed to the risk for strokes and heart attacks...but they were uncertain exactly why. Now they know that inflammation is the key ingredient. Each of these medical conditions and health habits can damage the walls of an artery. The damage leads to inflammation. When infective germs and an aggravating medical condition or health habit combine, they produce a double-whammy of inflammation, increasing the risk of stroke, heart attack and other complications.

Long-term infection and inflammation can turn atherosclerosis deadly, forming "soft cholesterol" and "vulnerable plaque."

It's bad enough that infection and inflammation create cholesterol plaque in the first place. But inflammation turns particularly nasty when it creates "soft cholesterol" and "vulnerable plaque."

You see, the more infection and inflammation a mound of plaque contains, the more likely it is to have a pool of soft cholesterol embedded within it. Think of this core of soft cholesterol as the liquid center of a chocolate candy. Just as the shell of hard chocolate keeps the liquid center from leaking out into the candy box, the hard mound of cholesterol plaque keeps the soft cholesterol from leaking out into the bloodstream—and a good thing, too.

It turns out that soft cholesterol is a super clot-producer. The moment that any soft cholesterol comes into contact with the bloodstream, it immediately begins to congeal the blood, turning it into a clot.

Most of the time, the mound of plaque keeps soft cholesterol safely away from the bloodstream. But active inflammation can weaken plaque, making it vulnerable to rupture. All that's needed is a trigger to crack open the plaque and release the soft cholesterol within it.

Physical or mental stress triggers spasm within arteries, cracking open cholesterol plaque.

Because arteries are designed to react quickly to nervous stimulation, episodes of stress—both physical and mental—can trigger attacks of spasm within an artery. During spasm, the walls of the artery collapse inwardly, rapidly shrinking the diameter of the blood vessel. If the artery is diseased with atherosclerosis, the spasm will literally crush the mounds of cholesterol plaque, rupturing them. And studies show that the very presence of plaque makes an artery more likely to suffer an attack of spasm.

Plaque ruptured by spasm releases soft cholesterol, producing the blood clots that initiate strokes and heart attacks.

This is the endgame. When plaque has been ruptured by spasm, soft cholesterol leaks into the bloodstream, instantly creating a thick, viscous blood clot. If the clot is big enough, it can completely plug up an artery, shutting off the flow of blood to a vital part of the heart or brain. And if the clot doesn't dissolve quickly, a stroke or heart attack is sure to follow.

This new understanding of strokes and heart attacks has led to powerful innovations in treatment, detailed in the second part of this book. So let's move on and consider…

Part II: Preventing Strokes, Heart Attacks and the Symptoms of Alzheimer's Disease with WIN/WIN Therapy

As you can see, infection and inflammation are the chief villains behind strokes and heart attacks. Yet—because this fact was unknown until a few short years ago—*most treatments for cardiovascular disease do nothing to stop infection and inflammation.*

Imagine trying to cure pneumonia without killing pneumonia germs or preventing polio without a vaccine against the polio virus. This is precisely the problem with most cardiovascular therapies; they simply don't fight against the Heart Attack Germ, *Chlamydia pneumoniae,* or the other germs of cardiovascular disease and the inflammation they create. That's why so many of the current treatments—such as surgery and "risk reduction"—have met with limited success. Despite decades of costly improvements in the treatment of cardiovascular disease, *more than two million Americans will suffer a stroke or heart attack this year.*

Clearly, any effective treatment for cardiovascular disease *must* fight against infection and inflammation—and that's exactly what **WIN/WIN Therapy** does.

WIN/WIN stands for **Whip Infection** and **Weaken Inflammation**.

WIN/WIN Therapy is a combination of anti-infective/anti-inflammatory therapy that targets the Heart Attack Germ—*Chlamydia pneumoniae*—and the other germs of cardiovascular disease. WIN/WIN Therapy works hand-in-hand with the more conventional cardiovascular treatments that are truly beneficial.

WIN/WIN Therapy also protects you against many common treatments that seem helpful, but actually contain serious, hidden dangers that may increase your risk for stroke or heart attack. Every element of WIN/WIN Therapy is safe, painless, low in cost and available right now in clinics, hospitals and doctors' offices throughout the nation.

Here's how it works:

WIN/WIN Therapy attacks infection and inflammation, which is the key to preventing strokes and heart attacks.

By eliminating infection and inflammation before atherosclerosis begins, you can eliminate most strokes and heart attacks. But even if atherosclerosis is already present, studies show that reducing infection and inflammation reduces the risk of plaque turning deadly.

This anti-infective/anti-inflammatory therapy is in the forefront of medical treatments for cardiovascular disease. The scientific studies that confirm its benefits have only appeared in the last few years. Yet, at the time of this writing, the evidence is so compelling that 14% of cardiologists in a recent survey *are already treating their patients against infection and inflammation in an effort to control cardiovascular disease.* No doubt, by the time you read these words, the percentage will be much higher.

WIN/WIN Therapy uses antibiotics to safely and painlessly reduce the risk of stroke or heart attack.

Antibiotic and antiviral drugs are potent weapons against the bacteria and viruses that are linked to cardiovascular disease. For example, once it was suspected that strokes and heart attacks were linked to germs, studies were conducted to test the effectiveness of antibiotics in patients with heart disease. Several studies have found that *the use of antibiotics significantly decreases angina, heart attack, cardiac death, bypass surgery, angioplasty and other consequences of heart disease.* That's why

WIN/WIN Therapy uses antibiotic and antiviral drugs as a first line of defense.

WIN/WIN Therapy uses additional anti-inflammatory treatments to lower the risk for cardiovascular events.

Aspirin has anti-clotting properties. When aspirin is given to heart attack patients, the risk of a second heart attack is reduced. And a new class of cholesterol-lowering drugs called statins has also been shown to reduce the risk of heart attack. But the most recent studies suggest that both of these drugs have anti-inflammatory action, which is a key reason why they are beneficial.

WIN/WIN Therapy uses traditional treatments to further enhance the benefits of anti-infective/anti-inflammatory therapy.

Many current heart medications are extremely beneficial to patients with cardiovascular disease. Controlling key risk factors—such as hypertension, diabetes and smoking—can also make a difference. WIN/WIN Therapy combines these traditional therapies with anti-infective/anti-inflammatory treatments, achieving the maximum protection against strokes and heart attacks.

WIN/WIN Therapy reduces the need for dangerous surgical procedures such as coronary bypass and angioplasty.

As a surgeon, I can attest to the fact that all surgery is dangerous, expensive, time-consuming and painful. Surgery rarely cures a metabolic disease, and cardiovascular disease is no exception.

Much of the cardiovascular surgery performed today—such as bypass operations and balloon angioplasty—is unnecessary and can actually *increase* your risk of stroke or heart attack. In many instances, even when this type of surgery is successful, there is little proof that patients will live a longer, healthier life as a result of the operation. One of the chief benefits of WIN/WIN Therapy is that, by preventing the build-up of cholesterol plaque, you can avoid the many costs and hazards of cardiovascular surgery.

WIN/WIN Therapy replaces dangerous stress testing with a safe and painless method to measure your risk for a heart attack.

As mentioned previously, arteries can react to moments of physical or mental stress by collapsing into spasm, which creates the blood clots that trigger heart attacks. That's why testing your body's reaction to stress is a key indicator of your personal risk for a heart attack.

You may already be familiar with the "treadmill" type of stress test. Although the treadmill test has its uses, it has a number of problems as well—not the least of which is that...*it's dangerous.* So dangerous, in fact, that a doctor has to be in attendance when you take the test in case you suffer a heart attack from the stress of the treadmill!

Instead of a treadmill, WIN/WIN Therapy uses the safe and painless "Sit-Down Stress Test." This test easily and accurately detects coronary spasm, which serves as a valuable aid to assessing your personal risk for a heart attack.

WIN/WIN Therapy explains why lowering your "risk factors" is seldom enough to prevent strokes and heart attacks and, in some cases, may actually do more harm than good.

Many of the steps people take to protect themselves from heart disease—such as low-salt diets and vigorous exercise programs—can end up damaging their health. With its emphasis on infection and inflammation, WIN/WIN Therapy places "risk reduction" into proper perspective and shields people from the dangers of many popular therapies.

WIN/WIN Therapy is leading the way to a healthy future where most strokes and heart attacks are eliminated through vaccination.

I believe that, starting with the therapy presented in *The Heart Attack Germ*, strokes and heart attacks will meet the same fate as poliomyelitis, another infective disease. Just as polio was eradicated in the 1950s by vaccination, strokes and heart attacks will also be eradicated once a vaccine is developed that immunizes people from the germs of cardiovascular disease. This will be the ultimate victory for WIN/WIN Therapy.

And now…

A Special Word about The Heart Attack Germ and Alzheimer's Disease

Alzheimer's Disease is a devastating illness—a progressive degeneration of the brain that leads to death. No doubt, it's unexpected that Alzheimer's—a neurological disease—should be included in a book about strokes and heart attacks. But everything you've learned so far about the infectious/inflammatory nature of cardiovascular disease has implications for the treatment of the symptoms of Alzheimer's.

New research indicates that there is an association between inflammation, strokes and Alzheimer's disease. When brain arteries become diseased by inflammatory atherosclerosis, it can lead to strokes and "mini" or "silent" strokes—strokes so small that they are often unnoticed by the victim or his family. The cumulative effect of just a few strokes—even small, silent strokes—can lead to the symptoms of Alzheimer's: progressive memory loss, impaired judgment, personality changes and eventual death.

Furthermore, research indicates that *Chlamydia pneumoniae*—the Heart Attack Germ—and the other germs of cardiovascular disease can infect the arteries of the brain. These infections are most pronounced in the parts of the brain damaged by Alzheimer's.

Consequently, we now have a link between the germs of cardiovascular disease and Alzheimer's: germs infect the brain arteries, infection leads to inflammation, inflammation leads to atherosclerosis, atherosclerosis leads to strokes, which leads, finally, to the symptoms of Alzheimer's. And just as with strokes and heart attacks, studies suggest that anti-inflammatory therapy has a protective effect against the symptoms of Alzheimer's.

"Is It Really True?"

Despite all I've said about infection, inflammation and cardiovascular disease in this opening chapter of *The Heart Attack Germ*, you might be thinking to yourself, "Is it really true? Can an infectious germ really lead to a stroke or heart attack? Can antibiotics really be used to treat heart disease?"

I can understand your doubts. It is only within the past few years that the first reports of germs causing heart disease—and being treated with antibiotics—have been reported in the popular media. *Dateline NBC* did a story on the subject and articles have appeared in several mass-media publications such as *The New York Times, The Wall Street Journal, The Washington Post, The Los Angeles Times, Discovery Magazine, Reader's Digest* and others.

For most readers, however, this will be their first in-depth introduction to an idea that catches everyone by surprise the first time they hear it. But your cardiologist is well aware of the subject; for the last several years it's been *the* hot topic in cardiovascular journals the world over. *The Heart Attack Germ* is the first book to reveal to the general public what researchers have discovered and reported on in professional medical journals. Reading this book will put you well ahead of the curve in the treatment for cardiovascular disease.

In addition, this book reflects the sum of my experiences as a physician and surgeon during more than fifty years in private practice. I hope to enliven the cold medical facts of cardiovascular disease with all the humanity, knowledge and hands-on experience that half a century of healing can bring. I've been using the principles of WIN/WIN Therapy in my own practice for most of the last decade. I can honestly say that the best way to safely and painlessly reduce your risk for stroke, heart attack and the symptoms of Alzheimer's disease can be found in this book, *The Heart Attack Germ.*

An important point to remember as you read this book: atherosclerosis is an inflammatory, and often, infectious, disease. Therefore, treating atherosclerosis—and cardiovascular disease in general—always requires the care of a physician. Always consult your physician before starting or changing any medical treatment.

Perhaps the most persuasive way to illustrate that germs and inflammation *really do* lead to cardiovascular disease is to begin with the remarkable story of the germ most associated with strokes and heart attacks—the Heart Attack Germ itself…

2

The Chlamydia Story

Science has only recently discovered that germs are a major source of strokes and heart attacks. There are several germs linked to cardiovascular disease, but none more important than *Chlamydia pneumoniae*, the Heart Attack Germ.

The first thing I need to tell you about the Heart Attack Germ is how to pronounce it. So, repeat after me:

Kluh-MID-ee-uh New-MOAN-eye-A

Don't worry if you don't get it on the first try. Most of the time, I'll refer to it simply as *Chlamydia* or its common abbreviation, *Cp*.

And since *Cp* is a germ, I should probably explain a few things about germs in general and the infections they cause.

To begin with, an ***infection*** is the invasion by, and the multiplication of, disease-producing ***microorganisms*** within the body. A microorganism, or ***germ***, is a form of life so small that it can only be seen with a microscope. Germs that have a high probability of causing disease are called ***pathogens***.

Most pathogens come in two distinct flavors—***bacteria*** or ***viruses***. Bacteria are actual living cells, capable of metabolism, growth and reproduction. Viruses, however, are *not* alive—they are microscopic containers of genetic material, 20 to 100 times smaller than bacteria. Viruses exist as parasites, invading cells and taking over the reproductive machinery for themselves to create new viruses.

Chlamydia pneumoniae, the germ most often implicated in strokes and heart attacks, is an unusual germ because it's a combination of flavors. It's a type of bacteria, but it shares one important characteristic with viruses: it's a parasite.

This means that *Chlamydia* germs cannot live on their own. They grow, feed and are sheltered in the cells of humans and animals while adding nothing to the survival of their host—a characteristic they quite possibly share with your brother-in-law. Adding injury to insult, these microscopic freeloaders inflict the body of their host with a wide assortment of diseases.

The Chlamydia Family and the Many Diseases They Cause

Chlamydia pneumoniae is only one species of bug in the genus *Chlamydia*, which contains three distinct species of bacterium. Each species causes different types of disease.

For example, **Chlamydia trachomatis** is a type you may already be familiar with, especially if you're a woman. *C. trachomatis* is responsible for pelvic inflammatory disease, a sexually transmitted illness that may result in ectopic pregnancy or sterility. It also causes several other diseases including blindness, reactive arthritis and proctitis. (What's proctitis? Believe me, you don't want to know.)

A second species of the *Chlamydia* germ, **Chlamydia psittaci**, is found in animals, chiefly birds, but it can be transmitted to humans. **Parrot Fever**, a pneumonia-like sickness, is caused by human contact with parrots or parakeets infected with *Chlamydia psittaci*.

The third species, *Chlamydia pneumoniae*, is the one we're interested in. Up until now it has primarily been known as the cause of both upper and lower respiratory infections such as pharyngitis, bronchitis and, as the name suggests, pneumonia—*especially* pneumonia.[1,2] It's thought that 10% of all pneumonia cases are caused by *Cp*.[3]

In addition to atherosclerosis, *Cp* is associated with other cardiovascular illnesses such as myocarditis, pericarditis and endocarditis, which are all diseases of the heart.[4,5] It's been implicated in certain neurological diseases, such as encephalitis, meningitis and multiple sclerosis, and it is also suspected to aggravate asthma.

Whew!—this germ gets around. All in all, *Cp* has distinguished itself as a top-notch pathogen and a model of morbidity.

To a bacteriologist, the story of the discovery of *Cp* makes for fascinating reading, worthy of several chapters. But my son and co-author, Russell, has assured me that the number of bacteriologists out there is considerably limited, so I'll deep-six those chapters and spend just a few paragraphs describing the highlights of…

Chlamydia Pneumoniae—A Bug's Life

The germ *Chlamydia pneumoniae* was discovered in 1965 by Dr. Thomas Grayston. The discovery was an accident—Grayston wasn't looking for anything new; and once he found the germ, he wasn't even sure what he had.

Grayston was in the Far East searching for *Chlamydia trachomatis* which, as mentioned above, can lead to loss of vision. While in Taiwan testing a vaccine against the bug, Grayston collected a germ sample from the eye of a boy who was going blind. Unable to identify the bacterium as *trachomatis*, the germ he was searching for, he stored the sample away.

Flash forward to 1978 and—of all places—northern Finland, where an outbreak of pneumonia hits two Finnish communities. Researchers studying the outbreak think the pneumonia is from a strain of *Chlamydia psittaci*, which causes parrot fever. The trouble is, there is no evidence that any birds are involved in the transmission of the epidemic. What they eventually discover is that the germ seems to be closely related or identical to the unusual strain of *Chlamydia* that Grayston collected in Taiwan.[6] Hmmm…

Flash forward again to 1985. By this time, Grayston has discovered, much to his astonishment, that this unusual strain of *Chlamydia* is infecting students at the school where he teaches, the University of Washington, causing pneumonia, bronchitis and pharyngitis. He believes that this strain of "human" *psittaci* is spread from person to person, without a bird or animal host.[7] Grayston concludes that this type of *Chlamydia* deserves its own name—*Chlamydia pneumoniae*.

Back to Finland again for the breakthrough discovery. Finnish researchers, who are testing blood samples for the newly discovered *Cp*, are stunned to find that a high percentage of the blood drawn from heart disease victims at Helsinki Hospital is testing positive for the germ. Patients with coronary arteries clogged by the cholesterol plaque of atherosclerosis showed an infection rate of 50%. Among patients who suffered a heart attack, 68% of them show *Cp* infection. Both these numbers were significantly higher than the general population.

Can you say "risk factor?"

That's certainly what the Finnish researchers said, although they probably said it with a thick Finnish accent. They set up a prospective experiment called the **Helsinki Heart Study** to determine if chronic *Cp* infection could be a significant new risk factor for the development of coronary heart disease. After analyzing the data from a 5-year trial, they concluded that it could.[8]

This was the beginning of the Heart Attack Germ.

Grayston and other researchers in America and around the world begin their own studies, setting off an explosion of data, nearly all of which confirmed the Finnish study. The conclusion was inescapable: there was a definite link between infection with *Chlamydia pneumoniae* and cardiovascular disease. Not only was *Cp* involved, but several other infectious microbes were also independently associated with cardiovascular disease.

The Chlamydia Bombshell and its Aftermath

Explosions often mark the beginning of revolutions, and that's exactly what happened in the world of medicine as a result of the new data about the Heart Attack Germ. Let me take a few paragraphs to explain how significant these studies were.

In the 19th century, medical knowledge of disease was largely *descriptive,* based on categorizing symptoms. By describing the physical similarities and differences between, say, various types of skin lesions, doctors were able to distinguish measles from chicken pox. Treatments were also based on description—certain medicines or treatments produced certain results.

But merely being able to describe a disease does not mean we understand the cause of it, or that we understand why certain treatments achieve certain results. It wasn't until the end of the 19th century, when the ***germ theory of disease*** was developed, that we really understood the origin of things like measles and chicken pox (both of which are caused by viruses).

Up until a few years ago, modern medicine had a 19th century view of atherosclerosis, the disease characterized by the deposition of cholesterol plaque within the arteries. Our knowledge of atherosclerosis was mostly descriptive—what it looks like, at what age it appears in the body, the consequences of having it, etc. Our knowledge of treatment was also descriptive—improve your diet and you're less likely to suffer from atherosclerosis; lower your high blood pressure and the risks associated with atherosclerosis are lessened. But nobody knew the *cause* of atherosclerosis. Or why certain treatments worked as they do. With our knowledge of atherosclerosis stuck in the 19th century, is it any wonder that cardiovascular disease is still the leading cause of death as we enter the 21st?

In medicine we attach three distinct labels to the causes of disease—"Infective," "Non-infective" and "We Don't Know." Up until now, atherosclerosis was firmly in the "We Don't Know" column. Then suddenly, almost overnight, research into *Cp* kicked atherosclerosis into the "Infective" category and the revolution began.

The discovery of The Heart Attack Germ changed everything. Paradigms shifted. The inexplicable became explicable. The conventional wisdom became unwise. Researchers the world over smacked their collective foreheads and shouted, "Of course!"

Unfamiliar, exotic terms such as "bacteria" and "virus" began to appear in cardiology journals. Med school professors began to utter never-before-heard words like "contagious" and "antibiotics" in their atherosclerosis lectures. Legions of bypass surgeons began to contemplate the meaning of the phrase "out of work."

It truly was an explosion. So much new research was done in so short a time that it became clear that the current medical therapy was deeply flawed. If medical therapies such as bypass surgery, balloon angioplasty and other cutting-edge treatments were *really* effective in preventing strokes and heart attacks, then why the rush to investigate an infectious cause? Why would dozens of researchers from medical clinics, university departments and hospitals from Japan to Argentina leap into investigating the Heart Attack Germ and other possible infectious agents?

The very fact that the explosion of studies and experiments took place underscores the dissatisfaction with current theory and treatments; *you don't rush to find an answer to a problem that is already solved!*

Clearly, the problem of strokes and heart attacks was not being solved by the current treatments that medicine had to offer. That's why researchers were so eager to study *Cp* and the other infectious agents. At last, here was a *cause* of atherosclerosis, not just a description of it.

Know Your Enemy

When it comes to infectious germs, every physician is a firm believer in "Know Your Enemy" and the known facts about the Heart Attack Germ—even apart from the role it plays in strokes and heart attacks—are truly remarkable.

In the space of a decade, *Chlamydia pneumoniae* went from being an obscure germ to being recognized as *one of the most prevalent causes of disease known to man.*

It is well established that *Cp* infection can begin in childhood, even before a child is old enough to attend school.[9, 10] After age five, the rate of infection climbs rapidly up to the age of 15 years.[11] After that, there is a slow increase in the rate of infection throughout adult life. By the time you reach older adulthood, the odds are you've got the germ. Estimates of infection reach as high as 80% and beyond.

As one researcher puts it, "virtually everyone is infected with the *Cp* organisms at some time." (And a great many of us will be infected more than once.)[12] That's a pretty amazing statement considering that, just a few decades ago, *Cp* was completely unknown.

How can it be that this pathogen, which is now recognized as commonplace, could have remained hidden so long?

It turns out that most *Cp* infections are **subclinical**, that is, they show no symptoms.[13] This is a characteristic that's shared by other Chlamydial infections. For example, 50 to 70% of women infected with the sexually transmitted *Chlamydia trachomatis* show no symptoms.

Most *Cp* infections are the same way. Up to 90% of *Cp* infections are asymptomatic.[14] Even the acute phase of the illness is usually just a mild pneumonia, with no indications of disease. In cases where symptoms are present, the pneumonia can be mistaken for a simple case of the flu.

And like influenza germs, the Heart Attack Germ loves a crowd. The infection is contagious, spreading mostly through coughing and sneezing. The victim either inhales the germ as it is suspended in air, or infects himself after touching a surface where the germ lives, such as a tabletop.[15, 16] In conditions where people are living in close proximity, it is easily spread from person to person.[17] Outbreaks of this disease are common in groups of people, from families to military barracks.[18, 19]

It is also found in groups of the very young to the very old. *Cp* is often found in young children attending day-care, although they usually don't get very sick from it.[20] Outbreaks have also been recorded in nursing homes, too. Here, however, the disease is not so benign. If the infection results in acute pneumonia, it can cause serious illness and mortality among the residents, probably due to the reduced immunity of the elderly.[21]

Strokes and Heart Attacks are Contagious

Consider for a moment the enormous implications of the facts as I've outlined them here. The research pouring in from all over the world is confirming that the Heart Attack Germ is a major cause of strokes and heart attacks. Since *Cp* is a germ that is easily transmitted from person to person—so much so, that infections can reach epidemic proportions—that means that strokes and heart attacks are *contagious*, passed along like the flu or a cold!

In fact, for a long time, scientists noticed that the rate of strokes and heart attacks seemed to act suspiciously like contagious diseases—there are definite "seasons" for strokes and heart attacks and outbreaks seem to occur in particular geographic locations, just like infectious epidemics. As you'll discover later in the book, the latest research indicates that respiratory diseases do indeed influence the rate of strokes and heart attacks.

The infectious connection was a shocking realization to the early researchers of the Heart Attack Germ. It would be like suddenly finding out that all cancers were caused by contagious disease. This new understanding of *Cp* demanded a comprehensive rethinking about the true nature of—and a possible cure for—strokes and heart attacks.

At the time of the Finnish research, *Cp* was chiefly known as a cause of pneumonia. The researchers realized it was a very long leap to go from *Cp* infection to strokes and heart attacks. They were understandably puzzled that a germ whose chief illness was a mild case of pneumonia—a disease of the lungs—would be implicated in atherosclerosis—a disease of the arteries. They needed a theory…some way of explaining how an infection by a pneumonia germ could result in a stroke or heart attack.

As it turns out, the theory they needed was being developed at exactly the same moment in other parts of the world.

In order to understand that theory, we need first to take a moment and consider the essentials of cardiovascular disease. That's why I've made the next chapter…

3

A Refresher Course in Strokes and Heart Attacks

Before we can really explore how *Chlamydia pneumoniae* and other germs lead to cardiovascular disease, it's worth our while to spend a few moments to review the basic facts behind strokes and heart attacks.

If you're like most people, you already have a working knowledge of the subject. Thanks to extensive coverage in the media, Americans are familiar with a wide range of cardiovascular topics. And if you or a loved one is currently suffering from cardiovascular disease, I'm sure you know more about the subject than you've ever wanted to learn.

But because your medical knowledge has been gleaned from many different sources over the years, it may be fragmented and incomplete in spots. So this chapter is just to reacquaint you with the major topics and definitions of terms.

First up is...

The Cardiovascular System

I'm sure you remember all about the body's *cardiovascular system* from your high school biology class.

You certainly remember that the primary job of the cardiovascular system is to transport blood to, and from, every part of the body in a process called *circulation.* Blood carries oxygen, nutrients and other things that your body needs in order to function. The two largest constituents of blood are *plasma*, a liquid made mostly of water and salt, and *red blood cells*, whose main function is to transport oxygen.

The HEART and MAJOR ARTERIES

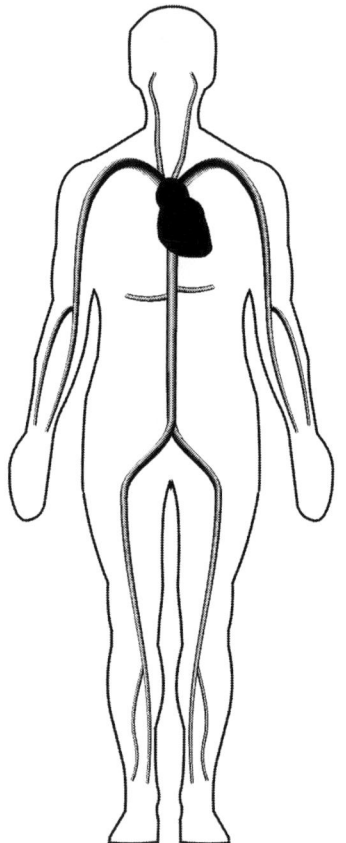

The cardiovascular system circulates blood throughout the body through a network of blood vessels. Strokes and heart attacks originate in the arteries of the heart and brain that are diseased by cholesterol plaque. Illustrated above is the heart and the major arteries of the body, which are often the site of plaque build-up.

There's no need to tell you that the center of the circulatory system is the heart, a strong and active muscle that, with every beat, pumps the blood and keeps it circulating through the body's blood vessels.

And, of course, you recall quite vividly the day your biology teacher explained that the blood travels through three different types of blood vessels.

First are the *arteries*, which carry the blood away from the heart. The main artery, the *aorta*, branches off into smaller and smaller arteries, carrying blood to every part of the body. The entire system of arteries is commonly referred to as the *arterial tree*.

The smallest blood vessels are the *capillaries*. For the most part, it's here where the blood interacts with individual cells, giving them what they need (such as oxygen and nutrients) and taking away from them what they don't need (such as carbon dioxide and waste products).

The capillaries turn into *veins*, which carry the deoxygenated blood back to the right side of the heart. The right side of the heart pumps this deoxygenated blood into the lungs, where carbon dioxide is exchanged for oxygen. This oxygen-rich blood travels back to the left side of the heart, which pumps it out to the rest of the body, and the cycle is repeated.

But since you already knew all that (you *did*, didn't you?), we can move on to defining a word you may not have heard before, but is a critical factor in strokes and heart attacks…

Ischemia

Proper circulation through the cardiovascular system is fundamental to your health. Inadequate circulation is responsible for nearly every symptom and danger associated with strokes and heart attacks. That's why medicine focuses so much attention on fighting the causes of poor circulation.

Any part of the body that does not receive an adequate amount of blood supply is said to be suffering from *ischemia*. In the world of

38   The Heart Attack Germ

strokes and heart attacks, sudden episodes of ischemia are produced in two different ways.

ISCHEMIA
HOW SPASM AND ATHEROSCLEROSIS REDUCE CIRCULATION

Ischemia is the loss of blood flow by an obstruction in an artery. A sudden episode of ischemia is the immediate cause of most strokes and heart attacks. Illustrated here are two common sources of ischemia - spasm and atherosclerosis.

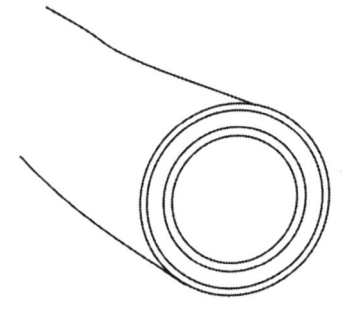

1. This is a cross-section of a normal artery, the way your artery *should* look - round and open, allowing blood to flow freely.

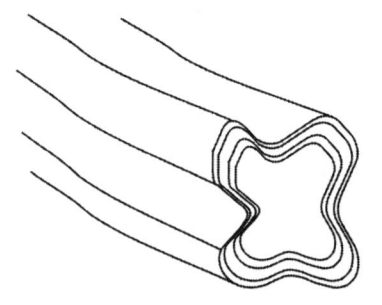

2. This is a cross-section of an artery in spasm, creating ischemia. The walls of the artery squeeze together in an irregular shape. The width of the artery is narrowed, reducing the flow of blood to your heart or brain.

ISCHEMIA
HOW SPASM AND ATHEROSCLEROSIS REDUCE CIRCULATION

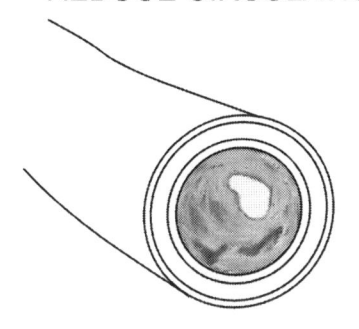

3. Atherosclerosis is the accumulation of cholesterol, inflammatory substances and other cellular debris into a thick plaque that lines the inside of arterial walls. Pictured here is an artery clogged with atherosclerosis. The channel of blood flow is irregularly shaped and very narrow, creating ischemia.

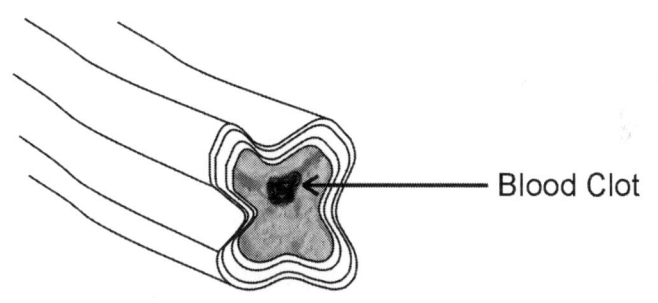

— Blood Clot

4. This is an artery suffering from both atherosclerosis and spasm, a deadly combination. Spasm can break open cholesterol plaque, creating a blood clot which may completely block the flow of blood through the artery, provoking a stroke or heart attack.

First is *spasm*, where the artery suddenly contracts and collapses inwardly. During spasm, the diameter of the artery dramatically reduces in size, restricting the flow of blood. Once an artery goes into spasm, the cells, tissues and organs that depend on blood from that artery begin to suffer, mostly because they become deprived of oxygen.

Ischemia can also occur when an object physically blocks the flow of blood through an artery. Most often, it is a **blood clot** or **cholesterol plaque** that is plugging up the artery. The complete obstruction of an artery by a blood clot or plaque is called an *occlusion*, which, like spasm, deprives the surrounding tissue of oxygen.

A **blood clot** is a jelly-like mass of congealed blood that is viscous enough to plug up an artery. When a clot develops, there are opposing chemical forces in the bloodstream that work to dissolve the clot. As a result, many blood clots don't last very long and the episodes of ischemia they produce are quickly resolved.

Cholesterol plaque, which is composed of many different substances besides cholesterol, has the appearance of a thick, yellowish paste that adheres to the inside of diseased arteries. It, too, can plug up an artery. We'll have much more to say about clots and plaque, but for now let's focus on why the occlusions themselves are so dangerous.

By reducing the flow of blood, occlusions reduce the amount of oxygen available to the cells, tissues and organs that are fed by the artery. Since the cells in your body demand a constant supply of oxygen, they are extremely sensitive to any reduction in the flow of blood.

Lack of circulation also prevents the blood stream from carrying away the byproducts of cells, resulting in a build-up of waste products. The build-up is unhealthy and one of the waste products, ***lactic acid***, is thought to be responsible for the painful symptoms of ischemia.

The seriousness of an ischemic episode depends on *where* the occlusion takes places and *how long* it lasts.

If an occlusion happens in a small artery, then only a small amount of tissue is damaged. But if occlusion occurs in a major artery, then a large section of tissue may suffer. So where the occlusion takes place can have a dramatic effect on its consequences.

Time is also a factor. If an occlusion lasts only a few seconds, then cells can recover from the loss of oxygen and there is no lasting damage. However, if the occlusion lasts for more than a minute or two, cells begin to die from lack of oxygen and tissue is destroyed.

Whenever a portion of an organ is destroyed by ischemia, it makes it more difficult for the rest of the organ to function properly. Over time, the health of the organ deteriorates from many small episodes of ischemia. Eventually, there comes a point when the organ can't take any more injury, and it ceases to function.

Then again, the entire organ may shut down from a single massive episode of ischemia, if the occlusion happens in a critical area.

Either way—bit by bit or in a single massive blow—the loss of circulation from spasm and arterial occlusions has a devastating effect on any organ, and the rest of the body suffers as a result.

The brain and the heart are organs that are especially susceptible to episodes of ischemia caused by spasm and occlusion. When these episodes last long enough to cause tissue death, they're known as...

Strokes and Heart Attacks

Right from the beginning I should emphasize that, while strokes and heart attacks always cause the destruction of tissues, they do not always cause the immediate death of the victim. Generally, strokes and heart attacks do their damage little by little, over the course of years, until their cumulative effect become life-threatening.

A *heart attack* is a sudden episode of ischemia that permanently damages a portion of the heart muscle. The loss of circulation is usually caused by an occlusion in one of the arteries that supply blood to the heart, although spasm in these arteries has also been known to cause heart attacks.

HEART ATTACK

Coronary Arteries

Blood Clot

Damaged Heart Muscle

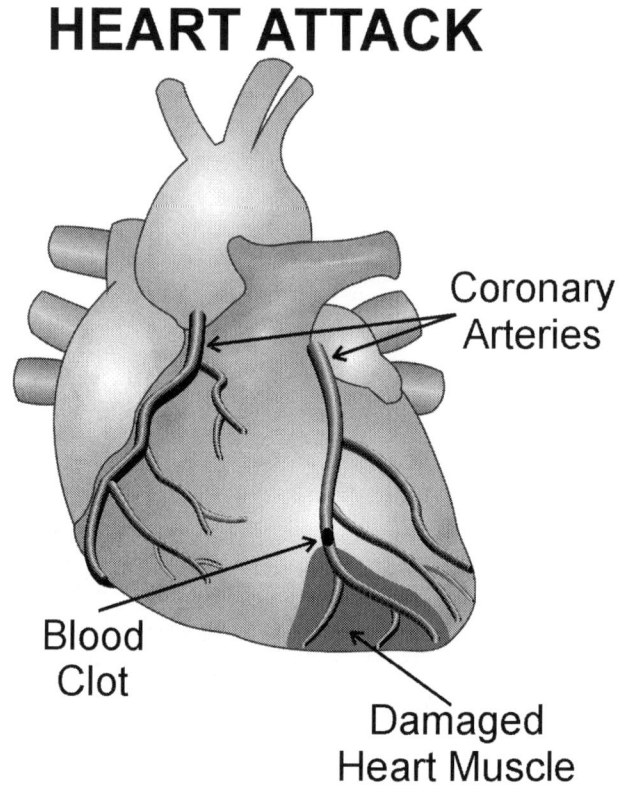

The coronary arteries provide a steady flow of blood that nourishes the heart and keeps it beating. A heart attack occurs when the blood supply inside a coronary artery suddenly becomes severely reduced or stopped altogether. The blood supply can be reduced by coronary spasm, the build-up of cholesterol plaque (called atherosclerosis), or from blood clots. The illustration above shows a blood clot obstructing the flow of blood through a coronary artery. This loss of circulation, called ischemia, damages a section of heart muscle provoking a heart attack, which weakens the heart's ability to beat.

STROKE

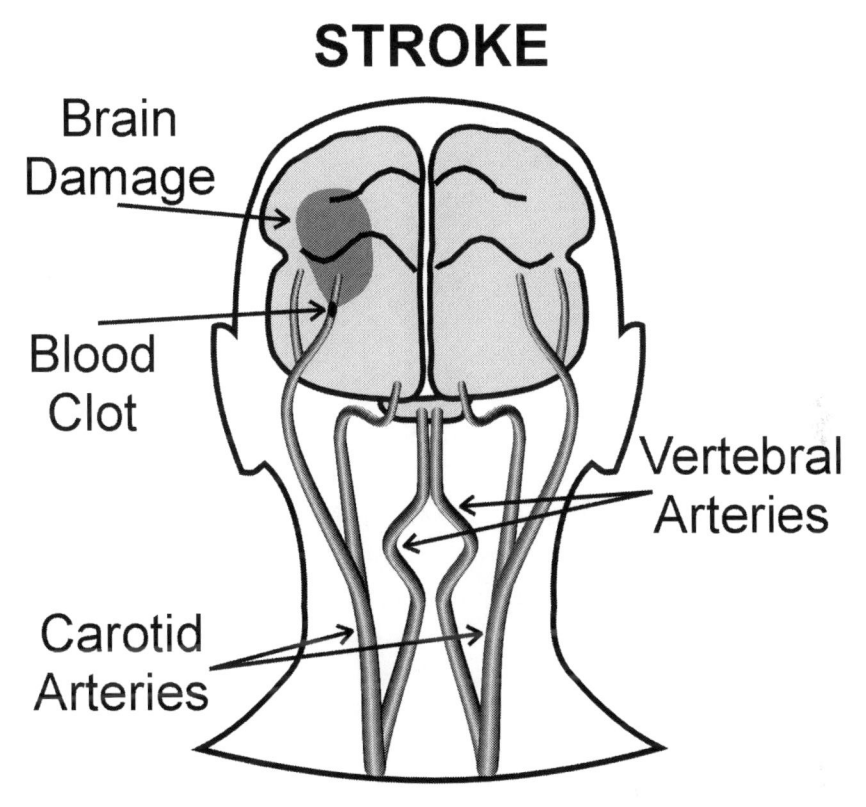

- Brain Damage
- Blood Clot
- Vertebral Arteries
- Carotid Arteries

Just like the heart, the brain also needs a steady supply of blood to function properly. There are four main blood supplies to the brain - two carotid arteries and two vertebral arteries. A stroke (or "brain attack") occurs when blood flow is severely reduced or stopped due to a sudden obstruction from spasm, cholesterol plaque or blood clots. The illustration above shows a blood clot obstructing the flow of blood to the brain, causing damage to brain tissue.

A heart attack is often called a *myocardial infarction,* or **MI**. *Myocardium* is the medical term for the muscle tissue of the heart and an *infarct* is an area of tissue that has died from lack of circulation. So "myocardial infarction" perfectly describes what happens during a heart attack—part of the heart muscle dies from a reduction in blood flow.

A *stroke* is a sudden episode of ischemia that permanently damages a portion of the brain. Just as with a heart attack, the loss of circulation is usually caused by cholesterol plaque or a blood clot occluding one of the arteries that supply blood to the brain.

Recently, the medical community has started referring to strokes as *brain attacks* to emphasize their similarity to heart attacks. The phrase hasn't really caught on yet—it sounds rather clunky to my ears—but it *does* make the point that the basic mechanism behind strokes and heart attacks is the same: the death of tissue caused by the sudden lack of circulation.

There's one more thing that needs to be pointed out about strokes. As mentioned above, strokes are usually caused by occlusions restricting circulation. But circulation can also be restricted if an artery bursts open and begins to bleed. A ruptured artery means that blood can no longer get to where it's needed. That, in turn, leads to the death of brain tissue. (And if blood begins to pool in the brain tissues next to the ruptured artery, the pressure from this pooling blood can also seriously damage the brain.)

So doctors use different terms to distinguish two types of strokes. *Occlusive stroke* describes loss of circulation to the brain from an obstruction in the artery. *Hemorrhagic stroke* describes loss of circulation to the brain caused by a bleeding artery. (To *hemorrhage* means to bleed profusely.) This book is concerned with the more common cause of strokes—occlusions. So, unless otherwise indicated, when I speak of stroke, I'm always referring to the occlusive kind.

And as long as we're on the subject of occlusions, now would be a good time to talk about the disease that most often causes the occlusions that lead to strokes and heart attacks…

Atherosclerosis

Atherosclerosis is a disease of the cardiovascular system. It is characterized by the deposition of cholesterol plaque in the innermost layer of arteries. The plaque, in turn, produces blood clots (in a process that will be discussed later). Often, in the last stages of atherosclerosis, the plaque becomes infiltrated with deposits of calcium, which hardens the plaque and makes the artery inflexible. This is why atherosclerosis is commonly referred to as **hardening of the arteries.**

Because atherosclerosis leads to occlusive cholesterol plaque and blood clots, it's the disease most often linked to strokes and heart attacks.

In many cases, the occlusion happens at the very spot in the artery where the plaque or blood clot originates. Often, however, plaque and clots will form in one part of the artery, then break loose and be swept away by the bloodstream until they lodge in another location. This type of wandering occlusive material is called an *embolus*. When an embolus finally lodges in a downstream artery, it becomes an *embolism*.

Atherosclerosis seems to like certain parts of the arterial tree more than others. As you might suspect, the arteries that supply blood to the heart and brain are common spots for atherosclerosis to develop. Let's take a look at each of these locations, which are…

The Hot Spots of Atherosclerosis

The first hot spots of atherosclerosis are the arteries that supply blood to the heart—the coronary arteries.

The heart is responsible for pumping blood to every organ of the body—even to itself. The heart's blood supply is delivered via the coronary arteries, which branch off directly from the aorta, the main artery that carries oxygenated blood away from the heart. The coronary arteries surround the heart, supplying blood to the heart muscle. There are two main coronary arteries—the *left coronary* and the *right coronary*—but they have many branches that circulate blood to different areas of the heart.

The coronary arteries seem particularly susceptible to the build-up of plaque and subsequent blood clots. It's not uncommon to find multiple branches of the coronary arteries completely occluded by plaque. When that happens, multiple areas of the heart muscle are destroyed by ischemia. Atherosclerosis of the coronary arteries is so common that it has its own name—*coronary artery disease* or ***CAD***.

The aorta itself is often diseased by atherosclerosis and may become occluded at several points along its considerable length. In addition, the walls of the aorta may be damaged by deposits of cholesterol plaque. When this happens, the weakened walls become abnormally wide, ballooning outward in an ***aortic aneurysm***. And, like an over-inflated balloon, the aneurysm can suddenly rupture causing massive bleeding that is often fatal.

One last fact about the aorta: despite its nearness to the heart, the aorta is a significant source of strokes in the brain. Emboli of blood clots and pieces of cholesterol plaque can break off from a diseased aorta and be carried along the bloodstream to the brain.

When it comes to strokes, however, the most common hot spots for damaging atherosclerosis are the four main arteries that supply blood to the brain—the left and right ***carotid arteries***, and the left and right ***vertebral arteries***. When atherosclerosis strikes these arteries, or their branches, the patient is said to have ***cerebrovascular disease***. All four arteries have numerous branches that feed circulation throughout the brain. As a result, strokes can occur in many different areas of the brain.

Long before a stroke or heart attack strikes, there may be signs of impending trouble. These early warning signs are…

The Symptoms of Atherosclerosis

Often, during an examination, a patient will complain of a symptom that seems far removed from strokes or heart attacks. But these symptoms are telltale signs that atherosclerosis is at work and may be afflicting the patient's heart and brain, though the patient is unaware of it.

For example, elderly visitors to my office often complain of pain in their legs after walking for a short time through the shopping mall or around the block. Upon resting for a few minutes, the pain goes away. This condition is called *intermittent claudication* and it's caused by cholesterol plaque narrowing the arteries that supply circulation to the legs.

When the patient is walking, there is an increased demand for oxygen to power the leg muscles and the narrowed arteries can't supply the need. Lack of oxygen and circulation produces a build-up of lactic acid, which causes pain in the muscle. When the patient rests, the need for increased oxygen diminishes, the build-up of lactic acid decreases, and the pain goes away.

Claudication is not the only symptom of atherosclerosis that seems far removed from strokes and heart attacks. *Impotence* may be a consequence of cholesterol plaque reducing circulation to the tissues of the penis. Even a symptom as simple as *cold hands or feet* can indicate atherosclerosis in the arteries that lead to the limbs.

All of these symptoms are an indication of cholesterol plaque clogging up the arteries on the periphery of the body—often called *peripheral artery disease*. Whenever I find evidence of peripheral artery disease, it's likely that the arteries of the heart and brain are also at risk for clogging up with plaque, and the patient will have to be carefully evaluated for coronary and cerebrovascular disease.

There are some symptoms, of course, that are obviously associated with coronary artery disease. The hallmark symptom is *angina pectoris*, often called simply, *angina*—a painful feeling in the chest that is caused by a lack of circulation to the heart.

The symptoms of angina vary greatly depending on the severity of the attack. If the episode is mild, angina can feel no more bothersome than a vague discomfort in the chest. During a severe attack, however, the victim may suffer a feeling of impending death from a crushing, suffocating chest pain that can radiate to the arms, jaw, back and elsewhere. One of my patients described the sensation as a giant hand gripping his heart—and squeezing hard.

The Symptoms of
ATHEROSCLEROSIS

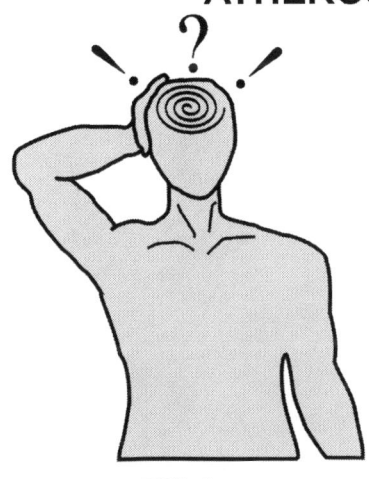

TIA

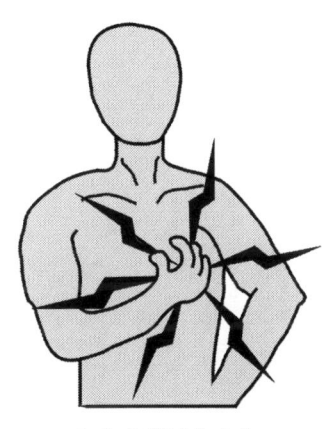

ANGINA

Atherosclerosis in the aortic, carotid or vertebral arteries can cause cerebrovascular ischemia, a deficiency of the blood supply to the brain. The medical name for this event is Transient Ischemic Attack or TIA. The attack appears suddenly, lasts generally from 2-3 minutes to under an hour, and then disappears leaving no residual effects. Common symptoms of TIAs are speech, vision and balancing problems, numbness or weakness of facial muscles, and mental confusion.

Atherosclerosis in the coronary arteries can cause myocardial ischemia, a deficiency of the blood supply to the heart. When this condition produces no obvious symptoms in the patient it is called silent ischemia or silent angina. Often, however, this condition is accompanied by angina pectoris, a sudden attack of chest pain accompanied by feelings of suffocation and impending death. An angina attack can be precipitated by physical exercise or strong emotions, but it can also occur during moments of rest.

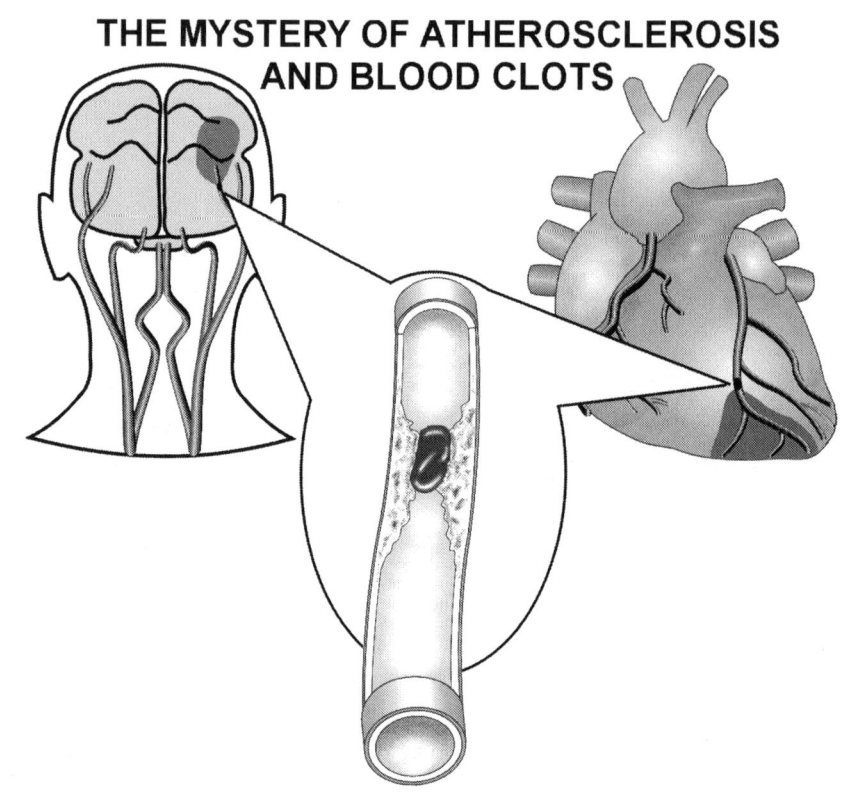

THE MYSTERY OF ATHEROSCLEROSIS AND BLOOD CLOTS

As the drawing above illustrates, both strokes and heart attacks are often caused by the same event - the sudden appearance of a blood clot that becomes snagged inside an atherosclerotic artery, shutting off circulation. For many years, it was unknown why blood clots so often formed at the site of cholesterol plaque, or how the artery itself became diseased by atherosclerosis. But as you'll discover in *The Heart Attack Germ*, both atherosclerosis and blood clots are closely linked to infection and inflammation within the artery. This new knowledge has led to a significant advance in the prevention of strokes and heart attacks.

It is thought that the pain of angina is the result of the same process that produces pain in claudication. Lack of adequate oxygen and circulation in the heart muscle leads to the build-up of lactic acid, causing pain.

Angina attacks are often divided into three categories.

First is *stable angina*. These attacks are called "stable" because the pattern of chest pain is predictable in terms of severity and frequency.

A typical case of stable angina is the patient who is never bothered by chest pain during times of rest; attacks come only when he physically exerts himself—for example, when he climbs a staircase. For this reason, stable angina is often referred to as *effort angina*—the attack comes when a physical effort is made by the patient.

In a patient like this, there is adequate circulation to the heart during times of rest. But during moments of physical exertion, when the amount of blood and oxygen needed to power the heart rapidly increases, the build-up of cholesterol plaque does not allow blood flow to increase. The result is predictable—large portions of heart muscle become starved for oxygen, resulting in the symptoms of angina.

Surprisingly, most patients suffering from stable angina are *not* at an immediate risk for a heart attack. Much more troublesome is the second type of angina—*unstable angina.*

Unstable angina attacks are not predictable in their severity or timing. The amount of pain they produce is variable and they can strike anytime—during moments of physical effort as well as during moments of rest. An attack can begin even while the victim is sleeping. Victims of unstable angina are at an increased risk for heart attack in the near future.

For a long time the cause of unstable angina was a mystery. Recently, however, it was discovered that an attack of unstable angina is due to the sudden appearance of a blood clot which briefly occludes the artery before being dissolved away.

Blood clots can suddenly form at any time in an artery diseased by atherosclerosis, which is why the angina attacks they cause are unpredictable. In addition, clots can vary in size and duration, which explains why the symptoms they produce vary in severity and length.

The third type of angina, called *variant angina*, is caused by spasm in the artery reducing the flow of blood to the heart. Studies indicate that the mere presence of plaque can induce episodes of spasm. And as you'll discover in later chapters, when spasm and plaque occur together, there is a great risk for strokes and heart attacks.

So much for the heart. Let's turn our attention now to the foremost symptom of atherosclerosis that is linked to the brain—*transient ischemic attacks*, often shortened to *TIAs*.

Transient ischemic attacks are aptly named; they are temporary, therefore *transient*, episodes of ischemia in the brain. The symptoms of TIAs have a rapid onset, but the attacks only last for a short time—from mere seconds to perhaps an hour in length. Since the attacks are of short duration, there is no lasting damage to brain tissue and symptoms quickly disappear. Common symptoms of TIAs are speech, vision and balancing problems, numbness or weakness of facial muscles, and mental confusion.

Similar in nature to the episodes of ischemia which give rise to angina, TIAs are caused by arterial spasm and occlusions briefly restricting circulation. Because these ischemic episodes can happen in different areas of the brain, the specific symptoms of a TIA depend on which part of the brain suffers the temporary loss of blood flow.

Angina and TIAs are tangible, often painful, evidence that atherosclerosis is slowly choking life from the body. The one virtuous quality of these symptoms is that they *are* evidence—evidence that something is wrong. It's as if an alarm has been tripped, alerting the victim to the presence of cholesterol plaque clogging his arteries. But atherosclerosis is not always so obvious. In many cases, the patient is a victim of…

Silent Atherosclerosis

Silent atherosclerosis is especially dangerous precisely because it is silent. With no indication that anything is wrong, the victim fails to seek medical attention that may prevent a debilitating stroke or fatal heart attack.

Astonishingly, *half of all people who die suddenly of a heart attack had no previous symptoms.* It's not uncommon for an artery to be 75% or more obstructed by cholesterol plaque, and yet the victim is totally unaware that he's suffering from severe atherosclerotic disease, which may, at any moment, kill or injure him.

When ischemia strikes the heart without the pain of angina, it's called *silent ischemia*. Even more ominous, a large percentage of victims suffer *silent heart attacks*, that is, a heart attack which produces either no symptoms or symptoms that are mistaken for other causes, such as indigestion. Patients can also suffer *silent strokes* (often called *mini-strokes*), which also produce no obvious symptoms.

Whether silent or with symptoms, all strokes and heart attacks cause the death of tissues. This damaged tissue leads to...

The Complications of Strokes and Heart Attacks

When a patient suffers a heart attack, many forms of heart trouble may follow. Perhaps the two most important troubling complications are *heart failure* and *heart arrhythmia*. Both of these conditions can be caused by damaged heart muscle.

The muscles of the heart need to be strong and flexible to provide the pumping action for circulation. When portions of the heart muscle are destroyed by ischemia, the heart loses its strength and flexibility, just as any muscle would. Patients with a weakened heart are said to be suffering *heart failure*.

Heart failure prevents the heart from pumping sufficient amounts of blood to the body. This causes many symptoms, such as shortness of breath, fatigue and swelling in the feet and legs. Because every part of the body is dependent on the heart, the whole body suffers when the heart begins to fail.

Heart attacks not only weaken the heart, they cause abnormal heartbeats called *arrhythmias*. Arrhythmias disrupt the flow of blood throughout the body because they disrupt the pumping action of the heart.

The pumping of blood through the heart is caused by the rhythmic contraction and relaxation of the heart muscle—in one word, the *heartbeat.* The heart muscle is responding to electrical stimulation from nerves located in the heart itself. So when a heart attacks strikes, ischemia not only kills muscle cells, it kills the nerve cells that tell the heart when and how to beat. If a critical portion of nerve tissue is destroyed, the electrical stimulation of the heart becomes erratic, which, in turn, makes the heart beat irregularly.

Often a patient will complain that he can feel his heart flutter or skip a beat. These symptoms are called *palpitations.*

But not all arrhythmias, including palpitations, are dangerous—in fact, arrhythmias are commonly found in healthy people. But if the rhythm of the heart changes as the consequence of a heart attack, then there is great cause for concern.

After a heart attack, arrhythmias may make the heart beat too slowly, causing the victim to become fatigued or even faint from insufficient circulation. Or arrhythmias may make the heart beat too fast, which, paradoxically, also leads to inadequate blood flow.

Sometimes, part of the heart muscle will beat so fast that it begins to quiver, causing portions of the blood to swirl around inside the heart instead of being pumped out. This turbulent, whirlpool motion creates blood clots, which may travel to the brain and cause strokes.

Just as the death of heart tissue leads to additional health problems, the death of brain tissue from stroke also has its consequences. Most often, the symptoms of stroke appear rapidly, within the span of a few minutes.

There are many possible symptoms of stroke—it all depends on which area of the brain suffers the damage. Parts of the body may be afflicted with sudden numbness, weakness or paralysis. The patient may have trouble talking or understanding speech. Loss of vision, dizziness or clouded thinking are additional complications. With therapy, there is a possibility of regaining the use of functions damaged by stroke, but often the damage is permanent.

Occlusive strokes rarely kill. Occlusive heart attacks, however, *do* kill—often with stunning swiftness—when victims suffer…

Sudden Cardiac Death

Sudden cardiac death is death due primarily from cardiac causes occurring less than one hour after the onset of symptoms.

Sudden cardiac death is provoked by a disturbance of the heart's electrical system that causes a critical portion of the heart muscle to shudder and vibrate. This quiver—called *ventricular fibrillation*—prevents the heart from beating. When this happens, the patient is said to be in *cardiac arrest*. Circulation is lost to every part of the body, including the brain, which is why the victims of cardiac arrest lose consciousness.

Ventricular fibrillation can arise from several different types of heart disease, but by far the most common cause is coronary atherosclerosis with its accompanying ischemia, heart attacks and arrhythmias. Often the patient will have a history of old myocardial infarctions before experiencing the final heart attack that leads to cardiac arrest.

Cardiac arrest is not the same as the actual death of the victim, which is usually defined as *brain death*. A patient may survive cardiac arrest, as long as his heart begins beating again before brain death occurs.

It's rare for ventricular fibrillation to stop of its own accord, however, which is why most victims perish unless there is immediate intervention to start the heart beating normally. Most of you are familiar with the defibrillator paddles in the emergency room that shock the heart back into its normal rhythms. Despite this and other medical advances, sudden cardiac death remains a leading cause of death, with very low survival rates.

After years of studying cardiovascular disease, doctors identified several factors that seemed to predispose an individual for the development of atherosclerosis. These are the well-known…

Risk Factors for Strokes and Heart Attacks

Most of you are familiar with the risk factors associated with strokes and heart attacks—*age, heredity, high blood pressure, high cholesterol levels, cigarette smoking, obesity* and others.

I'll have much to say about risk factors as the book progresses, but there's no need to focus on them just yet. The only thing to keep in mind at this point is that, while risk factors are important, they should not be mistaken as the only factors involved in the creation and progression of atherosclerosis. And simply controlling risk factors is no guarantee that you won't suffer a stroke or heart attack.

A Question for Extra Credit

This ends your refresher course in strokes and heart attacks. And you're guaranteed a passing grade if you can remember one simple fact: atherosclerosis creates the ischemic occlusions that lead to most strokes and heart attacks.

Now, here's a question for extra credit: What creates atherosclerotic disease in the first place?

Lucky for you this is an open book test! So just turn the page and consider the title of the next chapter…

4

The Response to Injury

Ever since atherosclerosis was associated with strokes and heart attacks, doctors struggled to understand the origin of this puzzling disease. Where does cholesterol plaque come from? Why does it adhere to the inside of arteries? Why are some people free of plaque, while others have arteries completely clogged with the stuff?

For decades, there was no satisfactory answer to these questions. But finally—at the beginning of this new century—science has discovered that the explanation to these and many other mysteries of atherosclerosis are contained in a single idea...

The Body's Response to Injury

Atherosclerosis begins—and is sustained by—the body's response to injury.

What exactly is a "response to injury?" Let me illustrate with a simple experiment that you, the reader, can perform at home.

Step 1

Find a dead person.

Step 2

Take a hammer and whack him on the thumb. What do you see? Well, if you followed Step 1 correctly, you won't see anything but the injury itself—a small, circular indentation on the thumb.

Step 3

Take the same hammer and whack *yourself* on the thumb.

Step 4

After you stop howling and skipping around the room, examine your thumb. What do you see?

Now you see much more than just the injury—you see your body's *response* to the injury. Within minutes, there is probably a nasty bruise beneath the thumbnail and the thumb itself may be hot, red and swollen to twice its normal size. You'd also expect loss of movement in the thumb joint and a throbbing pain, the last of which accounts for all that howling and skipping earlier in the experiment.

Step 5

Now, put down the hammer. Really…put it down. You're making me nervous.

So: the same injury, but two different results. What accounts for the difference? Only one thing: a living body. The bruise, the redness, the swelling, the pain—all of these symptoms are a living body's response to injury.

Life is the key distinction in the experiment above. A dead body is inert, incapable of responding to anything. But a living body automatically responds to injury.

We've all experienced the hard knocks of life. So it's no surprise that your body would respond to an injured thumb with heat, redness, swelling and pain. But perhaps you've never asked yourself *why* the body responds this way.

The body responds to injury with a single purpose in mind—to *repair the injury and restore the body to health*. All that painful heat, redness and swelling in your thumb is designed to (eventually) repair the damage of ruptured cells and tissues. Without this response, your thumb might never return to good working order.

This is an important point that bears repeating: *the purpose of the body's response to injury is to repair the injury and restore the body to health.*

Without this self-healing action of the body, life would be impossible. Day-to-day living requires a constant response to injury. Many thousands of cells from every part of the body die or malfunction in a day, either through injury or simply from wearing out. The body must always work to remove and replace these dead, injured and worn-out cells in order for health to be maintained.

An obvious example of this process at work is the cartilage in your knee, which makes up the joint between your leg bones. The cartilage is undergoing constant wear and tear from the stress of walking, running, bending, lifting weights and so on. If the cushioning tissues of the cartilage are not quickly replaced when they are injured or worn, the knee joint would stiffen painfully as the hard bones of the leg begin to scrape against one another. But the body automatically knows how to repair and restore the cartilage, and that keeps the knee flexible and pain-free.

Although there are many different ways for the body to be injured, the damage done by germs is of particular interest in the study of strokes and heart attacks. So let's examine…

Infectious Germs and the Injury They Cause

Germs are one of the chief causes of injury to the body.

Germs are considered *infective* when they are able to multiply and persist inside the body. Over time, multiplying germs injure the body. Bacteria usually do their damage by producing toxins that destroy cells and tissues. Viruses usually do their damage by destroying the structure of the cells they infect, which also destroys cells and tissues.

In either case, the end result is the same—cells and tissues die; this is the major injury of most infections. If too much damage occurs from infectious germs, the body may become irreparably harmed. In extreme cases, infection can lead to death.

Germs that have a high probability of causing disease are called ***pathogens***. Pathogens are often categorized by their ***virulence***, which indicates the degree to which a pathogen can cause illness. For example, all flu viruses are pathogens, but some strains of the flu are more virulent than others, causing a more serious degree of illness.

Infectious bacteria and viruses invade the body in numerous ways: through the lungs, a cut in the skin, bleeding gums, sexual contact—if your body had a second floor window, they'd climb through that, too.

The fact is, you are under constant assault from microorganisms that want to set up housekeeping in your body. Fortunately, your body is one tough landlord. It is constantly fighting off the invading germs, relentlessly tracking them down and killing them off, one by one, until not a single germ survives. How? It's all part of your body's response to injury…in particular, the response of your *immune system*.

The immune system is an exceedingly complex but potent collection of organs, tissues, cells and cell products designed to defend you against foreign invaders and repair any damage that they've caused. It would be impossible in a single chapter to touch upon all aspects of the immune system, so I'll limit our discussion to those parts of it that are most important to understanding strokes and heart attacks.

In order to restore the body to health, the immune system has two tasks it must accomplish. First, it has to destroy the invading germs. Second, it has to repair the damage they've done. We might as well begin at the beginning with…

Fighting Germs: Part I of the Response to Injury

How does the immune system fight against germs? Here's a look at a few of the key weapons in the immune system's arsenal.

The body's first line of defense against pathogens is a combination of physical barriers—such as the skin—and chemical barriers, such as the enzymes and acids of the mouth and stomach. Most germs never make it beyond this first line of defense.

Microorganisms that make it past these barriers are met by the body's *innate defenses*. The innate defenses are present in your body at birth and are non-specific—they defend against all pathogens, attacking them with ready-made, off-the-shelf weapons.

Chief among the innate defenses are the **white blood cells**. These cells roam the bloodstream like miniature versions of *The Blob*, surrounding and engulfing germs, and thus destroying them. The **lymphatic system**, a collection of interconnected vessels found throughout the body, also circulates white blood cells to the places where they're needed.

There are many different varieties of white blood cells, each assigned specific tasks to fight infection. **Neutrophils** are usually the first white blood cells to arrive at the sight of infective injury. They are the kamikaze pilots of the immune system—they dive after the invading germs, swallow them whole and secrete deadly chemicals that kill them, then die themselves from their own poisons a few hours later.

Sometimes an invading germ will make it past the innate defenses and the usual white blood cells become overwhelmed. When that happens, they send a message to the body: "Hey! The bad guys are winning! Send help!"

It's at that point that your body activates its *acquired defenses*. In contrast to the innate defenses, the acquired defenses are *not* present at birth. They are "acquired" only after you come into contact with a particular pathogen. Your immune system studies the germ, then designs specific weapons to destroy it.

I'll have more to say about acquired defenses as the book progresses. For the moment, however, it's enough to know that your immune system has many different ways of fighting off infections.

But eliminating germs is only half the job of your immune system. Once an infection is over, the body needs to repair and replace the cells and tissues that have been damaged. So let's continue on with…

Repairing the Damage: Part II of the Response to Injury

Nearly every injury to the body requires some measure of repair and replacement. Let me illustrate how it's done with a familiar example.

It's late at night. You should have been asleep hours ago. Instead, you're sitting up in bed reading *The Heart Attack Germ*, eagerly turning the pages of this fascinating book, when suddenly…Ouch! A paper cut!

If the cut is deep enough, there might be a thin line of blood across your finger, indicating that tiny blood vessels have been severed. Somehow, these blood vessels have to be repaired or the bleeding would never stop. Repairing this injury is, in large part, a responsibility of your immune system.

Initially, the body responds to the cut by producing a blood clot. The clot acts like a plug, stopping blood from leaking out of the blood vessel. But this is only a quick fix. The body needs to permanently repair the hole in the vessel. That's where the immune system comes in.

While scouring the area with immune cells looking for any stray germs that may have entered through the cut, the immune system rebuilds the artery in two ways. First, it stimulates cells near the cut to secrete special substances that link together like the girders of a skyscraper, creating scaffolding for new cells to latch on to. ***Collagen***, a tough white fiber, is one of those substances. Another important material is *elastin*, a flexible tissue which gives the artery elastic qualities.

Strands of collagen, elastin and other materials span the distance between one side of the cut and the other, joining the two sides together. Tissue like this, which tangle and cross-link together to form support for other cells, is called ***extracellular matrix***.

As the matrix is laid down, the immune system stimulates nearby cells to create replacement cells, rapidly filling in the gaps between tissue. This sudden proliferation of cells quickly replaces any tissues lost to injury. The result? In a few days, the cut is perfectly healed, with no indication that your skin or blood vessels have ever been damaged.

(By the way, matrix material such as collagen and elastin plays an important part in the creation of cholesterol plaque. Look for them to make a repeat appearance in the following chapters!)

No matter if it's a cut or a germ that destroys tissue, the same basic immune system process works to repair the damage.

Every second of every day, your body is responding to injury. With expert precision, your immune system and other mechanisms are responding to injury at exactly the right place, at exactly the right time with exactly the right remedies. And everything always works exactly as planned.

Right?

Well, not exactly.

When Good Immune Systems Go Bad—A Question of Balance

Occasionally, things go wrong. So wrong, in fact, that *the body's response to injury can be more dangerous than the injury itself.*

Sometimes the immune system kills more than just foreign germs; it can also mistakenly attack the healthy cells of your own body. Or, during the repairing phase, it can over-multiply too many replacement cells. Or it can over-stimulate the clotting factors in your blood, making your blood clot too easily. When things like this happen, dangerous new problems occur, which may turn out to be much worse than original injury.

How can it be that the mechanisms designed to protect you ends up hurting you?

Mostly, it's a question of balance.

Let's go back to that—ouch!—paper cut from a few paragraphs ago. Almost immediately after blood appeared on the skin, the blood began to clot. The clotting of blood is a necessary first step in response to a cutting injury.

Blood is a liquid, and the body maintains a delicate balance between the things that keep blood liquid (such as chemical substances like *heparin*) and things that make it clot (such as specialized blood cells called *platelets*). Upset this balance and a clot forms.

An injured artery is one of the things that upsets the balance. Platelets in the blood recognize the substances released from ruptured artery tissue and are activated to begin the process of clotting. At that point, the things that stimulate clotting win out over the things that inhibit clotting—the balance is tipped in favor of a clot to form. And a good thing, too. Otherwise, that cut on your finger might never stop bleeding.

Nearly every response to injury has dual forces like this at work—things that stimulate the response and things that inhibit the response. In most people, all these forces are properly balanced, ready to respond when injury pulls the trigger. Injury tips the balance one way; the countervailing forces respond and tip the balance back again. In this manner, the body can quickly respond to injury.

What would happen, however, if the forces were tipped too much in one direction? When it comes to the clotting process, the results can be extremely dangerous.

Hemophilia is an example of this. Hemophiliacs lack substances in the blood that stimulate clotting. Therefore, the things that promote bleeding are not properly balanced by the things that inhibit it. As a result, when hemophiliacs bleed, there is no counter-balance to stop the bleeding. So for people with hemophilia, even minor injuries can bleed excessively.

In contrast, some people are deficient in the substances that keep blood liquid. They form blood clots much too easily and the clots are not readily dissolved. As a result, they are much more likely to suffer the ill effects of blood clots.

As you can see, every response to injury must be well balanced. Anything that tips things too much one way or the other can lead to trouble.

This is especially true when it comes to the body's protective response to the germs that infect the arteries of the cardiovascular system.

When everything works as it should, the quick response of the immune system usually snuffs out infectious germs before they do too much damage. Occasionally, however, an infection may last a considerable amount of time. And as long as it does, the body keeps trying to counter-balance the infection with the products of the immune system. This is the key to understanding...

How the Response to Injury Creates Atherosclerosis

Most people assume that, when germs make you sick, it's the germs themselves that cause all the problems. But many diseases—including atherosclerosis—are made much worse by the body's *response* to the germ.

The sting of a bee is a vivid example of how the body's response can turn a minor injury into a life-threatening problem.

For most people, the venom of a bee sting produces a localized allergic response by the body—no more than a small, slightly painful bump that fades away after a few days. For some people, however, the body is hypersensitive to proteins in the venom, creating an exaggerated allergic response to the injury. Instead of localized swelling, the swelling may become extensive, with hives breaking out over the skin. In extreme cases, the entire body goes into shock—the victim has difficulty breathing, suffers vomiting, loses consciousness and may even die from loss of blood pressure.

In such a case, the balance of forces which respond to injury is pushed too far in one direction, affecting the entire body. Clearly, in a case like this, *the body's response to injury is far worse than the minor damage caused by the bee sting.*

The same is true when it comes to atherosclerosis—*the body's response to injury from cardiovascular germs is far worse than the minor damage caused by the germs themselves.* Unlike the massive, rapid response to a bee sting, however, the destructive response to cardiovascular germs is slow and small. But because the response lasts a long time, the danger grows with each passing day.

Cardiovascular germs often infect the artery for decades. Long-lasting infection constantly tips the balance of forces in one direction. Over time, the continual flood of immune cells pounding away at the same infected location begins to wreak havoc on the artery, setting in motion the build-up of cholesterol plaque. So, just like the sting of a bee, *the danger lies in the body's response to the injury, not in the injury itself.*

To understand in detail how the body's response to injury leads to atherosclerosis, we need to consider one more key factor…

5

Chronic Inflammation

Inflammation plays a critical role in the development of atherosclerosis; so much so, that atherosclerosis is now considered to be an *inflammatory disease*. Let's begin with an obvious first question…

What is Inflammation?

Inflammation is part of your body's response to injury—a localized, protective reaction to damaged tissue. Usually, there are five symptoms associated with inflammation: heat, redness, swelling, pain and loss of function.

Hmmm. Where have we seen these symptoms before? It had something to do with a hammer, didn't it?

Right! That experiment with your thumb in the previous chapter!

Sorry to bring up such a painful memory, but for several days your scarlet, throbbing thumb was an excellent example of inflammation at work. Thanks to the hammer blow, many of the cells in your thumb were injured, and as your body's immune system responded to the injury, it produced all the hallmarks of inflammation: heat, redness, swelling, pain and loss of function.

But you don't need to be whacked with a hammer to produce inflammation—you can get the same results from an infection. If you've ever suffered a cold virus, you're well acquainted with the heat, redness, swelling, pain and loss of function of a sore throat, all caused in reaction to the germ.

The point is, it doesn't really matter what type of injury you suffer—as long as cells are dying, the body's immune system usually responds to the injury with inflammation.

The symptoms of inflammation—swelling, pain, etc.—are largely produced by all the chemical activity going on as immune (and other) cells do their job. Most inflammation is localized around the site of the injury because that's where most of the activated immune cells are concentrated.

Now, on the face of it, inflammation seems like a bad idea. After all, who wants a body part that's hot, red, swollen, painful and unable to function? (Please feel free to make up your own punch line here.)

But, strange as it seems, these very symptoms are for our own good. The five hallmarks of inflammation are protective mechanisms designed to shield us from further injury.

Take pain, for instance. Admittedly, the pain of inflammation seems pretty darn undesirable. But the throbbing ache of, say, an inflamed toe reminds us not to walk on it, which might cause further injury to the toe and slow the process of healing.

When it comes to infection, the symptoms of inflammation work to destroy or dilute the agents of infection or to keep infection away from other parts of the body.

Each of the five hallmark symptoms provides some healing benefit to the body. That's why inflammation is desirable—it's a sign that the immune system is actively protecting the body and repairing damaged tissues. A strong inflammatory response to infection means that your body has discovered the invading germs and is fighting back. It is a perfectly appropriate *response to injury*.

The last thing you want is *no* inflammatory response to infection. People with immune deficiencies—such as the elderly or AIDS patients—show a diminished inflammatory response, indicating that they are unable to effectively fight off infection. As a result, every infection is a serious risk to their health.

So there are really only two options—suffer the painful but temporary symptoms of inflammation or succumb to the first infectious disease that takes hold in your body.

When the body suffers from infective disease, the infection and resulting inflammation are often categorized as either *acute* or *chronic*. The difference between acute and chronic is very important and it explains why the true cause of strokes and heart attacks has remained hidden for so long.

Acute and Chronic—Two Levels of Infection and Inflammation

The difference between the acute and chronic levels of infection and inflammation is not always clear cut, but *time* and *severity* are the key factors.

Acute infection and inflammation has a short and relatively severe course. *Chronic infection and inflammation*, on the other hand, takes place over a long time and does not usually cause sharp distress to the body. Perhaps the best way to distinguish between these two levels is with a concrete example.

During acute infection and inflammation, symptoms are usually obvious—often painfully so. Acute tonsillitis is a good illustration of this.

Most often, when streptococcal germs infect the tonsils, you *know* something is wrong. Your throat feels on fire because the tonsils are inflamed. (In fact, the word "inflammation" comes from the Latin *inflammare*, which means, "to set on fire.") When the doctor looks in your mouth, he can actually see the inflammation because the tissues in your throat are red and swollen. In addition to the localized inflammation, you can suffer general discomfort from the infection, including fever, chills, headache and fatigue. Add up all the symptoms of an acute infection and it's no secret to you or your doctor that you're ill.

That's because there is a high level of localized immune system activity within your body—infective germs are multiplying rapidly, destroying tissues left and right. The immune system is responding strongly with killer countermeasures all its own. Both germ and immune system are engaged in total war, which is why symptoms are so obvious. Once the infectious germs begin to die out and only a few are left alive in the body, the immune response begins to slacken as well. Eventually every germ is destroyed and the inflammatory response fades away.

In contrast to the total war of the acute level, the *chronic* level of infection and inflammation is more like a long-term series of minor skirmishes. That's because, after the initial acute infection, the pathogenic germs never completely die out; there's always a few hanging around the body. Although they are continuously present, the amount of infection they cause is small. Thus, the inflammatory response is small, producing no visible symptoms, like pain or swelling.

These bouts of **micro-infection** and **micro-inflammation** are essentially hidden—you're sick but you don't know it. These infections are subclinical because they're not detectable by clinical examination. So neither you nor your doctor may know that you're harboring an ongoing, infectious disease.

Why Acute Infection and Inflammation Turns Chronic

Infections become chronic because pathogenic germs are tough and wily opponents. They've been around a long, long time and have evolved effective strategies to protect themselves from the onslaughts of the immune system. They've learned how to hide out or hijack parts of the body to stay alive and multiply. Once established, a successful germ can elude your immune system for decades, always keeping one step ahead of total elimination.

And once an infection becomes chronic, inflammation becomes chronic too, because your immune system never gives up. It is programmed to track down and kill *every last germ*. It has to; even a single germ can multiply quickly and spread disease. So the immune system is always responding to an ongoing infection with a steady, low-level stream of the cells and chemicals that keeps the inflammation process going.

Consider again our experiment with the hammer and your thumb. After you whacked your thumb, the acute inflammatory process began. The thumb turned red and swelled, indicating a swift response to injury. After a few days, the body replaced and repaired the damaged tissue. With no more germs or injured tissue to react to, the immune response ceased, leading to the end of inflammation. Result: one healthy thumb.

Now imagine if, instead of giving your thumb a good whack with the hammer, you merely tapped the same spot on your thumb repeatedly—say, once a minute.

Every minute of every day.

For years on end.

What would happen?

What would happen, of course, is that the thumb would continually suffer micro-injury and never completely heal. The small, constant damage to the thumb would bring wave after wave of immune cells and their chemicals to the site, keeping the inflammatory process going.

This is basically what happens when an infection lingers. The pathogen's constant presence leads to the immune system constantly hammering away at the germ with chronic inflammation. And while acute inflammation is generally helpful to the body, *chronic* inflammation can do a lot of damage over time.

The Dangers of Chronic Inflammation

The cells and chemicals that the immune system uses to destroy toxic germs are, themselves, toxic; they destroy not only the germ but healthy tissues, as well. So when an infection lingers in the same spot, there is a risk that healthy tissues will be continually subjected to toxic substances from the immune system. It's the biological equivalent of "friendly fire" in warfare.

In addition, a lingering infection provokes endless stimulation of the immune system to repair and replace tissue—even when it's not needed. As a result, infected areas begin to swell with proliferating cells and extracellular matrix. This excessive tissue repair and replacement leads to *scar tissue*, a dense, fibrous tissue that replaces normal cells. Excessive scar tissue can disrupt the function of an organ or body part, causing new problems for the body.

All in all, chronic inflammation is simply too much of a good thing. Your response to injury is stimulated too much in one direction for an extended period.

Once chronic inflammation gets going, a vicious circle begins: as healthy tissue is damaged by the immune system, the body responds to the injury with even more inflammation. As a result, more healthy tissue is damaged, and the body responds with…well, you get the picture.

And that brings us back to a key point of the previous chapter: long-term infection and inflammation throws off the "balance of forces" that respond to injury. The constant build-up of inflammatory cells and chemicals by the immune system stimulate the protective mechanisms too much.

Again, the best way to explain how this process damages the body is with a few…

Examples of Chronic Inflammation

Tuberculosis, an infectious disease of the lungs, is an example of the damage done by chronic infection and inflammation.

The infectious germ responsible for tuberculosis is very good at fending off the immune system. It can reside dormant inside the lungs at the same location for years on end while the cells of the immune system repeatedly attack it.

Because the toxic cells and chemicals of the immune system are constantly bombarding the tuberculosis bacterium—day after day, year after year—the healthy tissues around the germ begin to suffer. When enough time has passed, large sections of normal lung tissue are destroyed and turned into scar tissue, which prevents the lung from functioning properly. In a fiendishly ironic twist, the injury to the body is not directly the result of the tuberculosis germ, *but of the immune system itself.*

There are other diseases that are caused by the immune system mistakenly attacking the body with chronic inflammation. **Rheumatoid arthritis** is a painful example of the damage that can be done by this type of error.

In fact, rheumatoid arthritis is often called *inflammatory arthritis.* The body mistakes the tissues of the joint as foreign substances and launches an immune reaction against them. Affected joints are attacked by a constant, low level of inflammation that can last for decades. The chemicals of inflammation damage the delicate membranes and cartilage tissues of the joint, leaving them full of inflexible scar tissue. The result of this chronic inflammation? A painful, crippling disease.

So: acute inflammation—good. Chronic inflammation—bad, because, over extended periods, the cells and chemicals of the immune system can damage healthy tissue.

With this key concept firmly established, we can at last turn our attention to strokes and heart attacks.

Chronic Infection and Inflammation as a Source of Atherosclerosis

For a long time, few people in medicine believed that atherosclerosis—the disease that leads to strokes and heart attacks—could be caused by infection and inflammation. You can't blame 'em. There were none of the classic symptoms of acute infection and inflammation: arteries clogged by cholesterol were not obviously inflamed; people with atherosclerosis didn't have fever or chills; no one could find a direct cause-and-effect connection between a particular germ and a heart attack.

Only recently, after significant advances in medical technology, was the truth finally revealed: atherosclerosis is a *chronic* inflammatory disease caused, in large part, by *chronic* infection of the arteries. Because of the low level of infection and inflammation, it was impossible to discover the connection—until now.

Highly advanced technology and rigorous studies have confirmed that the cholesterol plaque of atherosclerosis is a direct result of chronic inflammation of the arteries. In the next chapter, I'll explain in detail how this process occurs, but the basics have already been outlined above; think of cholesterol plaque as the "scar tissue" produced by chronic inflammation. The irony is that, just as with tuberculosis or arthritis, it is the inflammation itself—*the body's response to injury*—that causes most of the damage.

It's hard to imagine that such a hidden, small-scale process could have such terrible consequences. But think of it this way:

It takes thousands of years for the forces of wind and rain to crack and crumble a mountain. The process is invisible to the naked eye. Yet drop by drop, year by year the mountain is slowly cracked and fractured until the seemingly solid rock shatters in a massive, destructive landslide. The gentlest rain and softest breeze contribute to the eventual destruction of a great edifice.

Chronic infection and inflammation are like that. They are hidden processes, invisible to the naked eye. They do their damage slowly, over the course of decades, without obvious symptoms. Then one day—often without warning—the integrity of the body shatters. A coronary artery clogged by plaque suddenly becomes occluded by a blood clot. The next thing you know, you're lying on your back in the emergency room with the ER staff trying to shock your heart into beating again with electric paddles.

The best way to avoid this dramatic endpoint is to understand the starting point of…

6

Inflammatory Atherosclerosis

The discovery of inflammation's role in atherosclerosis changes everything. The fires of inflammation seem to illuminate every aspect of this disease, which was once shrouded in darkness and mystery. Here is a step-by-step outline of how the body's response to injury creates the cholesterol plaque that leads to strokes and heart attacks. Let's begin with...

A Few Facts about Atherosclerosis

Atherosclerosis is an ancient illness. It's difficult to assess how widespread this disease has been in the historic past, yet researchers have found signs of atherosclerosis in Egyptian mummies dating back over thousands of years.[22] Perhaps the reason atherosclerosis seems so prevalent in modern times is simply because humans are living longer. In early civilizations, people rarely reached old age. They often died young from other causes, before the ill effects of atherosclerosis manifested themselves. Generally speaking, atherosclerosis is found in animals that live a long time, such as elephants and primates.

For the most part, atherosclerotic disease is limited to the arteries; it is rarely found in veins. If you cut open a normal artery, you'll find a hollow tube composed of three distinct layers—the *adventitia*, the *media*, and the *intima*, the innermost layer. The intima is itself covered by a thin layer of cells called the *endothelium*, made up of *endothelial cells*.

Despite being only the width of a single cell, the endothelium acts as a barrier, keeping substances in the bloodstream from passing into the artery wall. It's also a very active layer of cells, controlling many of the functions of the artery. The endothelium produces substances that tell the artery when to contract or relax, it stimulates or inhibits the growth of cells in the artery wall, it stimulates or inhibits blood clots and it performs dozens of other tasks that are critical to maintaining the health of the artery.

SIMPLIFIED STRUCTURE OF THE ARTERY

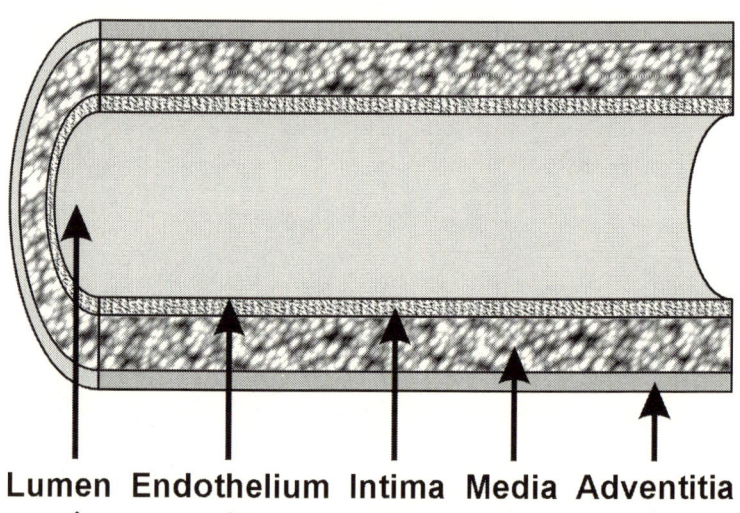

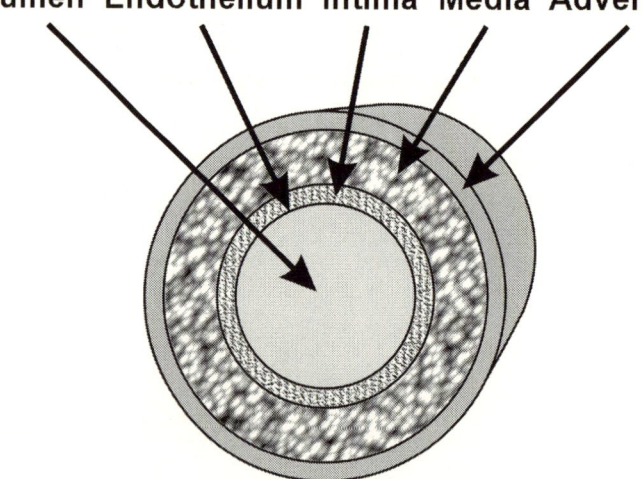

Lumen   Endothelium   Intima   Media   Adventitia

A CLOSER LOOK AT
THE ENDOTHELIUM

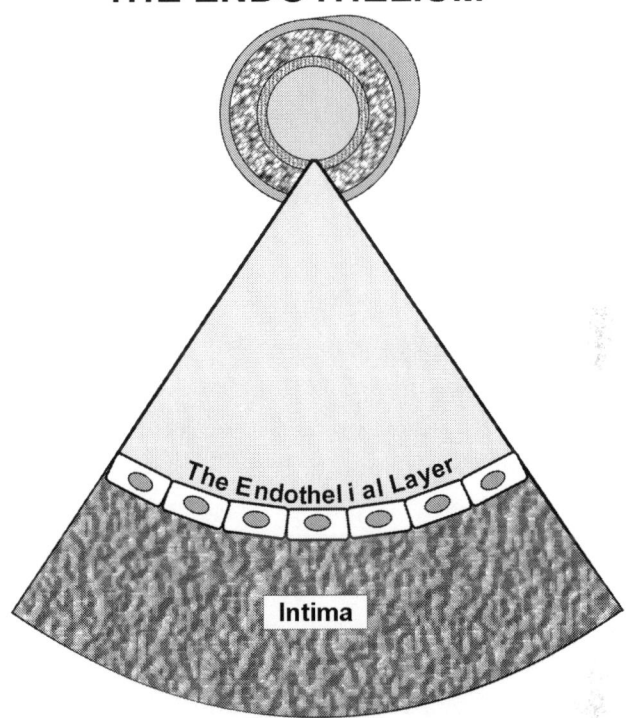

The Endothelial Layer

Intima

As the simplified illustration above shows, the endothelium, or endothelial layer, is a single layer of cells which cover the intima. A healthy endothelium regulates many of the key processes within the artery. When the endothelium becomes injured, however, it loses its ability to control the functions of the blood vessel and the health of the entire artery suffers. It's here, directly beneath the endothelial layer, that atherosclerosis gets its first grip on the artery. Ironically, the more the body tries to cure the injury with healing inflammation, the bigger the atherosclerotic lesions grow, creating mounds of cholesterol plaque and setting the stage for a stroke or heart attack.

Because the entire inside wall of the artery is lined with endothelial cells, it's these cells that are in direct contact with the bloodstream. As a result, endothelial cells are subject to injury from things in the blood such as germs, chemical substances and the swirling forces of the bloodstream itself. It all adds up to the endothelium being a prime location for injury to occur.

And an injured endothelium is bad news. It can no longer carry out the critical functions that keep the artery in proper health. In short, a healthy endothelium works to stop atherosclerosis, but a sick endothelium loses that ability.

With a sick endothelium, the barrier between the bloodstream and the artery becomes leaky, allowing substances into direct contact with the interior of the artery. An injured endothelium may cause the artery to contract too readily, or over-stimulate the growth of cells, or create too much clotting of blood. Injury and the inflammatory response upset the "balance of forces" which are key to keeping the artery healthy. These changes are so important that scientists use the phrase ***endothelial dysfunction*** as a shorthand way of describing any alteration of the normal function of the endothelium.

Endothelial dysfunction carries grave consequences. So keep an eye on this delicate layer of cells; injury and inflammation make the endothelium a hot spot for the formation of atherosclerosis.

For now, however, let's move on to the hollow space in the middle of the artery, called the ***lumen***. It's through here that the blood flows, like water though a garden hose. In a healthy artery, the lumen is smooth, round and open, allowing the blood to flow freely. This is the way you want your arteries to look.

If you cut open an artery diseased by atherosclerosis, however, you'll find that the layers of the artery are distorted, and a lumpy, yellowish paste called ***cholesterol plaque*** adheres to the interior wall of the artery. Often mixed in with the plaque are dark splotches of congealed blood and hard deposits of calcium. Not a pretty sight.

The very name "atherosclerosis" is a vivid description of this ugly mess. The word is derived from the Latin word *atheroma*, meaning, "a tumor full of pus that looks like gruel," and *sklerosis*, meaning "hardening."

The key thing to remember is that atherosclerotic plaque and its consequences interferes with the flow of blood through your arteries. Most of the bad effects of atherosclerosis stem from this single fact.

Atherosclerosis is not evenly distributed throughout the arteries. One artery may be totally clogged by plaque, while another, nearby artery remains healthy and open. Atherosclerosis forms into patches of disease called ***lesions***, which tend to grow in size and spread to other locations over time. In severe cases the entire length of an artery can be coated by lesions of atherosclerotic plaque.

In addition, atherosclerosis seems to like certain parts of the arterial tree more than others. As reported in an earlier chapter, atherosclerosis is common in the coronary arteries, which supply blood to the heart, and the carotid and vertebral arteries, which supply blood to the head and brain. The aorta is also a prime location for atherosclerosis to form.

Despite the fact that strokes and heart attacks are the leading cause of death in America, having atherosclerosis does not always condemn you to suffering a stroke or heart attack, even if the disease is rather extensive. For a long time, doctors didn't understand how this could be so. Isn't all atherosclerosis created equal?

Surprisingly, the answer is no.

Remember that the appearance of an occlusive blood clot is often the precipitating event of a stroke or heart attack. It turns out that some lesions are created in a way that makes them much more likely to produce these life-threatening blood clots. Why this happens depends, largely, on how inflammation shapes the course of the disease. So let's examine the birth and development of atherosclerosis, always keeping an eye on inflammation's lethal impact.

The Beginnings of Atherosclerosis—a Response to Injury

As stated before, atherosclerosis is the result of the body's immune system responding to injury—specifically, an injury to the endothelium, that thin layer of cells that lines the interior of your arteries. Exactly *what* is injuring the endothelium will be discussed later. For now, we'll focus on *how* the immune system responds to the injury.

As we learned in the previous chapter, one of the body's chief responses to injury is inflammation. In practice, that means surrounding the injured tissue with immune cells that are designed to produce inflammation. Perhaps the most important cells responsible for inflammation are ***macrophages***.

Macrophages begin life as a type of white blood cell called a ***monocyte*** that circulates in the bloodstream. When a monocyte drops out of the bloodstream and migrates toward injured tissue, it transforms itself into a macrophage.

Macrophages are very versatile, performing different tasks for the immune system: they surround and destroy germs; they signal the body to repair and replace injured tissue; and they secrete chemicals that orchestrate the immune response, giving them a role in both acute and chronic inflammation. So when macrophages gather in a group, it's a good bet that inflammation is in progress.

In fact, that's pretty much a defining characteristic of inflammation—where macrophages gather, inflammation flares.

Macrophages are able to move through tissue by squeezing between cells. This is how they manage to arrive at the site of injury, no matter where it occurs.

When an endothelial cell becomes injured, it uses a substance called ***adhesion molecules*** that turns the surface of the cell "sticky." Monocytes and other immune cells in the blood stream bump into the sticky cell surface and adhere to it, bringing immune system cells to the site of damage and beginning the inflammatory process.

Once clinging to a damaged endothelial surface, the monocytes burrow beneath the endothelial cell layer and turn into macrophages. The macrophages have a tendency to gather together, snuggling up beneath the endothelial layer and the intima of the artery. This new layer where macrophages gather is called the ***neointima***, appropriately named because it is the new, innermost layer beneath the endothelium.

Macrophages have one other special talent: under the right conditions, they soak up fatty compounds found in the bloodstream called ***lipids***. And—brace yourself—cholesterol happens to be one of these lipids.

Ding! Ding! Ding!

Those are the alarm bells that should be sounding in your head, right now. When it comes to strokes and heart attacks, anything that attracts cholesterol to your arteries can't be good!

But that's just what macrophages do. Thanks to the inflammatory response, macrophages gather together at the site of an injured endothelium, burrow into your artery and start soaking up cholesterol.

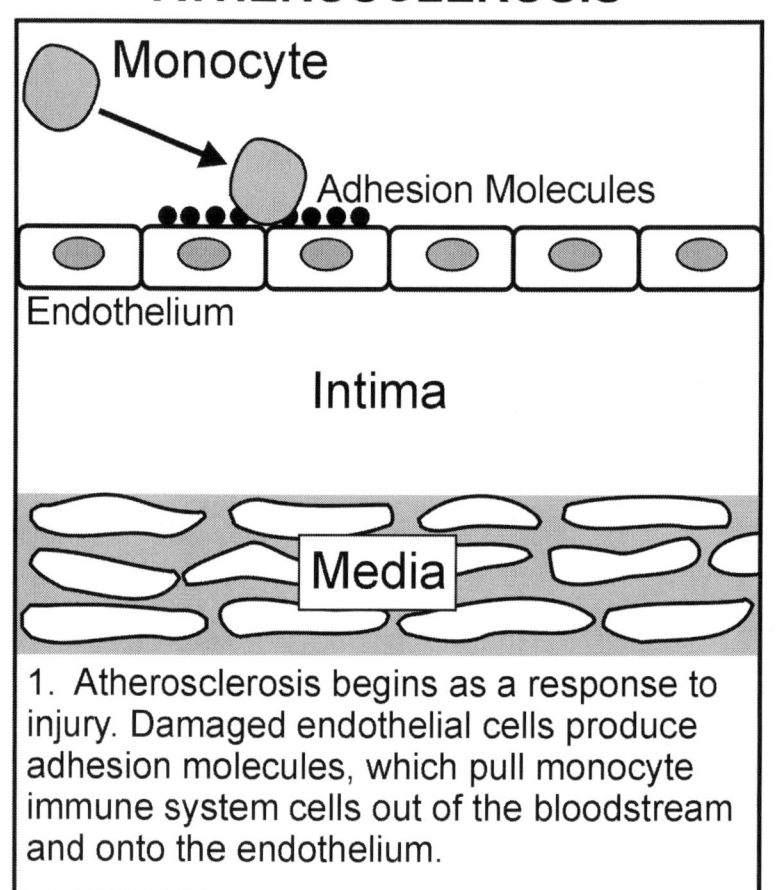

INFLAMMATION
AND THE BEGINNING OF
ATHEROSCLEROSIS

Monocyte

Adhesion Molecules

Endothelium

Intima

Media

1. Atherosclerosis begins as a response to injury. Damaged endothelial cells produce adhesion molecules, which pull monocyte immune system cells out of the bloodstream and onto the endothelium.

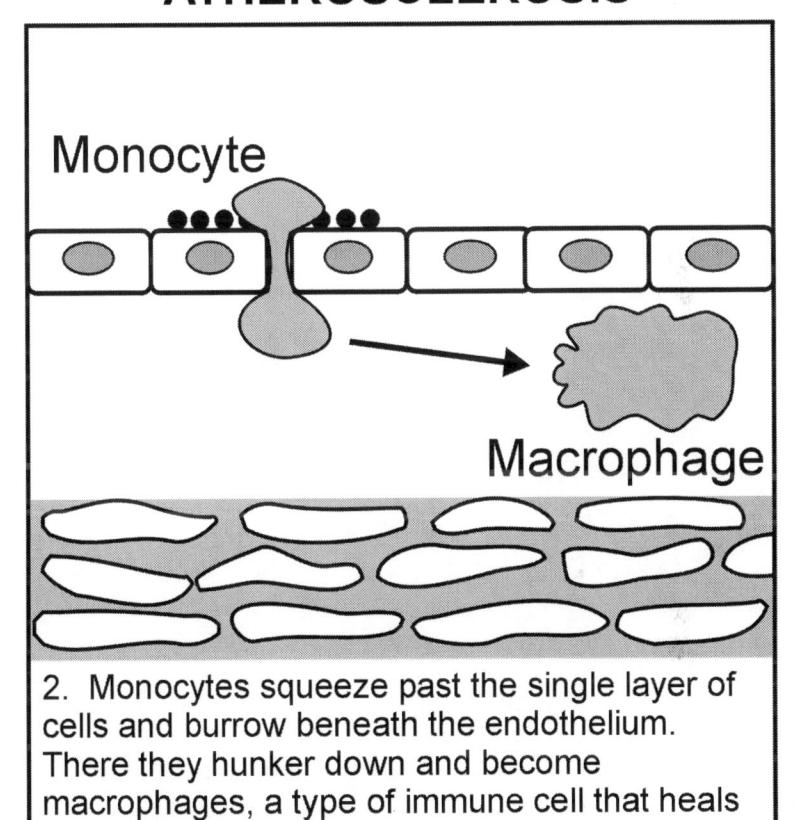

INFLAMMATION
AND THE BEGINNING OF
ATHEROSCLEROSIS

Monocyte

Macrophage

2. Monocytes squeeze past the single layer of cells and burrow beneath the endothelium. There they hunker down and become macrophages, a type of immune cell that heals damaged tissues through inflammation.

INFLAMMATION
AND THE BEGINNING OF
ATHEROSCLEROSIS

Cholesterol

Macrophage   Foam Cell

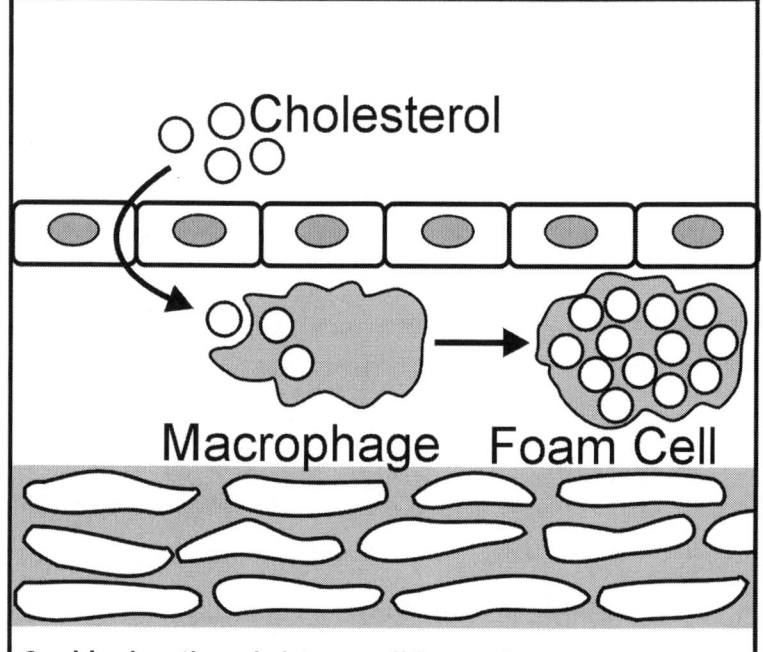

3. Under the right conditions, however, macrophages ingest fatty lipids such as cholesterol. They become a "cholesterol sponge" in the artery, soaking up so much cholesterol that they turn into "foam cells."

INFLAMMATION
AND THE BEGINNING OF
ATHEROSCLEROSIS

Fatty Streak

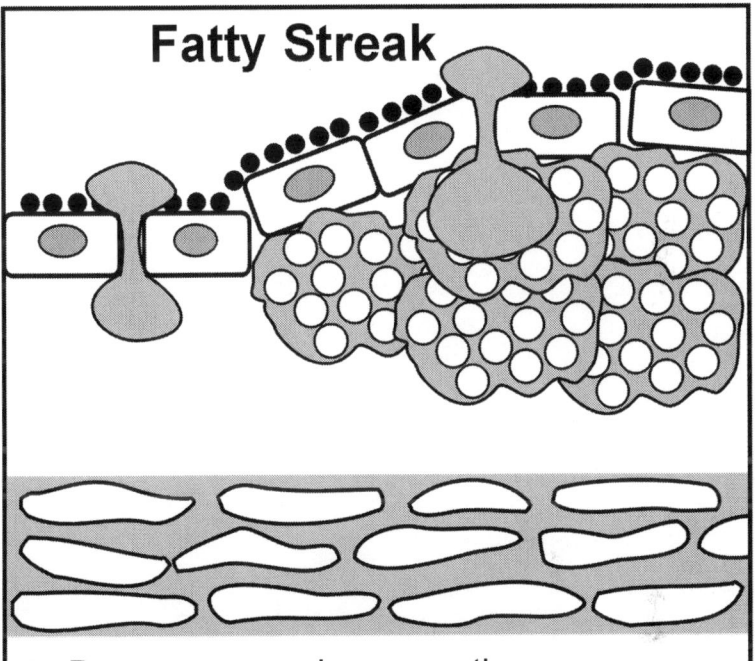

4. Damage spreads across the endothelium, recruiting more and more immune cells to the site of injury. Foam cells begin to pile up creating a pocket of chronic inflammation called a "fatty streak."

Now you know why the space between the endothelial layer and the intima is a hot spot for atherosclerosis. It's here that macrophages congregate, taking in cholesterol. And it's here that atherosclerosis gets its first foothold, forming into lesions of cholesterol plaque.

Scientists use a complex classification system to distinguish one type of atherosclerotic lesion from another. But for our purposes lesions can be classified as either *early*, **advanced** or **complicated**. Let's take a look at each.

Early Lesions

As the macrophages lodged in your artery take in more and more and fatty compounds, tiny bubbles of cholesterol and other lipids start to fill the cell. Under the microscope, the bubbles look like foam. For that reason, scientists named fat-filled macrophages *foam cells*.

So: a collection of macrophages, brought together by inflammation in response to injury, is now a collection of foam cells. These foam cells form in the neointima, positioned between the endothelium and the intima. This new layer of foam cells results in the first lesions of atherosclerosis—microscopic spots of disease on the artery.

These initial lesions appear surprisingly early in life. They are frequently found in infants and children, and in adults who are otherwise unaffected by atherosclerosis.[23] Because of their small size, they cause no symptoms.

Under normal circumstances, the healing properties of inflammation would handily repair and replace the injured cells that line the artery wall. With no more injury to react to, the body would stop sending immune system cells to the site and inflammation would simply fade away.

But for reasons you'll discover later in the book, injury continues along the artery wall and inflammation never dies down. It remains, turning into chronic inflammation.

More and more macrophages are drawn to the site, resulting in more and more foam cells. And that means that more and more cholesterol is deposited in the artery. Over time, foam cells collect into yellowish, cholesterol-rich *fatty streaks*. Although fatty streaks are visible to the naked eye, they are still too small to cause symptoms.

Fatty streaks start to appear during the teenage years—with a vengeance. Incredibly, one study found that 99% of 15-year-olds already have fatty streaks in the aorta. (As if acne isn't *enough* to deal with!)

Don't let anyone tell you that atherosclerosis is a disease of the elderly. The *symptoms* may take time to develop, but the disease itself begins early in life.

It's important to note that, at any stage, lesions can stabilize themselves temporarily or even permanently. There seem to be *pulses of growth* for atherosclerosis. It can lay quiet for many years, then suddenly burst into activity when properly stimulated. For some of us, atherosclerosis won't progress past the fatty streak stage—the disease becomes permanently stabilized. For others, however, fatty streaks evolve into…

Advanced Lesions

Advanced lesions, often referred to as **atheromas**, are characterized by the appearance of cholesterol plaque, the most prominent feature of atherosclerosis. As you might expect, plaque contains large amounts of foam cells, but plaque is more than just an overgrown fatty streak; plaque is a complex structure composed of many elements, most of them the result of inflammation.

Atherosclerosis, inflammation and endothelial dysfunction go hand in hand. When atherosclerosis gets a foothold on the interior of the artery, the endothelium can no longer regulate the proper balance of endothelial functions. So control is lost over things like the growth of artery cells and the clotting of blood, which has serious consequences for the progression of atherosclerosis.

As you know, inflammation stimulates tissues to regenerate and repair themselves. So it's not surprising to find that fatty streaks, which are constantly stimulated by inflammation, can become overgrown with extracellular matrix and cells from the artery wall.

In fact, chronic inflammation can make the smooth muscle cells and matrix of the intima begin multiplying so rapidly that they thicken and distort the artery, pushing the vessel wall outward into the lumen. This *intimal thickening* is a hallmark of atherosclerosis.

Not only does inflammation stimulate cells to multiply, it also recruits nearby cells to move into the site of injury. So as smooth muscle and endothelial cells multiply, they move from the artery into the lesion, integrating themselves into the structure of the fatty streak. And, in an added twist, smooth muscle cells begin soaking up cholesterol just as if they were macrophages. So now you've got a double-whammy inside the artery—both macrophages and proliferating smooth muscle cells turning into cholesterol-laden foam cells.

As a result of this movement and multiplication of arterial cells, and the continuing migration of macrophages to the lesion, the fatty streak grows. It changes its character, becoming more than just a collection of foam cells. The fatty streak transforms itself into a thick, yellowish mound of *cholesterol plaque*, which pushes into the bloodstream and spreads out along the artery wall. Plaque is the most visible sign of atherosclerosis. Whenever you see a photograph of atherosclerosis clogging up an artery, you're looking at cholesterol plaque.

The plaque itself is a mixture of nearly everything we have talked about so far—endothelial cells, smooth muscle cells, macrophages, foam cells, extracellular matrix and the debris of dead cells. But it's also chock full of additional inflammatory cells, such as *lymphocytes*, and inflammatory substances, such as *antibodies*, that the immune system keeps throwing at it.

The presence of lymphocytes in the lesion is another tip-off that inflammation is at work. Like macrophages, lymphocytes are a type of white blood cell that performs many functions during the course of inflammation. They usually don't arrive at the site of injury until *after* the initial stages of the immune response. So their presence in cholesterol plaque is a strong signal that the inflammation is chronic, i.e., lasting a long time.

The surface of plaque is shaped by the constant flow of blood that rushes past. The bloodstream smoothes the surface of the plaque like river water smoothes a pebble. The top of the plaque is covered by a layer of fibrous matrix tissue, which helps hold the mound together. This *fibrous cap* is made largely of smooth muscle cells and collagen, those tough white fibers which, you'll remember, are another sign of inflammation on the job.

Despite this motley mix of elements, most cholesterol plaques have an overall structure. If you sliced open the plaque, you'd find alternating layers of muscle cells and foam cells piled on top of each other like the layers of a cake.

The *shoulders* of the plaque are significant structural features. The shoulders are the points around the periphery of the lesion where it is attached to the artery. The thinnest—and thus, the weakest—parts of the fibrous cap are the shoulders. This area plays an important part in the eventual rupture of lesions.

As the plaque continues to grow, many foam cells undergo a dramatic change. Engorged by cholesterol and other lipids, foam cells burst open and die, releasing their fatty droplets into the spaces between the cells. This *extracellular lipid*, often called *soft cholesterol*, floats freely within the lesion and, over time, congregates into a pool at the core of the plaque.

As you'll discover in the next chapter, the size and makeup of this *lipid pool* (or *lipid core*) is critical to the life of the lesion. This is the pool of soft cholesterol that is most likely to create dangerous blood clots. At this stage, however, the lipid pool is still tucked safely away inside the mound of plaque.

Advanced lesions can become infiltrated with deposits of calcium in a process called *calcification*. Calcium is a mineral, the same substance that makes up a large portion of the bones of your skeleton. It can thoroughly penetrate a lesion, replacing dead cells and extracellular lipids, including the lipid core itself. Calcium has the same effect on lesions as it has on your bones—it makes them stiff and hard. In fact, this is where the term "hardening of the arteries" comes from. Lesions with deposits of calcium in them are often called *calcified plaques*. As a general rule, the longer the lesion survives, the more calcified it becomes.

Put all the elements above together, and you've got yourself a classic atheromatic lesion, a festering lump of cholesterol and inflammation simmering away inside the fragile lifelines to the heart and brain. Up until this point, atherosclerosis is "silent"—the disease progressing unnoticed by the victim or his physician. But now that the arteries of the heart and brain are becoming narrowed by cholesterol plaque, victims may begin to experience the first symptoms of atherosclerosis. Generally, the appearance of these symptoms begins around the age of forty, since that's when advanced lesions typically start to blossom.

Once a lesion enters the advanced stage, it has two paths before it. The lesion's plaque can become *stable*, in which case it holds together in one piece. Or the plaque can become *unstable*, splitting open and exposing its contents to the blood stream. Because unstable plaques are prone to rupture, they are often called *vulnerable plaques*.

The Three Stages of Atherosclerotic Lesions

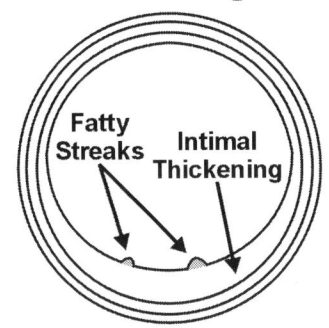

Early Lesions

One of the hallmarks of early lesions is the thickening of the artery intima at the site of injury and inflammation. It's here that foam cells filled with cholesterol congregate, clumping into small spots or threads of cholesterol plaque called fatty streaks.

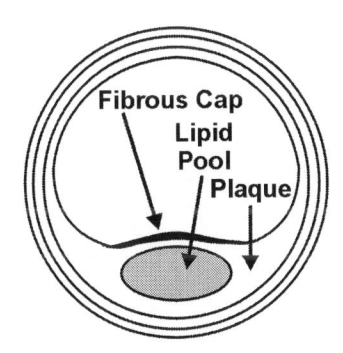

Advanced Lesions

Advanced lesions are characterized by a fibrous cap which forms over a protruding mound of cholesterol plaque. Often hidden in the center of the plaque is a lipid pool of "soft cholesterol" created by dead foam cells which have disintegrated, releasing all the fatty material they contained.

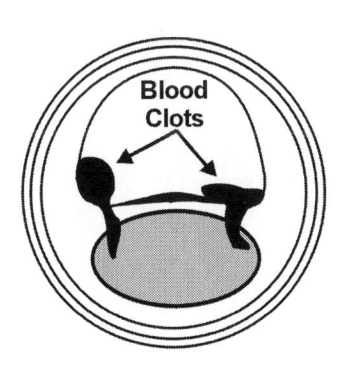

Complicated Lesions

A complicated lesion is an advanced lesion that has ruptured and formed blood clots. The fibrous cap has cracked and eroded, allowing cholesterol to mix with the bloodstream. This contact creates the blood clots that lead to strokes and heart attacks.

Advanced lesions made of vulnerable plaque progress to the third and final category of lesion…

Complicated Lesions

A healthy endothelium is ***antithrombotic***, that is, it tends to discourage clots from forming on the artery wall. But when injury and inflammation strike, and the endothelium becomes dysfunctional, the endothelium loses its ability to discourage clotting. It becomes ***prothrombotic***, that is, tending to promote the creation of blood clots.

Not only does an injured endothelium lose its ability to stop clots from forming, injury stimulates the production of substances that makes blood clot much more easily than it ordinarily would. Injured endothelial cells produce *tissue factor*, a type of protein that initiates blood clotting at the site of injury.[24]

This prothrombotic environment in the artery is bad news. It's a critical step toward the clots that will eventually lead to stroke or heart attack, and its most visible sign is the *complicated lesion*.

A complicated lesion is an advanced lesion that has ruptured and formed blood clots.

The plaque of a complicated lesion is no longer the smooth mound of an atheroma. Tears and fissures have cracked the surface of the plaque. When blood in the bloodstream seeps into the cracks, the prothrombotic substances in the plaque makes the blood clot. These clots plug up the tears and fissures in the plaque, creating a rough and bumpy covering to the lesion

The lesion is said to be "complicated" by layers of clotted blood, which are enveloped within the plaque and coat its surface. In sum, a complicated lesion looks exactly like what it is—a bloody mess.

Once lesions become complicated, the severity of atherosclerosis can increase dramatically. Suddenly, a disease that has taken decades to develop, races off in a spurt of growth. More and more new lesions spread throughout the arteries and old lesions increase rapidly in size as layers of clotted blood adhere to—and are enveloped by—cholesterol plaque. As the lesion grows in size, the diameter of the artery becomes narrower and narrower.

The narrowing of an artery is called *stenosis*. An artery can become so clogged with plaque that it completely stops the flow of blood. One way doctors try to determine the severity of their patient's atherosclerosis is by measuring how much an artery has been stenosed by plaque. But studies show that simple narrowing is only half the story. Much more important is the presence of…

7

Vulnerable Plaque and Blood Clots

To understand the serious consequences of vulnerable plaque and blood clots, you need to understand the meaning of...

Coronary Events

A *coronary event* is a shorthand term describing any acute symptom of coronary artery disease, such as an episode of angina or a heart attack. Not too long ago, doctors believed in a simple equation: the more an artery was narrowed by plaque, the more coronary events a patient suffered. Recent research, however, suggests otherwise.

It turns out that the majority of coronary events happen in arteries that are only mildly to moderately narrowed by plaques. Researchers came to the conclusion that *the vulnerability of plaque to rupture and produce blood clots was more important than the degree of arterial narrowing as a cause of coronary events.*

This is an important distinction. It suggests why some people with clogged arteries suffer few symptoms, while others with only mild narrowing can become dangerously ill. This paradox is partly explained by...

Collateral Circulation

It turns out that the heart is not completely helpless in the face of plaque build-up in the coronary arteries. As long as the occlusion of a coronary artery doesn't happen *suddenly* from a blood clot, there is a way for the heart to lessen the dangers of clogging and eventual occlusion.

When the body senses that areas of the heart are slowly being weakened by a gradual loss of circulation, it can respond to the injury. In a process called *collateral circulation*, the body stimulates the growth of new blood vessels. These new arteries branch out into the injured area, connecting up with the weakened heart muscle. These tiny vessels provide a detour for blood around the narrowed artery, restoring circulation to the areas of the heart that are suffering.

In effect, the body has performed its own natural bypass operation. So even if a coronary artery becomes completely blocked by plaque, these newly formed blood vessels can keep the heart going.

This natural bypass can be surprisingly effective. In many instances, patients lead active lives—even engaged in vigorous exercise such as running or jogging—without being aware that one or more of their coronary arteries may be severely clogged with plaque.

As long as the narrowing of an artery takes place over an extended period, the body has time to respond with a natural bypass that keeps the heart muscle supplied with blood. But arteries that occlude *suddenly*, due to ruptured vulnerable plaque and blood clots, create an emergency situation. There is no time for the body to respond with collateral circulation.

This is why—as stated in the last chapter—not all atherosclerosis is created equal. Vulnerable plaques are much more hazardous than stable plaques. Although they comprise only 10–20% of all lesions, vulnerable plaques are responsible for 80–90% of all acute coronary events, such as angina and heart attacks.[25]

With this new understanding of plaque's different degrees of danger, the medical world focused its attention on discovering what makes plaque vulnerable and why ruptured plaques so readily produce blood clots.

I know the suspense is killing you, so I'll come right out and tell you what the researchers found: chronic inflammation is the reason why plaques become vulnerable. It is also the reason blood clots form so easily from ruptured plaques.

Once again, it seems chronic inflammation makes all the difference. Here's an in-depth look at how chronic inflammation does its dirty work. We'll start by considering…

Stable and Vulnerable Plaques

By definition, vulnerable plaques rupture and stable plaques don't. Stable plaques are relatively inactive, growing slowly in size over the years or even regressing in size somewhat. In contrast, vulnerable plaques are active—they rupture repeatedly, changing their shapes and increasing rapidly in size.

Researchers suspected that the difference in activity between stable and vulnerable plaques could be explained by the differences in their structure and composition. After completing numerous studies, that's exactly what they found. But more than that, they discovered that most of the structural differences could be traced directly to the effects of chronic inflammation. Here's why.

Stable plaques are stable due to three main factors.

First, stable plaque is largely *fibrous* in nature. It is made up mostly of smooth muscle cells and matrix tissue, with relatively small amounts of macrophages and foam cells. Fibrous tissue created by chronic inflammation is typically dense and cohesive. Because stable plaques are made of these tougher materials, they're not prone to rupture.

Second, the fibrous caps of stable plaques tend to be on the thick side, giving them extra protection against the forces in the artery that would tear the plaque open. These caps are rich in smooth muscle cells and matrix, which gives the cap its strength.

Third, the pool of lipid at the core of stable lesions is relatively small, which means it is less disruptive to the integrity of the plaque. Plaque is a rather solid substance, but the lipid core is a soft semi-solid. Lipid cores are weak spots in the structure of lesions. So the smaller the weak spot, the less likely it is that a lesion will break open.[26]

Conversely, the larger the weak spot, the more likely it is that a lesion will break open. Studies suggest that when the lipid pool makes up more than 50% of the size of the lesion, the plaque becomes especially vulnerable to rupture.[27]

These are the main qualities of stable plaques. As you might expect, vulnerable plaques have the exact *opposite* characteristics.

They are not primarily fibrous in their makeup; they lack large amounts of smooth muscle cells and connective tissues. Instead, they contain an overabundance of macrophages and foam cells, making them more prone to erode, fissure and rupture. They tend to have thin, weak fibrous caps making them easier to tear open. And the lipid core at the center of the lesion is large in size, disrupting the integrity of the lesion. Taken together, these factors greatly increase the risk of rupture.

VULNERABLE PLAQUE AND BLOOD CLOTS

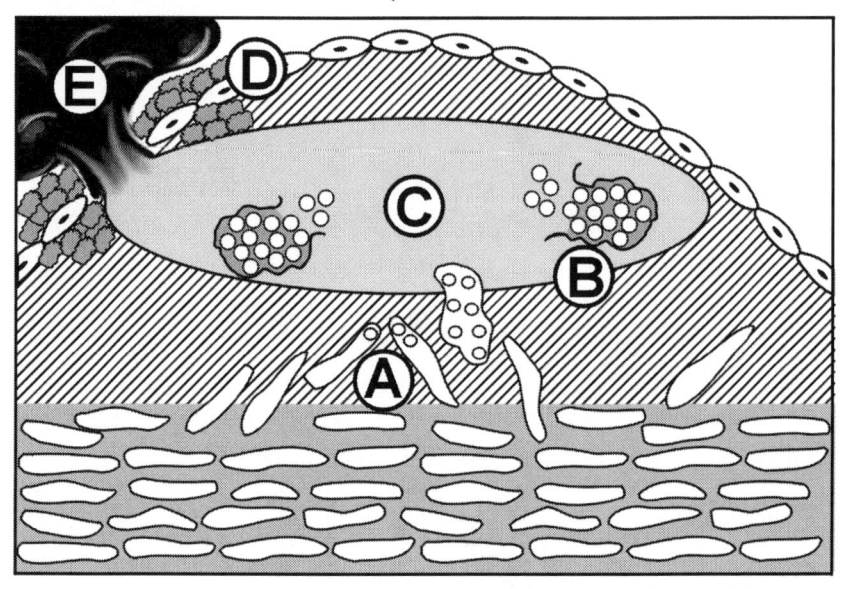

Compared to stable plaques, vulnerable or unstable plaques are more likely to rupture and create serious problems. In the vulnerable plaque pictured above, smooth muscle cells from the media (A) are moving into the lesion and turning into foam cells. Along with macrophage foam cells (B), they will burst open and die, releasing their cholesterol droplets into the lesion. Over time, these fatty droplets congregate into a pool of "soft cholesterol" (C) in the center of the lesion. Meanwhile, macrophages and other inflammatory immune system cells (D) gather together beneath and on top of the surface of the lesion, dissolving away the fibrous cap which holds the lesion together. With the cap completely eroded at the shoulder of the lesion, soft cholesterol leaks out into the bloodstream, creating a blood clot (E), which may lead directly to a stroke or heart attack.

Why do macrophages and foam cells weaken plaque and make it vulnerable? Is it simply because they are not as "strong" as connective matrix and smooth muscle cells?

No. It's more than that. The presence of macrophages and foam cells plays an *active role* in undermining the integrity of plaque. Chronic inflammation weakens the plaque, making the fibrous cap turn thin and easy to break open. Simply stated, *vulnerable plaques are prone to rupture because chronic inflammation actively weakens cholesterol plaque.*

At first, this may seem like a contradiction. After all, inflammation is responsible for building up the lesion in the first place. How can it be responsible for tearing it down as well?

The answer is found in the dual nature of inflammation—it both builds up and tears down tissues in a process called...

The Remodeling of Arteries

If you've ever had a kitchen remodeled, you know that remodeling is a two-step process. The first thing the installation crew does is tear down and haul away the damaged or unwanted structures—cabinets, shelves, walls, floors, etc. Then new structures are manufactured, pieced together and set into place.

Inflammation follows the same two-step process when it remodels damaged arteries. It tears down the tissues that are injured—dismantling them and hauling them off—and then directs the rebuilding of the artery with new cells and matrix material.

How does inflammation accomplish this tearing down and building up? In large part, it's done with substances manufactured by the inflammatory cells of the immune system, such as macrophages and lymphocytes.

Take macrophages, for example. These immune cells secrete many different chemicals during the course of inflammation. Some of these chemicals are toxic; when they touch nearby cells, they destroy them. In this way, macrophages "tear down" tissue.

But macrophages also secrete other substances that have the *opposite* effect. They act as a signal for nearby cells to either proliferate or start creating new matrix material. In this way, macrophages stimulate other cells to "build up" the surrounding tissue.

Science still has much to learn about this process, but we know some of the key substances that influence the course of inflammation.

When white blood cells, such as monocytes and macrophages, begin their inflammatory work they release special proteins called **cytokines**. Among their many functions, cytokines attract more white blood cells to the site of inflammation, which, in turn, keeps the inflammatory process going. But cytokines can also damage endothelial cells, which also works to keeps inflammation smoldering in the artery. In addition, cytokines encourage smooth muscle cells to move to a certain spot and proliferate. In this way, cytokines are thought to be a factor in the "building up" and "tearing down" of the artery wall.[28]

I've singled out cytokines because they make a repeat appearance later in the book and I wanted you to be familiar with the name. But there are other substances that inflammation uses to orchestrate the inflammatory process, and many of them play a role in the remodeling of arteries.

When inflammation proceeds according to plan, this two-step combination of "tear down" and "build up" works in harmony to remodel an artery—the familiar "balance of forces" that responds appropriately to injury.

But as we've already seen, *chronic* inflammation throws these forces out of balance. The long-term presence of macrophages and other immune system cells in the artery wall can produce too many substances such as cytokines that stimulate the proliferation of cells. This overstimulation of the tissue "build-up" phase is largely responsible for the growth of lesions.

The chronic presence of macrophages and other immune cells can also produce too many chemicals that "tear down" tissues, as well. And this is the reason why plaques become vulnerable to rupture.

In sum, inflammation is responsible for both building up atherosclerotic lesions and tearing them down by dissolving the fibrous cap.[29] It's still uncertain exactly how inflammation switches from the "build-up" phase to the "tear-down" phase, but collections of macrophages seem to be a key to dissolving the fibrous cap.

Macrophages are not evenly distributed throughout inflamed lesions. They tend to gather together in colonies, causing concentrated knots of inflammation, often within and underneath the fibrous cap. They also love to hang out on the edges of the lesion—the shoulders of the plaque—where the lesion is attached to the artery. It's here where the cap is usually the thinnest, thanks in large part to the toxic chemicals produced by macrophages.

Macrophages secrete a variety of enzymes that degrade and weaken matrix material such as collagen and elastin. Right away, you know that's bad news for the stability of plaque. After all, it's matrix material that holds the fibrous cap together.

Studies have found that when active macrophages gather together within and underneath the fibrous cap, these enzymes eat away at the cap, digesting collagen and elastin. This causes sections of the cap to become thin and weaken. It's been shown that plaque tends to break open at the places where the fibrous cap is weakest. So with sections of the cap literally dissolved away by macrophages, the plaque becomes vulnerable to rupture.

The shoulders of the plaque—the points where the plaque joins normal tissue—are especially vulnerable to this type of macrophage activity. The shoulders are the thinnest part of the fibrous cap to begin with. As inflammation eats away at the cap, the shoulders are typically the most likely to break open. One study found that 63% of ruptures occurred in the shoulders of the plaque.[30]

Additional inflammatory cells, such as lymphocytes, weaken plaque in a different way. Collagen fibers, which give the cap its strength, are manufactured by smooth muscle cells. But the chemicals secreted by lymphocytes inhibit smooth muscle cells from manufacturing collagen.

As a result, areas of the plaque inflamed by lymphocytes have fewer collagen fibers, weakening the plaque. Once again, inflammation has increased the risk of rupture.

In these and other ways, the chemicals produced by chronic inflammation work to destroy the structural integrity of plaque, making it vulnerable to breaking open. As if that wasn't enough, inflammation also has a hand in creating the deadly product of ruptured plaques...

Blood Clots

Once plaque has ruptured, blood clots take center stage in the story of strokes and heart attacks. Unlikely as it seems, blood clots, too, have their origin in inflammation.

As you may remember from the previous chapter, blood clots are a response to injury. Most of the time, the injury is a cut or bruise to a blood vessel. The response to injury generally happens like this:

When the wall of a blood vessel is damaged, interior substances, such as collagen, are exposed to the bloodstream. *Platelets*, small specialized cells found in the bloodstream, bump into the collagen and are activated to turn sticky. More and more platelets become stuck to one another, forming a plug against the vessel wall.

The combination of sticky platelets and injured tissues signals the body to begin the *coagulation cascade*, the process that turns blood from a liquid to a semi-solid. During this process, plasma, the fluid in which blood cells are suspended, turns into a gel at the site of injury. In addition, *fibrinogen*, a protein, is chemically transformed into a meshwork of fibers called *fibrin*. Red blood cells become trapped in the fibrin net and a blood clot is born—a semi-solid, jelly-like mass that helps seal up the vessel wall.

Medically speaking, a blood clot is called a *thrombus* and the process that forms the clot is called *thrombosis*. Any substance that produces clots is called *thrombogenic*.

Just as there are forces in the body which *create* clots, there are forces in the body that *inhibit* clots from forming or dissolves them away once they are no longer needed. When properly balanced, these opposing forces make sure that we neither bleed nor clot ourselves to death.

Early in the game, the endothelium plays a large part in this process. As we've previously noted, a healthy endothelium tends to prevent clots from forming on the artery wall. But an endothelium afflicted with inflammation turns dysfunctional, losing its ability to stop clots from forming.

So: blood begins to clot when it is exposed to substances which tip the "balance of forces," setting off the response to injury of coagulation and thrombosis. There are many substances in the body that can tip blood toward clotting. As it happens, some of the most potent clot-producing substances are concentrated inside atherosclerotic lesions, especially the lipid core.

For example, *tissue factor*, a substance released by cells when they are injured, is a very powerful stimulant of the coagulation cascade. It turns out that the macrophages and foam cells found in chronically inflamed cholesterol plaque are rich sources of tissue factor, making them thrombogenic. That's why you never want blood to come into contact with cholesterol plaque, especially the lipid pool, which is loaded with tissue factor and other procoagulative material.[31]

Fortunately, the fibrous cap found on lesions effectively separates blood from the plaque inside. But if the cap ruptures, then blood will be exposed to the thrombogenic material that makes up the interior of the lesion.

What happens next depends on a number of factors.

If the rupture is small, such as a microscopic crack or superficial erosion, then the amount of coagulation is small—just enough to plug up the crack or erosion. Once the crack is plugged, smooth muscle cells and matrix begin to multiply and the fissure is healed over. This is how vulnerable plaques grow in size. By continually building layers of coagulated blood and plaque, the artery becomes increasingly narrowed.

Because the amount of coagulation is small, the victim feels no symptoms when his vulnerable plaque cracks or erodes. Most plaque ruptures are small, like this. As a result, many people are lulled into thinking that—simply because they feel well—they are not suffering from steadily advancing cardiovascular disease.

The fact is, *half the people who die from a sudden heart attack had no previous symptoms.* Despite leading active, vigorous lives, numerous small and unnoticed episodes of ruptured plaque set the stage for the trouble to come.

And that trouble comes in the form of a *large* rupture that produces a large blood clot in an artery already narrowed by smaller episodes of ruptured plaque.

When ruptures are large, the blood is exposed to more of the inflammatory material that leads to coagulation. This, in turn, leads to a bigger blood clot. This is especially true if the lipid core is exposed.[32, 33]

Now you know why "unstable" angina is generally considered more serious than "stable" angina. Stable angina is usually the result of simple narrowing in the artery from plaque. But unstable angina involves ruptured plaques and blood clots, creating a much more dangerous environment for the kind of sudden occlusions that lead to serious injury.

The life span of a clot is critical to the severity of the occlusion. The longer the clot exists, the greater the damage from occlusion. Fortunately, because of the body's "balance of forces," there are substances in the blood that immediately set to work dissolving clots formed from ruptured plaque. If the clot dissolves quickly enough, the episode of angina is short lived.

But, as you'll soon discover, there are many reasons why the forces that work to dissolve clots may be out of balance with the forces that create them. Under these conditions—or simply because the clot is too large to begin with—a blood clot may last a long time, creating a dangerous occlusion that ultimately leads to a stroke, heart attack or sudden death.

In this chapter, most of our discussion has centered on the arteries of the heart. But nearly all the lessons we've learned can be applied to the arteries of the brain, as well. The same basic mechanisms of inflammation, ruptured plaque and thrombosis create the occlusions that lead to Transient Ischemic Attacks and strokes.

Summing up, inflammation is responsible for more than just the build-up of cholesterol plaque; it also creates the most dangerous consequences of atherosclerosis—vulnerable plaque and blood clots.

In the strictest sense, the rupture of plaque is an unpredictable event; it's simply impossible to say with certainty when an actively inflamed lesion will break open. Often, however, there are specific conditions under which plaques are much more likely to split apart. These conditions are known as…

8

The Triggers of Strokes and Heart Attacks

A Definition of Triggers

As we've seen, vulnerable plaques tend to cause more acute cardiovascular events than stable plaques. Therefore, being able to identify a particular lesion as either vulnerable or stable would be a big help in assessing a patient's personal risk for stroke and heart attack. Unfortunately, while medical tests such as angiography and ultrasound can detect the presence of plaque, they can't yet distinguish vulnerable lesions from stable ones.

This may change in the future. Remember that one of the hallmarks of inflammation is heat. Since vulnerable, inflamed lesions are hotter than surrounding tissue, new techniques are being developed that measure the temperature inside arteries. In this way, the presence of "hot spots" would indicate lesions of vulnerable plaque in the artery.[34] As of right now, however, the only way to identify vulnerable lesions is by the symptoms they produce when they rupture—and that's too late in the game to achieve the full benefits of early detection.

Moreover, no one can predict with certainty *when* a particular plaque will break open. But there are circumstances under which the likelihood of rupture increases dramatically.

It's thought that vulnerable plaques spontaneously rupture of their own accord when episodes of localized inflammation become so intense that they dissolve away the fibrous cap, exposing the interior of the lesion.[35] This is a hidden process, which is why it's so difficult to predict when a rupture will take place.

But it's also believed that plaques often break open in response to particular forces in the artery. These forces are called *triggers* because their presence kicks off the sequence of rupture and blood clots that directly initiates a stroke or heart attack.

In the last chapter, we discussed several things that make a plaque likely to break open—a thin fibrous cap, a large lipid core and chronic inflammation in and around the plaque. All these factors can *predispose* a plaque to rupture, but it's triggers that *precipitate* the actual event.

Think of triggers this way: when you're sick with a cold, you are more susceptible to sneezing. But just because you are more susceptible, doesn't mean you sneeze constantly. Only periodically, when conditions are right, does your body trigger a sneeze.

It's the same idea with strokes and heart attacks. When your arteries contain vulnerable plaque, you're more susceptible to strokes and heart attacks—but that doesn't mean you suffer these events on a constant basis. Only when conditions are right does your body trigger a plaque to rupture.

Most often, these cardiovascular triggers are created by the influence of...

The Sympathetic Nervous System

Many years ago, doctors noticed that many heart attacks happen when the victim is engaged in a particular type of activity. From these observations, the concept of triggers was born.

For example, moments of heavy physical exertion and sexual activity seem to increase the risk for heart attack. Both of these moments are marked by stimulation of the *sympathetic nervous system*, a part of the nervous system that regulates the actions of the heart, blood vessels, glands, and other parts of the body. The sympathetic nervous system reconfigures the body for intense physical effort by making changes such as…

- increasing blood pressure
- increasing heart rate and responsiveness
- opening up blood vessels in the heart
- constricting blood vessels in the skin
- directing blood to skeletal muscles
- opening up airways in the lungs

…and other adjustments that help the body cope with increased physical demands.

The heart and blood vessels can undergo tremendous changes when the sympathetic nervous system is activated. The interior walls of the body's arteries feel the effects of increased blood pressure, a rapid heartbeat and a strong, pounding pulse. These changes may be the very things that trigger a vulnerable plaque to rupture.

If you've ever held a dirty dish under the faucet or sprayed a sidewalk clean with a high-powered nozzle, you know that rushing fluid can exert a powerful force. Inside an artery, blood is a fluid with the same ability to exert force on anything in its path—especially cholesterol plaque.

When plaque first appears, it has a low profile on the artery wall; the force of the blood pushing against it is relatively small. But as the plaque grows and layer upon layer piles up, the plaque pushes into the bloodstream, feeling the full effect of the blood rushing past.

Once a fissure develops in the plaque, the fluid forces in the bloodstream can push and tug at the opening, peeling it away and exposing the interior of the lesion.

The mere presence of plaque also creates *turbulence* in the bloodstream—little whirlpools and squirting jets of blood. Turbulence can increase the amount of force acting upon a particular area, working to dislodge pieces of plaque from the artery wall and creating occlusions.[36]

Turbulence

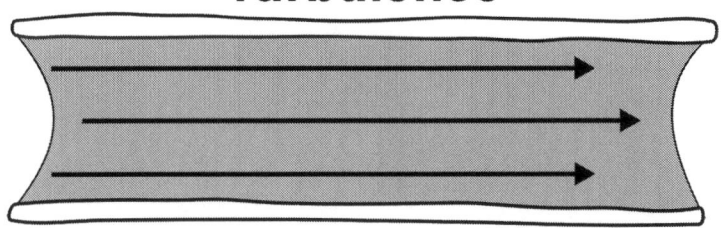

1. In a healthy artery, the flow of blood progresses smoothly.

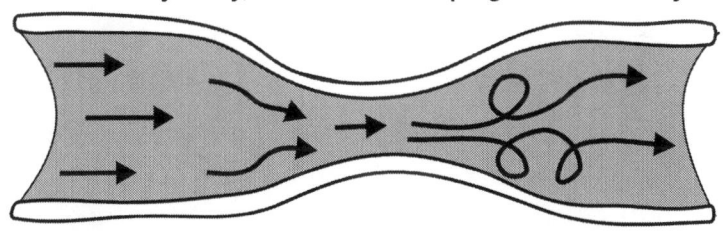

2. However, in an artery constricted by spasm, the bloodstream becomes turbulent. As the drawing above illustrates, beyond the narrowing there's a squirting action in the blood, creating little swirls and whirlpools. The force of the turbulence may damage the endothelial lining of the blood vessel, setting the stage for atherosclerosis.

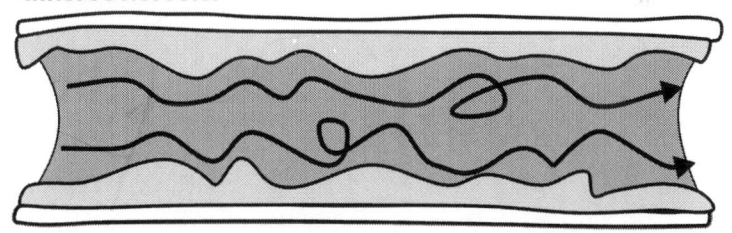

3. And atherosclerosis itself can create turbulence. The swirling forces in the bloodstream can dislodge pieces of plaque or promote plaque rupture, both of which lead to occlusions in the artery and the possibility of a stroke or heart attack.

Increases in blood pressure, pulse rate and pulse strength during moments of sympathetic nervous system activation are all believed to enhance the forces that can tear open vulnerable plaque. Whether these forces are sufficient to tear open a plaque depends on both the strength of the force and the vulnerability of the individual lesion. A lesion that remains whole during normal circumstances may break open under the increased forces of sympathetic nervous system activity.

Intense physical effort can be a trigger for strokes and heart attacks. This fact often leads to confusion about the benefits and dangers of physical activities such as running, exercising or lifting weights. Many of my patients hear two conflicting messages from the health care industry. On one hand, they're told that physical exercise is good for the heart and arteries. On the other, they're told that physical exercise is a trigger for strokes and heart attacks. So what are they supposed to do?

The answer depends largely on the cardiovascular health of the individual patient. If the patient is usually sedentary and suffering from atherosclerosis, then stimulation of the sympathetic nervous system from sudden, intense physical exercise may trigger vulnerable plaque to rupture. But, if the patient's arteries are clear of atherosclerosis, the risk is greatly lessened because there's no plaque for the stress reaction to trigger into a stroke or heart attack.

Of course, the patient may be totally unaware that his arteries are suffering from advanced atherosclerosis or some other limiting cardiovascular problem. (Remember, an artery can be occluded up to 75% yet produce no symptoms.) That is why you often hear the cautionary phrase "Check with your doctor before starting any exercise program." Only a thorough cardiovascular examination will reveal the presence of plaque or some other problem that may cause trouble when the body undergoes the physical changes brought about by exercise. I'll have more to say about exercise and the cardiovascular system in the next chapter about risk factors.

It seems as though any strong increase in the activity of the sympathetic nervous system can cause a triggering event. But physical activity is not the only thing that kicks the sympathetic nervous system into action. The body responds to a much broader range of stimuli, and this reaction is often referred to as...

Stress

Stress is the sum of the body's reactions to adverse influences. These influences can be external to the body—such as heat or cold—or they can be internal, such as an infection or an emotional reaction to something in the environment.

The definition of stress has become so elastic in modern times that it's often stretched into a meaningless concept. For our purposes, however, it is reasonable to say that anything that strongly stimulates the sympathetic nervous system can be considered stressful.

It's important to note that stress is often an entirely appropriate reaction by the body. At other times, the stress reaction can be inappropriate or inadequate. Under these conditions, long periods of stress upset the proper functioning of the body, leading to illness.

I'm sure you've heard the words "*fight or flight*" before. It's a phrase that describes a collection of bodily responses to situations that provoke fear or anger. These responses—a quickened pulse, a rising blood pressure and an increase in body metabolism—are an ancient survival mechanism that prepared our bodies for physical action, such as facing down a pack of jackals or fleeing a man-eating tiger. These changes are—as you might expect—caused by the stimulation of the sympathetic nervous system and are an entirely appropriate stress reaction, designed to prepare you for getting out of trouble.

Apart from the ravenous mosquitoes on the patio of my South Florida home, however, modern man rarely encounters animals that wish to eat us. And yet, many times a day, the "fight or flight" response by the sympathetic nervous system is kindled within us by the common occurrences of everyday live. The stimulus may be nothing more dangerous than a peeved boss at work, or an obnoxious driver who cuts you off on the road. Yet your body responds to these emotional stimuli as if they were life or death situations, kicking the sympathetic nervous system into gear. This, of course, is an entirely inappropriate stress reaction.

Much of the stress response is caused by a sudden increase in the bloodstream of *epinephrine* (more commonly known as *adrenaline*), a hormone secreted by the adrenal glands, which are located above the kidneys. Normally, there are only small amounts of epinephrine in the bloodstream. But during moments of excitement or other strong emotions, epinephrine production increases dramatically. It floods into the bloodstream, creating the physical changes in our body that prepare us for fight or flight.

So the body's reaction to stressful influences can be both appropriate or not appropriate, depending on the circumstances. Either way, however, the stress reactions of high blood pressure, a rapid heartbeat and a strong, pounding pulse are exactly the types of things that may cause a vulnerable plaque to rupture.

A key thing to notice is that these stress reactions happen prior to any physical activity of the body. The stress is not caused by physical demands on the body—such as exercise or sexual activity—but by an emotional or mental state that precedes physical action. Recently, there's been a rising interest in these non-physical stressors that may act as a trigger for stroke and heart attack. One type of stressor is called…

Acute Mental Stress

Acute mental stress is felt as a short, sharp moment of heightened emotional turmoil.

Acute episodes of mental stress, such as anger, are strongly felt but typically don't last a long time. We all have flashes of anger or shocking surprise, but we don't tend to be angry or surprised all day long. And we're always aware of these emotionally stressing moments. In fact, their emotional wallop tends to make them memorable events. When angered, we often say that something "makes our blood boil"—an indication that we feel the strong physical changes that the sympathetic nervous system is making to our heart and arteries.

It's not surprising to find that moments of anger and other acute mental stresses can be triggering events for strokes and heart attacks.[37] A recent study found that "middle-aged men who outwardly express their anger on a regular basis have more than twice the risk of stroke compared with their more even-tempered peers." And worse—the same report found the stroke risk was six times greater for men with a history of heart disease.[38]

In sum, it's thought that 32,000 heart attacks are caused by bursts of anger each year in the United States.[39] Other studies have found that many diverse types of acute mental stress—from speeding tickets to earthquakes—increase the risk for cardiovascular troubles.[40, 41] All of these moments of intense, emotional stimuli can rouse the sympathetic nervous system, causing the rupture of plaque.

As you might expect, these episodes of acute mental stress are also triggers for angina, that painful, crushing feeling in the chest. Angina, of course, is the result of ischemia, too little blood flowing through the heart muscle. It turns out that the ischemia that accompanies mental stress is often the result of…

Arterial Spasm

A *spasm* is the sudden, involuntary contraction of a muscle. All muscles are susceptible to spasm, and arteries, which are essentially long tubes of muscle, are no exception. There's even a special name for an episode of spasm that strikes a blood vessel—*vasospasm.* When vasospasm strikes a coronary artery, the result is ischemia.

Muscle spasms in general can exert tremendous force on the body. If you've ever suffered a severe leg cramp in the middle of the night, you've experienced firsthand just how powerful spasm can be. In fact, a tetanus infection can produce muscle spasms so strong that they crack the bones of the spine.

When the muscle that makes up an artery goes into spasm, the blood vessel contracts with surprising strength. In a matter of moments, the diameter of the artery shrinks dramatically. If the spasm is strong enough, the vessel is crumpled flat like an empty tube of toothpaste, and the flow of blood through the artery is reduced to a trickle.

Prolonged spasm in a coronary artery can cause cardiac damage by reducing circulation to the heart muscle, creating painful angina. There have been cases where spasm alone was sufficient to cause a heart attack, but this rarely occurs. Simple spasm in a healthy coronary artery usually does not increase the risk of death.[42]

But recent evidence has shown that spasm combined with atherosclerosis is a deadly mixture that can lead to unstable angina, arrhythmias, heart attack and sudden cardiac death. In my own practice, I consider spasm to be the most dangerous trigger of acute cardiovascular events. Here's why.

When spasm occurs in a coronary artery containing vulnerable plaque, the force of the contraction can be so great that it literally crushes atherosclerotic lesions within the artery.[43, 44] Vasospasm splits open the hard cholesterol plaque and the lipid core of the lesion spurts out like the white of a cracked egg. Once study called the process a "volcano-like eruption" as spasm squeezes the plaque and soft cholesterol gushes out into the bloodstream.[45] As you know, clots may form in response to the soft cholesterol, creating an occlusion that turns into angina, stroke or heart attack.[46] Or the clot may become incorporated into the plaque, further narrowing the artery and advancing the disease.

If the artery remains constricted, the potential for occlusion is great because the artery, already narrowed by plaque, is further narrowed by the ongoing spasm. This increases the likelihood that the clot will get snagged in the artery, stopping the flow of blood.

Spasm is perhaps the most potent trigger the sympathetic nervous system creates when it undergoes stress. All things considered, the *last* place you want spasm to appear is in your coronary arteries…and yet these very arteries seem particularly susceptible to spasm.

All arteries are designed to both contract and expand their diameters to meet the needs of the body. It is an integral and necessary part of their function. The contraction of a blood vessel's diameter is called ***vasoconstriction***, while the enlargement of the diameter is called ***vasodilation***.

During "fight or flight" preparation, the arteries near the body's surface tend to constrict, shutting down the blood supply to the skin, causing it to turn pale. Among other reasons, it's a way for the body to protect itself against bleeding during injury if a "fight" should happen. At the same time, the arteries of the larger muscles dilate, allowing plenty of blood to flow to the legs in case the "flight" option is in order!

So the constriction and dilation of arteries are not abnormal—it happens all the time, often with surprising swiftness. Think how quickly a blush of embarrassment can cover a face, turning it beet red within a split second. This blush is caused by the almost instantaneous dilation of blood vessels of the face. This rapid change is not in response to any great physical effort, but is caused totally by the person's emotional state, which illustrates how emotions alone can cause profound changes in the body's cardiovascular system.

The coronary arteries of the heart also seem to have a hair trigger for contraction and expansion…and with good reason. The demands for blood flow to the heart muscle can change at a moment's notice.

One second you may be casually strolling through your place of work. The next second, you may be racing up a flight of stairs when you realize you're late for a meeting. The sudden shift in activity requires your heart to pump faster, placing a great demand for oxygen to your heart muscle. To meet the immediate need, the sympathetic nervous system instructs the coronary arteries to rapidly expand in size allowing more blood to flow to the heart.

Once you reach the meeting room and plop down in the chair, there is no need for your heart to pump faster. So now your coronary arteries shrink in diameter, reducing the flow of blood to your cardiac muscle.

In this way, the body makes sure that the heart gets the proper amount of circulation. In a normal coronary artery, then, stress opens up the artery, allowing blood to flow. In an artery diseased by atherosclerosis, however, stress causes *the exact reverse to happen*—the coronary arteries constrict in spasm, shutting down the flow of blood to the heart and potentially rupturing plaque.[47]

This is an important point that bears repeating: *stress tends to open up healthy coronary arteries, but in arteries diseased by atherosclerosis, stress creates spasm that produces ischemia and may rupture plaque.*

For a long while, the reason why this deadly reversal takes place was a big mystery. And while the exact mechanism is still not fully understood, it's becoming clear that atherosclerosis and its accompanying inflammation damage the normal constricting and dilating functions of the artery.[48]

When any part of the body is diseased, it tends to lose at least part of its normal functions. The ability of an artery to constrict or dilate depends in part on a healthy endothelium, that thin layer of cells that lines the interior of arteries. When the endothelium is injured, it can no longer react properly to the stimuli that it receives.[49, 50] It may become hypersensitive to stimuli, or even react the opposite way that it should, such as telling the artery to constrict when it should be telling it to open wider.[51, 52]

And if there's one thing we *know* injures the endothelium, it's atherosclerosis. After all, atherosclerosis makes its home in the endothelium, radically changing the health of the inner artery. There is evidence that the inflammatory nature of atherosclerosis produces substances that damage the endothelium and make it become vasoconstrictive.[53, 54] The destructive effects of atherosclerosis are blamed as a reason why arteries under stress collapse into spasm when they should be opening up to the flow of blood.[55]

The bottom line: atherosclerotic plaque is more than just a passive player, waiting for a triggering force to rupture it. It actually carries the seeds of its own rupture by promoting the very spasm that will crack it open, kicking off a stroke or heart attack.

And while an attack of spasm may begin as a reaction to stress, it may not end there. It's my belief that the sudden appearance of a blood clot acts like a foreign object in the artery, irritating it into a second wave of spasm.

Think of what happens when a speck of dust gets in your eye and you'll know what I mean; the muscles of the eye react so violently to the foreign object that they clamp down in a vigorous contraction and it's very difficult to keep your eyelids open. In an artery that is already hypersensitive to constrictive stimuli, the presence of a sudden blood clot acts much the same way as a speck of dust, triggering the artery into spasm. The clot becomes locked inside the narrowed artery, prolonging the occlusion and increasing the risk of damage to the heart or brain from loss of blood flow.

STRESS and SPASM

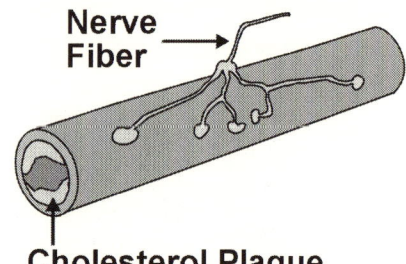

Nerve Fiber

Cholesterol Plaque

Stress is often a trigger for strokes and heart attacks. An artery is designed to react quickly to moments of stress by contracting or expanding in response to the signals it gets from the many nerve fibers that connect to it.

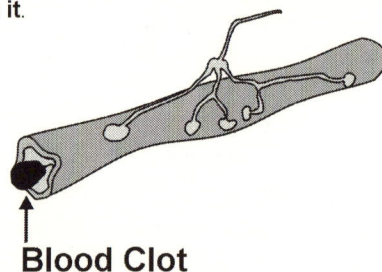

Blood Clot

When an artery is diseased with cholesterol plaque, it's much more likely to contract in spasm as a response to stress. The force of the spasm cracks open the plaque, producing a blood clot.

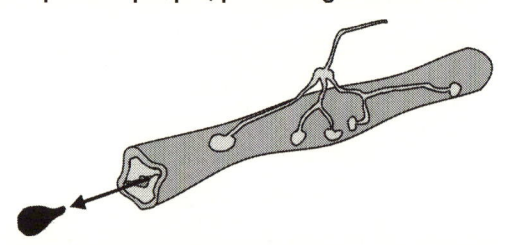

The clot can occlude the artery at the site of spasm or be swept away by the bloodstream, causing an occlusion further down the artery. Either way, the result may be a stroke or heart attack.

But the problem of spasm isn't confined to the dramatic, painful events of angina, stroke and heart attack. Spasm combined with atherosclerosis can cause dangerous ischemia to the heart muscle without the victim even being aware of it. This new idea has come about as a result of studying a slightly different type of mental stress...

Chronic Mental Stress

Acute mental stress is usually pretty easy to recognize because of the strong outbursts of emotion that accompany it. ***Chronic mental stress*** is not so vividly apparent or easily explained.

On a small scale, chronic mental stress accompanies many of the tasks that we attend to every day. These tasks usually involve some level of frustration or mental effort—solving an arithmetic problem, speaking in public, memorizing facts for an important test and so on.

On a larger scale, chronic mental stress is best understood as a "stonewall worry," that is, the state of your mind when it is confronted by a problem that seems to have no ready solution, such as loneliness, relationship troubles or depression.

As its name implies, chronic mental stress lasts a long time, or has constantly recurring episodes. The effects of chronic mental stress on the body are much the same as other stressors: a rise in blood pressure, increased heart rate, and ischemia caused by arterial spasm, although physical stress typically provokes a larger response in all these categories.

In contrast to the short outbursts of acute mental stress, chronic mental stress involves a long-term activation of the sympathetic nervous system. So while chronic stress may not be as strongly felt as acute episodes, it will affect the cardiovascular system over a much more extended period of time.

In the past, researches tried to provoke coronary spasm and ischemia in their subjects with strenuous exercise stress tests, which put a large physical burden on the heart and arteries. But in the past few years, scientists discovered they could reproduce these same stress reactions in subjects who were engaged in mental tasks such as arithmetic tests, word games, memorization, public speaking, and so on.

They found that these rather simple tasks could trigger attacks of spasm and ischemia in patients suffering from atherosclerosis in their coronary arteries. Approximately 50% of patients with coronary artery disease will suffer ischemia when given a mental stress test.[56] And it's estimated that half of all patients who suffer ischemia during exercise testing also suffer ischemia during mental stress testing.[57]

In addition, it was discovered that patients who showed ischemia during mental stress testing also had a higher prevalence, longer duration, and more frequent episodes of ischemia during the common activities of daily life.[58, 59]

For example, one study attempted to assess the risk of ischemia attacks triggered by the typical emotions of daily living. The researchers monitored the hearts of 132 patients with coronary artery disease for 48 continuous hours. At the end of the study, they concluded that an episode of chronic mental stress—which included feelings of tension, frustration and sadness—more than doubled the risk of ischemia in the following hour.[60]

Now, think of how many times you feel tense, frustrated or sad during the course of a day and compare that with the number of times you engage in strenuous physical exercise. It's clear that a good many people with coronary artery disease are likely to experience spasm and ischemia far more often as a consequence of the innumerable daily mental and emotional stresses of life, rather than large, physical ones. So, in the end, mental stress may be a more likely trigger for plaque rupture and subsequent damage.

But the effects of chronic mental stress are not so easily seen. Instead of painful angina, it seems that mental stress if more likely to result in "silent angina" or, more properly, "silent ischemia" in patients with coronary artery disease.[61, 62] People suffering an attack of silent ischemia feel no painful symptoms, even though their heart is starving for oxygen. One study concluded that up to 75% of ischemic attacks in patients are silent.[63]

But even though an episode of ischemia during mental stress may be silent, the victim is still at risk. A patient's ischemic response to mental stress predicts his outcome for coronary artery disease. As one study put it, "The presence of mental stress induced ischemia is associated with significantly higher rates of subsequent fatal and nonfatal cardiac events."[64]

In fact, it appears that mental stress may actually promote the build-up of atherosclerosis in the body. One study found that men whose sympathetic nervous systems respond strongly to mental stress have a high likelihood of developing atherosclerosis in the carotid arteries.[65] Another study measured the effect of mental stress on women and found the same thing; subjects who had an exaggerated stress response to simple tasks such as giving a speech or tracing an image in a mirror had an acceleration of atherosclerosis in their carotid arteries.[66]

(Plaque in the carotid arteries, of course, is a source of strokes. But the carotids are often considered a marker for atherosclerosis throughout the body—if your carotids have atherosclerosis, it's likely your coronary arteries do, too. That's why many studies measure disease in the carotids to make generalizations about the presence of heart disease and the risk of heart attack.)

Why do people with an exaggerated response to mental stress seem to promote the build-up of atherosclerosis within their arteries? Once again, the answer seems to be *inflammation as a response to injury*.

Researchers suspect that the cardiovascular changes brought on by mental stress—a rise in blood pressure, increased heart rate and especially arterial spasm—damages the lining of the artery.[67] This begins the process of repair and inflammation that can generate or accelerate atherosclerosis.[68]

So the role of chronic mental stress in cardiovascular disease is twofold: it acts both as a *risk factor for promoting atherosclerosis* and as a *trigger for rupturing plaque*.

There are two more areas of study that strongly reinforce the role of mental stress as a trigger for strokes and heart attacks…

Circadian Rhythms and Stressful Dreams as Triggers

One of the first things I noticed when I began my medical practice was the amount of emergency phone calls I would get from patients in the early hours of the mornings, especially on Mondays and Tuesdays.

Typically, a patient would awaken with pain or discomfort in his chest at about three o'clock in the morning. He'd take some antacid, go back to bed, wait an hour or two, but continue to get worse. Finally his wife would call me on the phone and, hearing the symptoms, I'd send him to the emergency room, where an hour later I'd walk in and find him being treated for a heart attack by the ER staff.

I've lost track of the amount of times this scenario played out in my younger days. Early on, I wondered why heart attacks seemed to happen so often in the morning, when the patient (and I!) was at rest or even asleep. It seemed at odds with the then-current belief that most heart attacks are triggered by strenuous physical exertion.

It turns out that heart attacks follow a *circadian rhythm*. A circadian rhythm is a daily cycle of biological processes and activities. It's been established that the factors which influence the triggering and severity of strokes and heart attacks—such as blood pressure, heart rate and the tendency for blood to form blood clots—show a daily increase during the early morning hours. It's also been shown that ischemia, stroke, heart attack and sudden cardiac death occur more frequently in the morning hours after awakening.[69]

Researchers now believe that the activation of the sympathetic nervous system during sleep and awakening account for the triggering of these acute cardiovascular events. Among the triggering factors, perhaps none is more significant than the fact the coronary artery spasm occurs most often during times of rest, between midnight and the early morning hours.[70] Since we know that mental stress can induce coronary spasm, is it possible that mental stress plays a role in triggering strokes and heart attacks while the victim is asleep?

Many researchers believe that it does, in the form of dreams during **REM sleep**. REM stands for **Rapid Eye Movement**. When the eyes twitch and move during sleep, it's often a signal that the subject is dreaming. Research has determined that it's during REM sleep that the body undergoes elevated pulse rate, increased brain activity and other physical changes.

REM sleep is often called *paradoxical sleep* because the body seems to be deeply at rest, yet the state of brain activity is similar to that of wakefulness. Studies indicate that surges in sympathetic nervous system activity during REM dream sleep have the potential of triggering ischemic episodes and cardiac arrhythmias, which can trigger heart attacks.[71,72]

There's another factor that adds stress to the heart during nighttime. In one more apparent paradox, your heart may have to work harder when you're resting compared to when you are standing upright. When the body is in the reclining position, the heart becomes flooded with blood and it has to work harder by about 1/3 to pump it out. (If you've noticed, patients in cardiac Intensive Care Units almost always lay in their beds in a semi-upright position—rarely fully reclined—for this very reason.) With the heart already working harder because it's horizontal, the stage is set for increased susceptibility to cardiovascular triggers during sleep.

Often we are not aware of the amount of acute emotional stress that dreams provoke in us while they are happening. We can suffer many moments of nighttime anguish and distress, yet upon wakening these anxiety-producing dreams are largely forgotten, evaporated by the morning sunlight.

One of the few times when we are aware of the amount of stress that can occur during sleep is when a dream is so disturbing that the body's stressful response to it shocks us back into consciousness. Who hasn't awoken from a particularly vivid nightmare to find his heart jumping, his pulse racing and his body bathed in a cold sweat, all indications of intense activity by the sympathetic nervous system? Our minds may forget most of these dark moments of stress, but our bodies do not.

Day and night, the effects of mental stress accelerate the process of cardiovascular disease or trigger an actual attack.

Because of the serious consequences that mental stress causes for patients with atherosclerosis, I take the time to administer a mental stress test during examinations in my office. I've found this test to be extremely valuable. It alerts me to patients who have an exaggerated response to stress and are therefore at increased risk for cardiovascular disease. The test is very good at revealing coronary spasm and ischemia, even if the patient seems healthy and has no symptoms. I'll talk more about this test in a later chapter.

For now, it's enough to know that strokes and heart attacks can be triggered by the simple tasks of everyday living—you don't have to be shoveling heavy winter snow or chasing after a rush-hour bus to be at risk for plaque to rupture. You don't even have to be awake!

Finding out who is or is not susceptible to such triggers is an invaluable aid for the prevention of strokes and heart attacks and, as you'll see in Part II of this book, that's exactly what WIN/WIN Therapy does.

9

Risk Factors—Old and New

In the stories of Sherlock Holmes, the master criminal Professor Moriarty was often the hidden figure behind the many evils that Holmes encountered. In much the same way, chronic inflammation is the Moriarty of cardiovascular disease—it always seems to be the hidden figure behind every evil in the story of strokes and heart attacks.

Take this chapter, for instance; this is supposed to be a chapter about risk factors but, before long, the conversation will turn once again to inflammation. That's because chronic inflammation plays a key role in the creation of the traditional risk factors…and several new ones, as well.

Let's begin by considering…

The Problem of Traditional Risk Factors

When a patient comes to see me in my office, he usually has two big questions on his mind:

> *How likely am I to get a stroke or heart attack?*

…and…

> *What can I do to prevent them?*

Most likely, as a reader of *The Heart Attack Germ*, these questions are uppermost in your mind, as well. As you've probably discovered, however, finding answers to these questions is maddeningly difficult.

Until recently, a book such as this would have attempted to answer these questions by discussing the well-known *risk factors*—cholesterol levels, smoking, obesity, and so on. It's widely believed that the more risk factors you possess, the more likely you are to suffer a stroke or heart attack. It's also felt that by lowering your risk factors—for example, through diet or exercise—you also lower your risk for cardiovascular disease.

The trouble is, there are so many exceptions to the risk factor rules that predicting which individual will or will not suffer a stroke or heart attack is simply not possible.

I've had many patients who lived their lives like Winston Churchill: smoking, drinking, overweight, rarely exercising—in short, breaking all the rules for cardiovascular health. And they lived to a ripe old age like Churchill, who died peacefully in his sleep two months after his 90th birthday.

Other patients lived the "Jim Fixx" lifestyle. Fixx practically invented the jogging craze with his book "The Complete Book of Running," which extolled the benefits of exercise as a part of healthy living. Despite his efforts, Fixx died at the early age of 52 from heart disease—while jogging. On autopsy, they found three of his major coronary arteries clogged with cholesterol plaque. All that exercise and "healthy living" did not prevent plaque from clogging the arteries of Jim Fixx.

As the contrasting lives of Churchill and Fixx demonstrate, risk factors are not sure predictors of cardiovascular disease. In fact, studies show that nearly half of all patients with cardiovascular disease have *no known risk factors*.

So, early in my career, when patients asked me *How likely am I to get a stroke or heart attack?* and *What can I do to prevent them?*, medical science gave me little more than vague generalities to offer. Clearly, there was something else beyond mere risk factors that determined the course of cardiovascular disease. As a doctor dedicated to improving the health and longevity of my patients, I was determined to discover what that "something else" might be.

Thanks to the recent advances in medical research and my own years of personal observation and study, I now know the reason why the old risk factors only partially explain the problem of strokes and heart attacks. And why a *new* set of risk factors points the way toward WIN/WIN Therapy.

The Development of Traditional Risk Factors

The concept of risk factors began about 50 years ago. When I attended medical school, back in the 1940s, I rarely heard my professors talk about strokes and heart attacks. They didn't know much about them so there wasn't much to say.

In fact, doctors of the time often didn't know a heart attack when they saw one. They used to say that people dropped dead from "acute indigestion" because severe heart attacks are often accompanied by chest pain and vomiting.

Back then, strokes and heart attacks were not even considered to be diseases. They were just part of the aging process, a consequence of growing old. If you lived long enough, you got strokes and heart attacks, just like you got liver spots.

There were no treatments, other than morphine to relieve pain. No intensive care units. No cardiac rehabilitation centers. No belief that heart attacks could be treated or prevented. The general feeling was, "Well, people have to die of *something*, don't they?"

Slowly, things began to change. We got better electrocardiograph machines, which showed the relationship of heart attacks to irregularities in heart rhythms. As a result, new medicines were created to control the rhythm of the heart. Eventually, we discovered the role of blood clots in strokes and heart attacks and created medicines to dissolve them or prevent them from forming.

The thing that really got our attention, however, happened in the 1940s and 50s when people of middle age started showing up in the emergency rooms suffering heart attacks. Up until then, cardiovascular disease was largely a problem for the elderly. No one could figure out why there was a sudden rise is death among the middle-aged. So several large medical studies were established to track the course of cardiovascular disease in the population. It is from these studies that we developed the concept of risk factors.

Perhaps the most important project was the *Framingham Heart Study*, which was designed to track the health of men and women who appeared to be free of heart disease. A large number of subjects were recruited and the progress of their health was followed for decades. More than 1,000 scientific papers have been based on the Framingham study and it's from this research that much of our knowledge about risk factors was formed.

Smoking was one of the first risk factors to be discovered. The evidence was pretty clear that people who smoked had a higher risk of developing cardiovascular disease. It also became clear that people with diabetes and high blood pressure were also at increased risk. Over time, elevated cholesterol levels, obesity, family history and lack of exercise were identified as additional risk factors.

Even though the idea of risk factors was a medical advance, researchers knew that risk factors alone were not the full answer to predicting strokes and heart attacks. There was something else that was fundamental to the development of atherosclerosis, but nobody knew what it was.

With the rise of advanced medical technology and investigative techniques, however, the risk factors themselves began to reveal the answer. So let's consider the most well-known of…

The Traditional Risk Factors

Traditional risk factors can be placed into two categories: Non-changeable and Changeable.

Non-changeable Risk Factors cannot be modified to reduce their risk. *Changeable Risk Factors*, however, *can* be modified in some way—either by behavior or medical treatment—to reduce the amount of risk they present. The traditional risk factors are categorized as follows:

Traditional Risk Factors	
Non-Changeable	**Changeable**
• Increasing Age • Male Gender • Heredity	• High Blood Pressure • Diabetes • Cholesterol Levels • Smoking • Physical Inactivity • Obesity

Here's a closer look at each group, beginning with the Non-changeable Risk Factors.

Increasing Age

For cardiovascular disease, increasing age is a certain risk factor. The older you get the more likely you are to suffer a stroke or heart attack.

Atherosclerosis can begin as early as childhood, but the symptoms, strokes and heart attacks resulting from atherosclerosis generally don't appear until middle age. After the age of 55, the risk of stroke doubles every ten years.[73] And nearly four out of every five deaths due to heart disease occur in people older than age 65.[74]

Male Gender

As a general rule, the risks of cardiovascular disease are greater for men than for women. From the ages of 34 to 74, the risk of death from stroke is 30% greater for men and the risk of death from coronary heart disease is two to three times greater. After age 75, however, the differences disappear and the risks tend to be the same for both men and women.[75]

Heredity (Family History/Race/Ethnicity)

Heredity plays an important role in strokes and heart attacks, but cardiovascular disease doesn't always follow the hard and fast outlines of genetic inheritance. Most of the time, genetic factors work in combination with other factors to affect the course of disease.

Here's an example of what I mean. If you plant an acorn in an open field, its genetic inheritance will likely instruct it to grow into a massive oak tree. Plant that same acorn in a small pot on your kitchen windowsill and—despite its genetic inheritance—the acorn will never grow into a massive tree. In both instances, the genes exist for a massive tree but, for the acorn in the pot, environmental factors come into play that don't allow the genes to fully express themselves.

The same is true of the body. Just because you have a certain genetic inheritance for disease, doesn't always mean that these genes will fully express themselves into actual sickness. Other factors in the body and the environment are brought into play, which influence the course of disease. Keeping this fact in mind, there are some broad generalizations we can make about the role of heredity and cardiovascular disease.

If a primary relative, such as a parent, grandparent or sibling, has early heart disease (defined as before age 55 in men and 65 in women), your risk for heart disease increases dramatically. For example, if your father had a heart attack before the age of 55, you are 12 times more likely to have a heart attack compared to others without that family history.[76] And a recent study found that half the people who had a close relative suffering from coronary artery disease had the disease themselves.

Many of the people in the study didn't even know they had diseased coronary arteries until a cardiovascular examination revealed it.[77]

The relationship between family history and stroke is a little murkier, but it's generally thought that your risk of stroke is influenced by this factor. For example, the Framingham Study found that people with a family history of stroke were at an increased risk for stroke themselves.[78]

A family history of other key risk factors—such as high blood pressure, high cholesterol and diabetes—also increases the risk for stroke and heart disease.

Cardiovascular disease seems to follow racial and ethnic groups, as well. Population studies have found that the rate of stroke and death from heart attack is significantly higher among blacks than whites.[79, 80, 81] And one study found that Mexican-Americans have a lower rate of heart attacks and heart disease despite having an increase in unfavorable risk factors.[82]

Now we can turn our attention to the Changeable Risk Factors.

High Blood Pressure (Hypertension)

Liquid blood in your arteries exerts pressure against the vessel wall. If the amount of pressure is too high, it can damage the lining of the artery. By measuring the amount of pressure in your arteries, the doctor can tell a number of things about the state of your cardiovascular system and potential problems down the road.

To help you understand the concept of blood pressure, imagine that you're standing in the back yard with a garden hose in your hand—the end of the hose is open, no nozzle attached. With the faucet running at just a trickle, the pressure in the hose is low. Water flows from the end of the hose with a lazy gurgle before plopping to the ground.

Now imagine placing your thumb over the end of the hose, covering the opening completely. Immediately, water begins to back up within the hose. Within seconds, you can feel the water pressure rising behind your thumb, exerting a strong force on it. Suddenly, your thumb can no longer contain the force and a jet of water under high pressure spurts from the hose traveling several feet before falling to the ground.

The lesson here is that, by narrowing the opening of the hose with your thumb, you increased the resistance to the flow of water, and that increased the water pressure. In the same manner, anything that narrows the arteries in your body—such as atherosclerosis or vasoconstriction—will restrict the flow of blood and make your blood pressure rise.

So high blood pressure often means that there is a higher than normal resistance to the flow of blood through the circulatory system. Much of the time, the cause of high blood pressure can't be determined, a condition called *essential hypertension*. The rest of the time, high blood pressure can be traced to a specific cause, such as atherosclerosis in the arteries or kidney disease.

Blood pressure—which is measured in millimeters of mercury (mm Hg)—has two numbers associated with it, usually written as "x/y." The first number—called the *systolic pressure*—is the higher number because it's measured at the point where the heart is squeezing blood out of the heart and into the arteries. (As you can imagine, anything that is squeezed is put under a higher pressure.) The second number—called *diastolic pressure*—is the lower of the two because it's taken at the point where the heart relaxes and blood flows back into the heart, relieving pressure in the cardiovascular system.

In a healthy patient, blood pressure usually falls within a normal range of values. When a doctor measures one or both of the numbers at a higher than normal level, it's called hypertension or high blood pressure.

So what numbers qualify as high blood pressure? High blood pressure is defined as a systolic blood pressure greater than 140mm Hg and/or a diastolic blood pressure of greater than 90mm Hg. Generally speaking, the higher the numbers, the higher the risk associated with hypertension.[83]

A study published in the American Heart Association journal *Circulation* underscores this fact. Researchers found that, compared to men with normal values, men who have blood pressure numbers of 160/90 are "more than two times more likely to have fatal or non-fatal stroke, twice as likely to die of any cardiovascular disease, and 78% more likely to have a fatal or non-fatal heart attack."

But even if the systolic number is "borderline high"—between 140 and 159—the men had a "42% increased risk of fatal and non-fatal stroke; 56% higher risk of death from cardiovascular causes, and a 26% higher risk of fatal and non-fatal heart attack."[84]

So every increase above normal blood pressure seems to exact a price in cardiovascular health. Fortunately, taking drugs that reduce blood pressure can significantly reduce cardiovascular illness and death.[85]

Diabetes Mellitus

Diabetes mellitus is a disease caused by the body's inability to utilize carbohydrates, which includes sugar.

The ***pancreas*** is a long gland that sits behind the stomach. One of its functions is to produce insulin, a hormone that allows the tissues in you body to absorb sugar, the fuel that gives them their energy. If the pancreas fails to create insulin (called *Type I diabetes*) or if the tissues in your body are unable to use insulin adequately (called *Type II diabetes*), then sugar begins to build up in the blood and urine. This condition causes a number of health problems such as kidney disease and failing vision. Diabetes tends to run in families and tends to strike people who are overweight, inactive or more than 45 years of age.

Diabetes has long been recognized as a risk factor for strokes and heart disease. Nearly three-quarters of people with Type II diabetes end up dying from cardiovascular disease.[86] Diabetics have two to four times the risk for developing heart disease and two to four times the risk of dying from heart disease and stroke, compared to non-diabetics.[87]

Cholesterol Levels

We've touched briefly on cholesterol when discussing atherosclerosis, but now it the time to take a closer look at this important player in strokes and heart attacks.

Cholesterol is a fatty substance found in many foods such as dairy products and animal fat. Along with ingesting cholesterol, humans can manufacture their own supply in the liver. Cholesterol is vital for the proper functioning of the body because it is a key ingredient in the membranes of cells.

Cholesterol has to travel through the bloodstream to get where it's needed in the body. But cholesterol, like other fatty substances, can't be dissolved in the blood. So cholesterol attaches itself to special proteins called *lipoproteins,* which transports the cholesterol through the bloodstream.

The type of lipoprotein that the cholesterol is attached to makes a big difference in atherosclerotic disease.

If too much cholesterol is carried by *low-density lipoprotein*, or *LDL*, it is more likely to be deposited inside arteries, creating cholesterol plaque. That's why LDL is often referred to as "bad cholesterol."

However, if cholesterol is carried by *high-density lipoprotein*, or *HDL*, then it is more likely to be transported away from the artery wall and, eventually, out of the body. That's why HDL is often called "good cholesterol."

A simple blood test can determine the level of LDL and HDL in your blood. Typically, doctors advise that a total cholesterol number on a blood test should be below 200 and the LDL number should be less than 130.

Cholesterol Ratios are helpful tools to determine the risk that cholesterol poses to your health. The *Total Cholesterol/HDL Ratio* is arrived at by dividing the total cholesterol number by the HDL number. Ideally, the result should be below four.

The *LDL/HDL Ratio* divides the LDL number by the HDL number. This time, the result should be below about 2.5. If these numbers are on the high end of the scale, it's an indication that you are more susceptible to cholesterol being deposited in your arteries and, hence, more at risk.

So what are the risks attached to cholesterol levels? A "high" cholesterol number is considered anything above 240. People with cholesterol levels of 240 or above run twice the risk of heart disease compared to a "normal" level of 200.[88]

Smoking

Cigarette smoking is another major risk factor for cardiovascular disease. In fact, more smokers die of cardiovascular disease than any other smoking-related illness, even lung cancer.[89] In one study of middle-aged men, the rate of coronary artery disease was three times greater for smokers compared to nonsmokers.[90] And in a combined study, the overall risk of heart attack and cardiac death was increased three-fold for heavy cigarette smokers.[91]

Smoking is also a risk factor for strokes. Smokers have twice the risk for stroke compared to nonsmokers.[92]

Smokers who quit the habit can reduce their risks considerably. Within a few years of quitting cigarettes, the risk of coronary disease and stroke is reduced to the level of nonsmokers.[93, 94]

Physical inactivity

Compared to active people, people with a sedentary lifestyle have nearly twice the risk of developing heart disease.[95]

But don't think that you have to be a marathon runner or an iron man contestant to qualify as "active." The latest studies show that regular moderate exercise—such as brisk walking—can significantly reduce the problems of cardiovascular disease.[96] As one example, a study found that, for women, merely walking briskly for 30 minutes a day reduced their risk of heart attack and stroke by 53%.[97] So even a small amount of moderate exercise every day can be beneficial.

Obesity

Obesity is an excessive accumulation of fat beyond the physical requirements of the body. The effect of obesity on cardiovascular health is often related to the magnifying effect that excess weight has on other risk factors, especially if the weight is carried in the waist area.

But obesity itself may be an independent risk factor. A report based on the Framingham study found that, for women, weight gain was independently associated with coronary artery disease, stroke and death from cardiovascular disease.[98] Even small amounts of weight gain can hurry the rate of development for cardiovascular disease.[99]

There are several additional points to be made about these traditional risk factors.

First, one type of risk factor is often associated with several others. For example, obesity is associated with an increase in hypertension, cholesterol levels and diabetes, all of which are independent risk factors for cardiovascular disease.[100] So it's very common to find people having multiple risk factors at the same time.

And that leads to a second point: people with multiple risk factors are at an increased risk for cardiovascular disease. The combined effect of two or more risk factors is greater than the sum of the individual risks. So even small rises in more than one risk factor can significantly increase the overall risk of cardiovascular disease.[101]

Which leads to a third point: reducing the risk in one area can reduce the risk in others.

For example, regular physical activity can have a beneficial effect on blood cholesterol levels, diabetes, obesity and blood pressure, and these improvements reduce the overall risk of cardiovascular problems.

So modifying the risk factors that are amenable to change—losing weight, controlling hypertension, stopping smoking, exercising and so one—may prevent a stroke or heart attack in your future.

Or it may not.

That's the maddening thing about risk factors. They only tell part of the story.

Half of the people with cardiovascular disease have none of the traditional, changeable risk factors. So no amount of exercise, cholesterol lowering or weight loss would have made any difference in their cardiovascular illness.

Moreover, people are tempted to think that—by lowering their risk factors—the numbers and percentages attached to the lowered risks will apply to them as individuals. But these figures apply only to groups as a whole. They make no prediction about what will or will not happen to you, personally. It is a cruel fact that percentages of risk mean little to someone who actually develops cardiovascular disease; when you get a stroke or heart attack, you get it 100%.

So medicine was stuck with risk factors that were far from perfect in their ability to explain or predict cardiovascular troubles. But once atherosclerosis was revealed to be an inflammatory condition, scientists took another look at the traditional risk factors from a different perspective. They began to wonder about…

The Connection between Traditional Risk Factors and Inflammation

If atherosclerosis is an inflammatory disease, then researchers concluded it was reasonable to suspect that the changeable, traditional risk factors might have something to do with inflammation.

They were right.

The most recent research has demonstrated that cholesterol, cigarette smoking, diabetes and hypertension injure the walls of arteries—specifically the endothelium—in many ways, creating endothelial dysfunction and chronic inflammation.[102, 103]

In Chapter Six, I took you through the many steps that lead to atherosclerosis—how the injured endothelium becomes "sticky" making inflammatory immune cells like monocytes adhere to it, how cells in the artery over-proliferate, how the blood is more likely to clot when the endothelium is damaged, and so on. It's now believed that the traditional risk factors work to promote atherosclerosis by these very mechanisms.[104]

By the same token, it's been shown that reducing hypertension, controlling diabetes, stopping smoking, and lowering cholesterol levels works to *improve* endothelial function, which may account for the reduction of risk that accompanies these favorable changes.[105]

Instead of detailing how each risk factor damages the artery and creates inflammation, let me focus on one particularly significant risk factor that will serve as an example for all of them...

Oxidized LDL

We've already found out that high levels of LDL cholesterol lead to an increased risk of cardiovascular disease. But new research has added a significant twist to the story.

Ordinary LDL is not easily absorbed into the artery to form cholesterol plaque. It is only when ordinary LDL undergoes a chemical transformation called *oxidation* that it is then easily deposited inside arteries.

What is oxidation? Oxidation is a chemical process that combines a substance with oxygen. Oxygen readily combines with many substances and oxidation occurs around us all the time. For example, many of the garden tools in my garage are covered with rust, which is an example of oxidation. In the case of the tools, oxygen combines with the iron in the metal blades producing *iron oxide*, the chemical name for rust.

When conditions are right, molecules of LDL cholesterol undergo oxidation in the body. Once that happens, cholesterol is transformed into *oxidized LDL*, an inflammatory substance.

Inflammatory is the key word, here. (Isn't it always?)

Oxidized LDL is *cytotoxic*, which means it can kill or injure healthy cells.[106] In this way, oxidized LDL cholesterol provokes the inflammatory response when it comes into contact with the tissues of the artery wall. By provoking inflammation, oxidized LDL becomes a super plaque-producer, helping to set into motion the chain of events that leads to the deposition of cholesterol plaque inside the artery.

Here's a quick rundown of how oxidized LDL can turn into cholesterol plaque—a familiar story of inflammation as a response to injury that we outlined in Chapter Six.

First, LDL becomes oxidized in the body. This process can take place within the cells of the artery, including endothelial cells. But oxidized LDL happens to be toxic to these cells, so the endothelial layer becomes injured by the oxidized cholesterol.

This begins the process of inflammatory repair. Oxidized LDL stimulates the surface of the injured endothelium to turn sticky, attracting immune system monocytes to the site of injury to begin the healing process. The monocytes arrive and turn into macrophages, just as they should.

Here's the kicker…when LDL cholesterol is oxidized, it turns into a favorite meal for macrophages. They much prefer oxidized LDL compared to ordinary LDL. They can't get enough of the stuff and gorge themselves on all the oxidized LDL cholesterol they can hold. The ingestion of oxidized LDL turns macrophages into foam cells, a crucial step on the road to building cholesterol plaque.

Oxidized LDL inhibits the macrophages from moving around. Like bumps on a log, macrophages simply hunker down on the artery wall and soak up the oxidized cholesterol, turning into foam cells. This loss of movement accounts for the foam cells collecting together into fatty streaks. Smooth muscle cells also begin to gorge themselves on oxidized LDL, also turning into foam cells and contributing to the growth of the lesion.[107, 108, 109]

The normal forces that regulate artery health break down as endothelial dysfunction enters the picture. By now, the lesion is well down the road to the chronic inflammatory process that leads to plaque build-up and rupture, ending in strokes and heart attacks.

Oxidized LDL is now recognized as a potent agent that promotes atherosclerosis. Lately, there's been much interest in employing the so-called ***antioxidant vitamins***—chiefly ***vitamin E***, ***vitamin C*** and ***beta-carotene*** (which the body converts into ***vitamin A***)—as a way to protect against atherosclerosis by inhibiting the oxidation of LDL cholesterol. A number of studies have suggested that dietary antioxidants have some protective function, but the jury is still out on whether taking antioxidant vitamins in pill form is beneficial or not.[110]

At any rate, oxidized LDL cholesterol appears to be a risk factor because it damages arteries and aggravates the inflammatory response of the body. The other traditional, changeable risk factors of hypertension, diabetes and smoking are also thought to be risk factors for the same, basic reason—they damage the arteries and create inflammation.

Since these traditional risk factors are so tightly bound to inflammation, scientists began to wonder if inflammation *itself* might be considered a risk factor. This idea quickly blossomed into…

The New Risk Factors

The *new*—or *non-traditional*—*risk factors* for cardiovascular disease are associated with inflammation.

Inflammation is a very complex process, often hidden from the naked eye. However, when inflammation occurs, several telltale immune system cells and inflammatory substances circulate in the bloodstream. Increasing levels of these cells and substances are a sure signal that inflammation is underway in the body. These *markers of inflammation*, which are detected by blood tests, can be used to predict the risk for developing cardiovascular disease and acute coronary events, such as strokes and heart attacks.

Some of these inflammatory markers are already familiar to you. Take *white blood cells*, for example—those immune system monocytes and macrophages we've been talking so much about.

A 1996 study of elderly men found that high levels of white blood cells in the body—a sign of inflammation—strongly correlates with an increased risk of coronary heart disease. The men with the highest levels of white blood cells had seven times the risk of dying from coronary heart disease within the next five years.[111]

White blood cells are just one example of a marker of inflammation that has been established as a cardiovascular risk factor. There are several more inflammatory markers—such as *interleukin-6* (a cytokine) and *serum amyloid A* (a protein that increases manyfold during inflammation)—that science has linked to increased cardiovascular risks. It's tempting to examine each and every one of these new, inflammatory risk factors, but in the interests of simplicity, I'll limit our discussion to the two substances that are considered the most important, beginning with…

Fibrinogen Levels

You may remember *fibrinogen* from Chapter Seven. Fibrinogen is a protein that aids in the coagulation of blood, turning blood from a liquid into a semi-solid. In other words, fibrinogen helps to create blood clots. People with high levels of fibrinogen are said to suffer from *hypercoagulability*, that is, their blood is more susceptible to clotting.

Levels of fibrinogen in the blood rise in the presence of inflammation. Therefore, higher than normal levels of fibrinogen is considered to be a marker of inflammation.

When injury strikes the body, the cells of the immune system release cytokines as part of the inflammatory response. The liver responds to the presence of cytokines in the body by producing fibrinogen and releasing it into the bloodstream. It's believed that a prime reason for rising fibrinogen levels in cardiovascular patients is the injury done to arteries from atherosclerotic disease.

When high levels of fibrinogen circulate through the body it's easier for blood clots to be produced. In people with atherosclerotic disease, this is a recipe for disaster—blood clots cause the occlusions that lead to strokes and heart attacks. So, when vulnerable plaques rupture, high levels of fibrinogen in the body increase the risk that blood will coagulate into clots, forming the occlusions in the artery that kick off strokes and heart attacks.[112]

High levels of fibrinogen are associated with many of the traditional risk factors for cardiovascular disease—increasing age, hypertension, diabetes, levels of both LDL and HDL cholesterol, obesity, smoking, physical inactivity and a family history for cardiovascular troubles.[113, 114] When high fibrinogen levels are combined with factors such as hypertension, diabetes and—especially—smoking, the risk for cardiovascular disease is significantly enhanced.[115]

By the same token, it's been shown that by reducing traditional risk factors—such as stopping smoking, losing weight and exercising regularly—the levels of fibrinogen are also reduced.[116]

Aside from clotting, fibrinogen may also promote atherosclerosis because it stimulates the movement and proliferation of smooth muscle cells, a prime factor in the growth of cholesterol plaque.[117]

All of these elements contribute to one, established fact: levels of fibrinogen in the body are strongly associated with the severity and extent of atherosclerosis in the heart and brain.[118] This association has led to fibrinogen levels being identified as a new, inflammatory risk factor for stroke and heart attacks.

Many studies support fibrinogen as an independent risk factor. For example, a 1999 study of male doctors found that men with high levels of fibrinogen had twice the risk for a heart attack compared to men with lower levels. The authors of the study concluded that "fibrinogen is associated with increased risk of future [heart attack] independent of other coronary risk factors."[119] A continuation of the Framingham Heart Study, called the *Framingham Offspring Study*, found that fibrinogen levels were higher among subjects with cardiovascular disease compared to those without disease, and fibrinogen was associated with traditional cardiovascular risk factors.[120]

In sum, when inflammation rises, the level of fibrinogen in the bloodstream rises as well, indicating a significant risk for cardiovascular disease. But there is a second, potentially more important, inflammatory risk factor that can predict future cardiovascular troubles…

C-Reactive Protein

Along with fibrinogen, another product of the inflammatory response is a special protein called *C-reactive protein* or *CRP*. Like fibrinogen, CRP is produced in the liver in response to the presence of cytokines in the body. Among other things, C-reactive protein aids immune cells in the removal of germs from the body.

As a general rule, CRP levels correlate to the amount of inflammation in the body—the more inflammation, the more CRP is present in the blood. Through testing, doctors can measure the amount of CRP in the bloodstream. Thus, they can be alerted to the presence, and strength, of inflammation in the body.

Bacterial infections tend to cause the highest CRP values, but the test is sensitive to any type of tissue damage that causes the inflammatory response, such as surgery or a traumatic injury to the body.

The CRP test has been around for many years, but I've never used it in the day-to-day work of my office. A big problem with the test is that it is nonspecific—any number of things could be causing your CRP level to rise. So, in a practical sense, its use as a diagnostic tool is limited.

But once the word began to spread in the medical community that atherosclerosis might be a chronic, inflammatory process, scientists began to take a new look at this reliable marker of inflammation.

It happens that the latest versions of the CRP test are very sensitive. They can detect very low levels of inflammation—in other words, chronic levels—which is just what you need in order to study the hypothesis that long-term, low-level inflammation is the source of atherosclerosis.

Scientists wanted to know if they could link chronically increased levels of CRP with cardiovascular disease. So they set up a number of studies to test the theory.

When the results came in, the studies did indeed establish a link between chronic CRP levels and cardiovascular trouble. The studies were able to predict who was at increased risk for strokes and heart attacks by looking at their chronic CRP levels. Most astonishing, however, was the conclusion that *chronic CRP levels predicted the risk of strokes and heart attacks even in people who seemed perfectly healthy.*

For example, one study—called the *Physician's Heart Study*—followed the course of apparently healthy men for a period of eight years. Those who showed the highest chronic CRP levels had a three-fold increase in risk of developing future myocardial infarction and twice the risk of developing a stroke, compared to men with the lowest levels. Importantly, high levels of CRP predicted the risk of a first heart attack up to eight years before it occurred—and these were men who had no history of cardiovascular disease.[121]

A second study was conducted among healthy, post-menopausal women. For women who had the highest levels of chronic CRP, the risk of developing any cardiovascular disease was increased five-fold and the risk for developing a stroke or heart attack was increased seven-fold.[122]

A third study found that raised levels of chronic CRP are predictors of coronary events in patients with both stable and unstable angina.[123] A fourth study found chronic CRP concentration strongly associated with coronary heart disease.[124] Fifth and sixth studies found that high levels of chronic CRP in apparently healthy men predicts future risk for developing peripheral artery disease.[125, 126]

The list goes on. The evidence has been so consistent and convincing that the association of chronic CRP levels to cardiovascular disease is cited as one of the most persuasive arguments that atherosclerosis is, essentially, a chronic, inflammatory illness.

It is also acknowledged that increased levels of chronic CRP are a long-term predictor of cardiovascular disease—even in apparently healthy people—especially when combined with cholesterol levels.[127]

The full story of C-reactive protein has yet to be written. Initially, CRP's association with atherosclerosis was thought to be only an indication that inflammation was present. But new evidence suggests that, once CRP appears, it helps attract white blood cells like monocytes to the artery wall, an important step in the growth of a lesion.[128] In other ways, CRP promotes inflammation and encourages blood to clot.[129, 130] So instead of being just a passive sign of inflammation, CRP seems to take an active role in the atherosclerotic process.

The measurement of CRP levels has leapt to the forefront of risk factors for cardiovascular disease. CRP testing is particularly useful for predicting the risk of healthy people with no symptoms. Later in the book, I'll explain how you can personally benefit from CRP testing, which is finally becoming available to the general public.

About the time that the new, non-traditional, inflammatory risk factors were being discovered, several drugs came into prominence for their ability to lower the risk of strokes and heart attacks...

The Anti-inflammatory Therapies of Aspirin and Statins

Although aspirin was discovered more than 100 years ago, its use as a therapy against cardiovascular disease has only occurred within the last two decades or so. Aspirin's first widespread use was, of course, as a pain reliever. Its second medical use was to relieve the swelling caused by arthritis or injury. But aspirin also had a third effect: it was known as a "blood thinner"—a substance that inhibits the blood's ability to clot.

Since clots are a main factor in strokes and heart attacks, tests were begun to see if aspirin could be used to reduce acute cardiovascular events. Over the years, many studies have concluded that aspirin is a very beneficial treatment for the dangerous consequences of atherosclerosis.

Aspirin reduces the risk of death by up to 23% if administered when a heart attack is suspected and for 30 days thereafter.[131]

For strokes and Transient Ischemic Attacks caused by occlusions, aspirin was found to reduce the combined endpoints of stroke, TIAs and death by 13% to 18%.[132] Two Canadian studies found that, after suffering a Transient Ischemic Attack, daily aspirin use reduced the risk of death or major stroke by almost 50%.[133]

And for patients who are suffering from unstable angina and previous heart attacks, daily doses of aspirin can reduce the risk of death and repeat heart attacks by up to 20%.[134]

While aspirin is beneficial to patients already suffering from coronary artery disease and its symptoms, it's still an open question whether healthy people can prevent future heart attacks by using aspirin.[135]

That's why, in my own practice, I don't prescribe aspirin for healthy people in the hopes of warding off future cardiovascular disease. But if the patient shows some carotid or coronary artery disease, I would definitely prescribe low-dose aspirin, perhaps once a day or once every other day. Providing, of course, that the patient doesn't have a problem that would argue against its use. For example, if I discover that the patient has clotting problems, using aspirin might aggravate internal bleeding. In this case, the risks of aspirin would outweigh its benefits.

There's one important property of aspirin that I haven't mentioned yet: aspirin works to reduce inflammation. Aspirin's potent anti-inflammatory effect makes it a favorite drug for the pain of arthritis, a chronic, inflammatory disease.

For a long time it was assumed that aspirin's blood-thinning ability was central to its achievement of limiting strokes and heart attack. But recent studies point toward aspirin's anti-inflammatory effect as another reason for its success.

A few paragraphs ago, I mentioned the Physician's Heart Study which showed how rising CRP levels can predict the risk of stroke and heart attack. As part of the study, the researchers also followed the effects of aspirin on the subjects. They discovered that aspirin worked best in the men with the highest levels of C-reactive protein. In raw numbers, the study found that aspirin reduced the risk of heart attack overall by 44%. But for men with the highest levels of CRP, the reduction in risk was by 55%.[136]

Since CRP is a sign of inflammation, the researchers concluded that part of aspirin's protective benefits might be due to its anti-inflammatory properties.[137]

The same anti-inflammatory effect has also been suggested for the risk-reducing properties of a relatively new class of cardiovascular drugs called *statins*.

Statins were designed to reduce the amount of cholesterol in patients with high cholesterol levels. Statins work by interfering with the liver's ability to make cholesterol.

Since cholesterol levels have been identified as a risk factor, scientists set up studies to examine whether reducing cholesterol levels with statins could reduce the risks associated with cholesterol.

The results were encouraging. The first large-scale study on the effect of statins on cardiovascular risk was the ***Scandinavian Simvastatin Survival Study***, whose subjects were middle-aged men with high cholesterol levels and a history of coronary artery disease. Over a period of about five years, the study found that a statin called *simvastatin* reduced coronary heart disease deaths by 42%, reduced nonfatal heart attacks by 37% and reduced the need for undergoing heart surgery (such as angioplasty and coronary bypass) by the same 37%.[138] In 1995, simvastatin was designated by the FDA as the first cholesterol-lowering drug approved for reducing deaths and preventing heart attacks in patients with a prior heart attack and high cholesterol.

A different type of statin, called *pravastatin*, was used in another landmark test called the ***West of Scotland Study***. The researchers of this study knew that statins could reduce the risk for a second heart attack. What they didn't know was whether statins could be effective in preventing a *first* heart attack in men in good health but with elevated cholesterol levels. So they designed this study specifically to answer this question.

Again, the results were encouraging. After five years, death from all cardiovascular causes was reduced by 32%. There was even a 22% reduction in the risk of death from any cause. And, like the Scandinavian study, the need for heart surgery was reduced by 37%.[139] In 1996, the FDA cleared pravastatin for use in the prevention of a first heart attack in patients with elevated cholesterol levels. Additional studies have shown that pravastatin reduced the rate of strokes in patients with coronary disease.[140]

One might think, of course, that the success of statins is due entirely to its ability to reduce cholesterol levels. But, like aspirin, statins may reduce cardiovascular risk by fighting inflammation.

A few years ago, a group of researchers studied whether inflammation after a heart attack is a risk factor for further coronary events and whether treatment with pravastatin could reduce that risk. Not surprisingly, they found that patients with the highest levels of C-reactive protein were more at risk from further events compared to those with the lowest levels.[141] But they also discovered that the levels of CRP were up to 38% lower in patients who were given the pravastatin compared to those who received a placebo. In other words, the pravastatin was responsible for lowering inflammation as well as cholesterol levels.

It's thought that the benefits of pravastatin, and perhaps other statins, is due in part because of its ability to reduce inflammation within atherosclerotic arteries. Previous studies suggest that pravastatin has an inhibiting effect on many of the inflammatory elements found in vulnerable plaque, thereby stabilizing the lesion and making it less prone to rupture.[142]

From start to finish, the traditional risk factors of strokes and heart attacks walk hand and hand with inflammation. So much so, that the new, non-traditional risk factors are *founded* on inflammation itself. And the most recent therapies of aspirin and statins seem to work, in part, on limiting the inflammatory process.

And yet...

We're still left with the fact that half of the patients with cardiovascular disease have none of the traditional risk factors. So something else besides cholesterol, hypertension, diabetes and so on, must be responsible for injuring arteries and provoking the inflammatory response. And that something is...

10

Bugs in the System: The Link between Infection, Inflammation and Cardiovascular Disease

As I've stressed in the previous chapters, it is injury and inflammation that lead to the build-up of cholesterol plaque. But the genesis of atherosclerosis is considered **multifactorial** because arteries can become injured and inflamed from several different sources.

Traditional risk factors provide one set of sources. But, as we've seen, the traditional risk factors do not fully account for the creation of plaque and its vulnerability to rupture. The "usual suspects" of cholesterol levels, diabetes, hypertension and the other artery-injuring risk factors account for only half the cases of cardiovascular disease. But recent evidence has pointed toward some very *un*-usual suspects for arterial injury: infectious germs—the microscopic bugs that afflict all of us, at one time or another.

In this chapter, we'll take our first in-depth look at how the germs of cardiovascular disease lead to strokes and heart attacks.

Infection and Systemic Inflammation

Inflammation is a response of the immune system—and few things provoke an inflammatory response stronger than the presence of germs in the body.

As previously mentioned, when bacteria and viruses invade the body they damage cells and tissues by either producing toxins or multiplying inside cells which are then destroyed when the new germs are released. The body's immune system is designed to heal this damage by destroying the invading germs while restoring and repairing the injured tissues. It accomplishes this with the familiar cells and products of the immune system.

In the past few decades, scientists have come to believe that infectious germs can act as the spark that ignites atherosclerotic inflammation. It's thought that these invading germs can create or accelerate atherosclerosis in two basic ways.

First, by directly infecting the artery wall, germs provoke the inflammatory response that leads to plaque build-up. In this case, inflammation is focused on a particular point in the artery. We'll deal with direct infections in the next chapter.

But infections that take hold elsewhere in the body may have a second, indirect effect on arteries, as well. When infectious germs begin to multiply—say, in the lungs—the body responds with inflammatory substances, such as C-reactive protein. These substances are released into the bloodstream creating *systemic inflammation*, that is, inflammation throughout the body.

As these inflammatory substances spread through the circulatory system, they may damage artery walls, provoking atherosclerosis. Or if lesions are already present, the increased inflammation may encourage plaques to destabilize and rupture. These "remote" infections can also elevate clotting risk factors, such as fibrinogen levels, so when plaques rupture, they are more likely to create blood clots. In these ways, infections outside the artery exert an indirect—but still damaging—effect that increases the risk for strokes and heart attacks.

Many studies have found just such a link between infection, systemic inflammation and cardiovascular troubles. The infections that cause *respiratory disease* and *gum disease* have been studied intensely for several years now, yielding significant insight into the cardiovascular risks of systemic inflammation. We'll begin by considering…

Respiratory Disease and the Risk for Stroke and Heart Attack

For our purposes, *respiratory disease* refers to contagious viral and bacterial infections of the respiratory system, such as pneumonia, influenza and bronchitis. These infections have been associated with an increased risk for stroke, heart attack and coronary death.

A 1996 Finnish study of nearly 20,000 middle-aged men and women found that chronic bronchitis was an independent risk factor for coronary artery disease. For men with chronic bronchitis the risk for heart attack was raised by 52% and the risk of dying from a coronary illness was raised by 74%, compared to men without the disease. The rate for women was lower but still significant—38% more likely to suffer a heart attack and 49% more likely to die from a coronary illness.[143]

A separate Finnish study that same year had a similar finding—men with chronic infections of the upper respiratory tract had a pronounced risk for heart attack.[144]

A 1997 German study reported that patients with chronic bronchitis in the preceding two years had a 2.2 times greater risk for stroke or TIAs.[145]

A study at the University Medical Center in Tel Aviv found that 24% of patients admitted to the hospital for stroke had some type of short-term, severe infection—mostly of the respiratory or urinary track—within the week prior to admittance.[146] An Italian study found much the same—20% of the patients admitted to a hospital for acute heart attack reported respiratory symptoms during the three weeks prior to admission.[147]

And a study from the United Kingdom of 9,000 patients concluded that respiratory infection is a risk factor for heart attacks. The risk for acute myocardial infarction was two to three times higher for patients who had a respiratory infection within about two weeks prior to their heart attack.[148]

Looking at the subject from a slightly different angle, a 2000 study from the University of Texas found that preventing respiratory disease with a flu shot can significantly reduce the odds of having a heart attack. When examining heart disease patients, the researchers found that patients who received a flu vaccination had a 67% lower risk for a second heart attack compared to patients who didn't receive the vaccine. The finding that flu shots have a preventive effect on coronary risk strongly supports the previous studies linking respiratory infection with stroke and heart troubles.[149]

Let's turn now to another source of infection and systemic inflammation that is linked to cardiovascular troubles…

Gum Disease and the Risk for Stroke and Heart Attack

Gum disease, medically referred to as *periodontal disease*, is caused by chronic bacterial infections around the teeth. Typically, gum disease is divided into two general categories: *gingivitis* and *periodontitis*.

When bacteria in the mouth multiply, they form a film of plaque on the teeth which, over time, turns into tooth *tartar*, a hard, yellowish deposit which adheres to the tooth surface. The constant presence of bacteria-laden plaque and tartar leads to *gingivitis*, a chronic inflammation of the gums characterized by swelling, redness and pain.

In severe cases, long-lasting infection from bacteria can lead to *periodontitis*, the destruction of gum and bone tissue by the presence of chronic inflammation. Since the bone of the jaws supports the teeth in the mouth, periodontitis is the main reason why people lose their teeth in their later years. It's estimated that periodontal disease is responsible for 70% of all adult tooth loss.

The progression of gum disease is a familiar story of chronic injury creating chronic inflammation.

The presence of mouth bacteria and the toxins they produce stimulates the immune system into action. Inflammatory substances are released at the site of injury in the gums to destroy the bacteria and repair injured tissue. But bacteria in the mouth can be very difficult to eradicate, so the immune system is constantly throwing inflammatory cells and chemicals at the same spot, often for decades. This chronic inflammation tears down healthy gum and bone tissue, resulting in tooth loss—a classic example of how inflammation, once it turns chronic, can do more harm than good.

Over the past 15 years or so, scientists have suspected that the harmful effects of chronic inflammation caused by mouth bacteria may not be limited to gum disease. Study after study was linking the presence and severity of gum disease to an increased risk of stroke and heart attack.

An early study from 1989 found that dental health was significantly worse in patients who suffered acute heart attacks.[150] This breakthrough study set in motion the examination of dental health and cardiovascular disease by other scientists.

When researchers analyzed the results from two long-term studies of men from the Boston area, they found that the men with the most bone loss from periodontal disease had a 70% increased risk for developing the symptoms of coronary heart disease. They found much the same increased risk for stroke.[151]

A 1993 study that followed nearly 10,000 subjects for more than a decade reported that patients with periodontitis had a 25% increased risk of coronary heart disease relative to those with minimal periodontal disease. For men under age 50, the risk was even higher.[152]

A German study of 166 stroke victims published in 1997 revealed that patients with poor dental status linked to gum disease were at 2.6 times greater risk for stroke and TIAs.[153]

A 1998 study of 400 elderly men who were patients at a Michigan VA hospital reported that the patients with the most extensive gum disease were four and a half times more likely to suffer coronary heart disease than the patients without gum problems. Subjects who saw a dentist at least once a year were four times *less* likely to suffer a stroke.[154]

And a 2000 study presented at an annual meeting of the American Heart Association found that 85% of the heart attack victims in the study had chronic periodontitis compared to only 29% of healthy volunteers. That means that heart attack patients are more likely to have severe gum disease.[155]

The good news in all this is that gum disease can be prevented through good oral hygiene: brushing, flossing and visiting the dentist on a regular basis—a small price to pay for preventing a stroke or heart attack!

The evidence linking oral health to cardiovascular disease has been so consistent over the years that I personally pay strict attention to my teeth, brushing frequently with a tartar control toothpaste and a liquid plaque remover...and I advise all my patients to do the same.

Here's one more interesting sidelight.

A 2000 study at an Australian dental school found that men who regularly took aspirin to prevent stroke and heart disease also achieved an unexpected benefit—they had significantly less periodontitis.[156] It seems that aspirin's anti-inflammatory effect, thought to prevent strokes and heart attacks, also alleviates the inflammation associated with severe gum disease—just one more example of...

The Link between Infection, Inflammation and Cardiovascular Disease

It's believed that the reason why both respiratory disease and gum disease are associated with strokes and heart attacks is because these chronic infections produce chronic, systemic inflammation throughout the body. This widespread inflammation stimulates atherosclerotic plaques to grow or rupture, and stimulates blood to clot more easily.

There is certainly evidence that supports this idea. Studies demonstrate that patients with chronic bronchitis have increased levels of C-reactive protein and fibrinogen in their blood.[157, 158] And studies have found that people suffering from periodontal disease also tend to have high levels of both C-reactive protein and fibrinogen—and possibly higher cholesterol levels and other inflammatory risk factors, as well.[159, 160, 161] All of these markers of inflammation are thought to influence the progression and stability of cholesterol plaque and, thus, raise the risk of stroke or heart attack.

So it appears that systemic inflammation caused by infectious disease poses a significant risk for cardiovascular disease. By preventing respiratory and gum diseases, it may be possible to prevent a significant number of strokes and heart attacks.

But recent evidence has added an unexpected twist to the story.

In 1999, Canadian researchers examined human carotid arteries diseased by atherosclerosis for signs of infection. To the surprise of many, they discovered that two of the germs that cause gum disease—the bacteria *Porphyromonas gingivalis* and *Streptococcus sanguis*—had infected the cholesterol plaque of the atherosclerotic arteries. Moreover, the germs were located within unstable sections of the plaque, which had ruptured and clotted over with blood.[162] Subsequent studies confirmed that gum disease bacteria is often found in cholesterol plaque, even infecting the artery wall itself.[163, 164]

There is now strong evidence that the germs of gum disease may be *directly* involved in the infection and inflammation of cholesterol plaque—perhaps even involved with the triggering of plaque rupture.

This new evidence fit perfectly with the radical rethinking of the cause and prevention of strokes and heart attacks that is the essence of The Heart Attack Germ—and the subject of the next chapter…

11

The Germs of Strokes and Heart Attacks

Early in *The Heart Attack Germ*, I introduced you to the bacterium *Chlamydia pneumoniae*, the infectious germ most associated with an increased risk for heart disease. Since its discovery, scientific institutions around the world have been searching for additional connections between infection and atherosclerosis. They were especially keen on discovering whether *Cp* or other germs might actually live and breed in the walls of atherosclerotic arteries and in the lesions themselves.

The reason to search the artery for infectious germs was obvious: infection in the artery would help explain why arteries become inflamed and why atherosclerosis is, essentially, an inflammatory disease.

The periodontal bacteria *P. gingivalis* and *S. sanguis* were not the first germs found in cholesterol plaque…they're only the latest. More than a decade of research has uncovered several germs that are associated with atherosclerosis, strokes and heart attacks.

Most of the research has centered around the following four germs:

Chlamydia pneumoniae

This is the Heart Attack Germ that we first considered in detail in Chapter Two. *Cp* is a bacterium that causes respiratory diseases such as bronchitis and pneumonia; most often, however, *Cp* produces no symptoms at all. At some point nearly everyone becomes infected by *Cp* and the infection can last for decades, often sparking to life again with renewed activity after a period of quiescence.

Herpes Simplex Virus (HSV)

This common, contagious virus creates blisters on the skin, particularly around the face and mouth. A *cold sore* (also known as a *fever blister*) is the most well-known symptom of HSV infection. In the course of a lifetime, nearly everyone will become infected by herpes simplex virus. Most people don't know they're infected because HSV often provokes no symptoms. And the immune system has a hard time eliminating HSV infections, so the virus remains persistent in the body and may flare up repeatedly.

Cytomegalovirus (CMV)

Cytomegalovirus infects nearly everybody; by age 60 it can be found in 90% of the population. Most often, people are able to handle CMV infections very well, suffering only mild symptoms such as fever and malaise or no symptoms at all. But if the CMV virus is transmitted from mother to baby during pregnancy, it can cause severe health problems for the child. And for patients with damaged immune systems, CMV infection can cause serious complications, or even death. Once contracted, CMV infection can last a lifetime with multiple episodes of reactivation of the virus.

Helicobacter pylori (H. pylori)

H. pylori is a bacterium responsible for peptic ulcer disease, a chronic inflammatory condition of the stomach. The germ lives in the protective secretions that coat the interior of the stomach, sheltering it from the digestive acids and enzymes that would destroy most other bacteria. The germ has been described as the most common bacterial infection in man, yet most *H. pylori* infections are asymptomatic, with only one in six people infected by the germ actually developing a peptic ulcer. Perhaps because they live in such a harsh environment, *H. pylori* bacteria are difficult to eradicate from the body. Without medical treatment, most victims suffer life-long infection.

Note that all four of these germs—*Cp*, HSV, CMV and *H. pylori*—share similar characteristics that are very important to the development of atherosclerosis:

1. Most everyone, in the course of a lifetime, will become infected by one or more of these germs.

2. Most people will not know they are infected because these germs often cause no symptoms.

3. The immune system has a hard time eliminating these infections, so the germs are persistent in the body and they may flare up repeatedly.

Together, these shared characteristics make *Cp*, HSV, CMV and *H. pylori* germs a hidden source of chronic inflammation—the chief instigator of atherosclerosis. And almost everyone will be exposed to the hidden, chronic inflammation from these germs because almost everyone will become infected by one or more of them.

Everything that we've talked about up to now—from inflammation as the body's response to injury through the new inflammatory risk factors of C-reactive protein and fibrinogen—has been to prepare you for this chapter. That's because nearly everything we've talked about so far can be associated with the germs of cardiovascular disease. So I'll constantly be referring back to our previous discussions to show how everything connects together.

One final note before beginning.

At the time of this writing, there are well over 150 scientific studies that have reported on an association between cardiovascular disease and chronic infection.[165] In this chapter and the next, I'll present evidence from many of these studies. But you should be aware that the evidence concerning cardiovascular infection is still controversial...and occasionally contradictory. One study may associate a germ such as *Chlamydia pneumoniae* with an increased risk of heart attack, while another, similar study may find no such association. And often, authors of a positive study make it a point to caution that, by itself, the positive study does not provide conclusive evidence and more research is needed.

The research into cardiovascular infection stands at the very edge of advanced medical theory and technology. Many of the tools used to explore cardiovascular germs—such as ***immunocytochemistry*** (a method of identifying infective agents in tissue samples) and ***polymerase chain reaction*** (which amplifies the presence of germ DNA in tissue samples) are very sophisticated, requiring great care to perform correctly. As of yet, there has been no standardization for these tests, which many believe accounts for the varying results.

In any new field of medical exploration, there is bound to be conflicting evidence and opposing viewpoints. I and hundreds of other doctors have concluded that the evidence compels us to take the safe, simple, and tried-and-true precautions to eliminate infection and inflammation as a source of cardiovascular troubles—which is exactly what WIN/WIN Therapy does as described later in the book.

So let's begin with the most researched germ of the bunch, the Heart Attack Germ itself...

Chlamydia pneumoniae

Here is a step-by-step outline of how *Cp* infection leads to strokes and heart attacks, based on the best evidence so far:

Chlamydia Germs Infect the Respiratory System

In our first discussion of *Chlamydia pneumoniae* back in Chapter Two, we found that *Cp* bacteria are contagious and often a cause of epidemics. The germ spreads easily from person to person through respiratory secretions, just like flu or cold germs. Sneezing and coughing flings the *Cp* bacteria into the air where it is inhaled by the next victim. Or the germ may land on a surface that is subsequently touched by the victim's hands. The bacteria are transmitted to the mouth or nose where they enter the respiratory system and multiply, causing the initial infection—most commonly pneumonia or bronchitis. Usually, the initial infection is so mild that the victim never even knows that he's picked up the germ.

Immune Cells Respond to Cp Infection in the Lungs

Once in the respiratory tract, the multiplying *Cp* germs infect the tissues of the lungs. The body responds to the injury with immune system cells, which arrive at the site of infection to deal with the invading germs. Remember—it's the job of the white blood cells, such as macrophages, to engulf and destroy harmful microorganisms.

But *Chlamydia pneumoniae* has a clever trick up its sleeve—you don't get to be one of the world's most successful pathogens by quickly falling prey to the body's immune system!

Recall that the *Cp* germ, although it is a bacterium, shares one important characteristic with viruses—it acts as a parasite. It lives inside human cells. In fact, *Chlamydia pneumoniae* can quite comfortably take up residence inside monocytes, macrophages and lymphocytes—the very cells that the immune system sends to destroy it.[166, 167, 168]

Usually, when immune cells surround and ingest a bacterium, they destroy the captured germ by dissolving it with digestive proteins. But the *Cp* germ creates a membrane around itself that protects it from being destroyed by the host cell. Safe inside its bubble, the *Cp* germ parasitically lives off of the host cell.

If you stop and think about it, it's a pretty audacious survival strategy—not only do the *Chlamydia* germs find a place to live and flourish, but they do it at the expense of their sworn enemies. Imagine a criminal on the "Ten Most Wanted" list hiding out inside an FBI office and eating his meals at the Bureau cafeteria—that's the "hide in plain sight" gambit that *Cp* germs use to protect themselves from the immune system.

Immune Cells Infected with Cp Spread the Germ throughout the Body

But the *Cp* scheme for survival doesn't end there. The body's immune cells become hijacked by the *Chlamydia pneumoniae* germs that they've swallowed. Or perhaps a better term would be "carjacked" because the *Cp* germs appear to use the infected immune cells for transportation.

The bloodstream acts as a freeway system for immune cells, and studies suggest that this is how *Cp* travels through the body.[169] When infected monocytes and macrophages enter the bloodstream, the *Cp* germs are picked up from the lungs and swept away to other organs and tissues, which they then proceed to infect. It's a bitter irony that the immune system—which should be protecting the body—is responsible for spreading the infection. It's as if the *Cp* germs were brazenly taking police cars to the scene of their next crime.[170, 171]

Immune Cells Transfer Cp Infection into the Arteries of the Heart and Brain

Often, germs and viruses prefer to infect one type of body tissue over another, say, nerve cells over muscle cells. *Chlamydia* germs seem to prefer the type of tissue that make up the lining of organs. The endothelium is just that type of lining.

As the immune cells infected with *Cp* circulate throughout the bloodstream, they bump up against the artery walls. Monocytes infected with *Cp* are more likely to adhere to endothelial cells and smooth muscle cells.[172] And studies demonstrate that macrophages can transmit the *Cp* germ to the artery wall by coming into direct contact with the cells of the endothelial layer.[173] Numerous other studies show that the major cells that make up the interior of an artery—endothelial cells and smooth muscle cells—are readily infected by *Chlamydia pneumoniae*.

One study found that, when smooth muscle cells are loaded with cholesterol, they become even more susceptible to *Cp* infection.[174] Therefore, it may be that *Cp* infection becomes more likely to take hold in an artery when prior lesions of atherosclerosis are present. These prior lesions may be the result of previous endothelial damage caused by the cardiovascular risk factors. Researchers have noted that the risk factors for both atherosclerosis and chronic infection with *Chlamydia pneumoniae* are much the same—age, gender, smoking, hypertension, heredity, physical activity, diet, stress, etc.[175, 176]

Cp Germs Linger in the Artery, Creating a Chronic Infection

Once a macrophage infected with *Cp* attaches to an artery wall, the germ can be transferred to neighboring cells. Studies show that *Cp* bacteria are able to replicate in the key cells of atherosclerosis—macrophages, endothelial cells and smooth muscle cells—allowing the germ to proliferate and spread from cell to cell within the artery wall.[177]

Chlamydia pneumoniae has one more ace in the hole for eluding destruction from the immune system. The germ has an unusual life cycle, with three distinct stages of development.

During the ***reticulate body*** stage, the *Cp* germ grows inside the host cell. During this phase, the germ in non-infective, unable to spread to other cells. Within 48–72 hours, however, the germ reaches the ***elementary body*** stage, where it replicates itself into infective spores. As the host cells dies and bursts open, the elementary bodies are released into the surrounding tissue, looking for new cells to invade—or sneezed into the air, looking for new humans to infect.

But there is an unusual third alteration when the germ transforms itself into a ***persistent body***.

During the persistent body phase, *Cp* bacteria become inactive, lying dormant inside an infected cell for long periods of time. In this state of "hibernation" the *Cp* germ is protected from attack by the immune system and most antibiotics.[178, 179]

Chronic Cp Infection Leads to Chronic Inflammation in the Artery

As a result of all this artful dodging, *Cp* germs can hide out inside the human body for extended periods, then reawaken and multiply once more, creating infective elementary bodies and releasing them to spread the germ to neighboring cells.

These periodic pulses of infection are difficult for the immune system to handle. By the time the immune system defenses respond to a new eruption of *Chlamydia* germs, many of the spores have infected new cells, starting the hiding and multiplying process over again.

The periodic pulsing of infection and immune response repeats itself endlessly, and this accounts for the long-lasting, chronic nature of *Cp* infection. The immune system never gets to finish the job, but is always reacting to new pulses of infection. It sends wave after wave of inflammatory cells and chemicals to the same spot in the artery, continuously responding to the injury caused by the lingering *Chlamydia* germ.

This continuous response is not good for the healthy tissues that surround the infected cells. Remember that the cells and chemicals that the immune system uses to destroy toxic germs are, themselves, toxic; they destroy not only the germ but healthy tissues, as well. So when an infection lingers in the same spot, there is a risk that healthy tissues will be continually subjected to toxic substances from the immune system or be stimulated to undergo harmful changes such as over-proliferation, enhanced clotting or the formation of scar tissue. It's a classic example of how the body's healing response to injury can be tipped too far in one direction, creating problems much worse than the initial injury.

The micro-infection caused by *Cp* bacteria produces no symptoms. Neither you nor your doctor can tell that your arteries are being damaged by a simmering infection. Yet the chronic, low-level inflammation that *Cp* creates is fundamental to the birth, progression and rupture of atherosclerotic plaque, which may lead—eventually—to strokes, heart attacks and sudden death.

Numerous studies have shown just how closely *Cp* infection follows the process of injury and inflammation that generates cholesterol plaque. Nearly every element of atherosclerosis we've discussed so far—from fibrinogen levels to foam cells to the rupture of lesions—has been associated with *Chlamydia pneumoniae* infections. So let's continue with the evidence, step-by-step.

Cp Lives in the Cells of Cholesterol Plaque

If you're going to make the argument that *Chlamydia pneumoniae* germs create arterial inflammation by directly infecting the vessel wall, you would expect to find *Cp* germs living in the cells of atherosclerotic lesions.

Sure enough, when scientists examined specimens of cholesterol plaque taken from the arteries of cardiovascular patients, they repeatedly found *Chlamydia pneumoniae* germs in endothelial cells and macrophages, and in smooth muscle cells that had migrated into the plaque. They've also found *Cp* in the smooth muscle cells and in small arteries below the plaque.[180]

Endothelial Cells Infected by Cp Turn "Sticky"

In our discussion of atherosclerosis in Chapter Six, I mentioned that, when endothelial cells become injured, they use substances called adhesion molecules to turn the surface of the cell "sticky." Monocytes and other immune cells in the blood stream bump into the sticky cell surface and adhere to it, bringing immune system cells to the site of damage and beginning the inflammatory process.

Several experiments show that, when *Cp* infects endothelial cells, the cells react to the germ by increasing adhesion molecules on the cell surface.[181, 182, 183]

"Sticky" Cells Infected by Cp Attracts Immune Cells to the Site of Injury

Further experiments reveal that, as a result of increased adhesion molecules, endothelial cells infected by *Cp* do indeed attract immune system cells such as neutrophils and monocytes to the site of infection.[184]

Since *Cp* infections can be persistent within the artery, it follows that chronic *Cp* infection may continually draw immune cells to the infected area—exactly the type of chronic, low-level inflammatory response that results in the formation of cholesterol plaque. It's thought that *Cp* infection does much of its dirty work simply by sustaining inflammation in the artery.

Monocytes Attracted by Cp-Infected Cells Pass through the Endothelial Layer

Again in Chapter Six, we learned that, once a monocyte arrives at the site endothelial damage, the monocyte burrows beneath the endothelial cell layer creating a new space that's a hot spot of early atherosclerotic development. Experiments with endothelial cells infected with *Cp* demonstrate that the germ induces just this sort of migratory action from monocytes.[185]

Cp Induces Oxidation of LDL Cholesterol

In Chapter Nine, we found that ordinary LDL cholesterol is not easily turned into cholesterol plaque. But when LDL becomes oxidized, it becomes a very potent plaque-producer. So the last thing you want is for LDL to become oxidized in the artery.

But that's just what *Cp* does.

Researches discovered that cells infected by *Chlamydia* germs induce the oxidation of LDL inside the cell. Which means that *Cp* infection creates one of the most dangerous elements of atherosclerosis.[186] This leads to another important development...

Cp Stimulates the Creation of Foam Cells

In Chapter Six we also learned that, when monocytes leave the bloodstream and burrow into the artery wall, they turn into macrophages. It's macrophages that really soak up oxidized

LDL cholesterol. And once they do, they turn into foam cells, the cellular engine that sucks cholesterol out of the bloodstream and piles it up on the artery walls.

It turns out that the presence of *Chlamydia pneumoniae* causes the formation of macrophage foam cells.[187] So not only does *Cp* induce LDL cholesterol oxidation, it stimulates the creation of foam cells that take the oxidized LDL into the artery—both key elements in the birth and growth of atherosclerotic lesions.

Cp Infection is Associated with Cholesterol Risk Factors

With the knowledge that *Cp* stimulates the creation of oxidized LDL and foam cells, it's not surprising to find that studies associate *Cp* infections with cholesterol risk factors such as high LDL and low HDL levels.[188, 189] Researchers believe that one way *Cp* might promote atherosclerosis is by adversely altering these types of cholesterol risk factors.

Cp Infection Induces the Proliferation of Smooth Muscle Cells

Recall also from Chapter Six that one of the hallmarks of atherosclerosis is "intimal thickening" caused by the proliferation and migration of smooth muscle cells in the artery. A recent study linked *Chlamydia pneumoniae* to this distinctive feature by demonstrating that *Cp* infection of endothelial cells induces the proliferation of smooth muscle cells.[190]

Cp Infection of Endothelial Cells Stimulates Blood Clotting

From Chapter Six we learned that the endothelium controls many of the functions of the artery, stimulating or inhibiting the events that take place within it. When a healthy endothelium is injured, it can no longer control these critical tasks, becoming "dysfunctional" and setting in motion the forces that lead to atherosclerosis.

For example, a dysfunctional endothelium releases tissue factor which promotes thrombosis and the adhesion of blood platelets to the artery wall, both of which are elements associated with the formation of cholesterol plaque.

A study released in 1997 found that endothelial cells infected with *Chlamydia pneumoniae* significantly increased both tissue factor procoagulant activity and the amount of platelet adhesion to infected cells.[191]

Cp Infection is Associated with Loss of Vasodilation

Another consequence of endothelial dysfunction is the impaired ability of the artery to relax or dilate. This diminished ability is linked to the formation of atherosclerosis and the susceptibility of arteries to go into spasm.

An animal study showed that *Cp* infection of the endothelium impairs the ability of the artery to relax, supporting the role of *Cp* infection in the development of atherosclerosis.[192]

Cp Infection is Associated with Elevated CRP Levels

In Chapter Nine we discovered that levels of C-reactive protein, an accurate marker of inflammation, can be used to predict the risk for stroke or heart attack, even in people who appear to have no cardiovascular disease. Elevated CRP levels are regarded as a new, inflammatory risk factor for cardiovascular disease.

Naturally, researchers were interested in finding if *Cp* infection could be associated with raised levels of CRP. Sure enough, a 1996 study from England found just such an association.[193] In fact, the risk of coronary heart disease is greater when patients suffer from both *Chlamydia pneumoniae* infection and high CRP levels, compared to just *Cp* infection alone.[194]

Cp Infection is Associated with Elevated Fibrinogen Levels

Like C-reactive protein, fibrinogen levels are considered a new, inflammatory risk factor for strokes and heart attacks. A high level of fibrinogen makes it easier for blood to clot, a clear danger to patients with vulnerable plaques.

A 1998 study associated *Cp* infection with increased levels of fibrinogen, thus implicating the *Cp* germ as a factor in blood clotting. The same study also noted that chronic *Cp* infection was common in patients with unstable coronary artery disease, a condition noted for the clotting of blood due to rupturing vulnerable plaques.[195] A second study in 2001 also found a connection between *Cp* infection and elevated fibrinogen levels.[196]

Cp Found in Early, Advanced and Complicated Lesions

From fatty streaks to advanced, complicated lesions, *Chlamydia pneumoniae* can be found infecting plaques at all stages of development, suggesting both an initiating role and an exacerbating role for *Cp* in atherosclerosis.[197]

Cp Infections Induce the Inflammatory Substances that Lead to Plaque Rupture

A quick refresher: in Chapter Seven we learned that the blood clots which lead to strokes and heart attacks are the result of rupturing plaques. Plaque becomes prone to rupture in the presence of macrophages that secrete various types of enzymes. These enzymes dissolve the fibrous cap, weakening it to the point of breaking open. One of the chief cap-dissolving enzymes are called the matrix metalloproteinases.

Now, here's the news. A 1998 study found that *Cp* germs can induce macrophages to produce the cap-dissolving metalloproteinases, thus implicating *Cp* germs in the rupture of plaque and the creation of blood clots.[198] A later study, from 2001, confirmed that *Cp* infected plaque released matrix-dissolving metalloproteinases.[199]

Cp is highly prevalent in unstable versus stable plaques

A 2000 Brazilian study looked at the amount of *Cp* germs in stable plaques compared to the ruptured, fatal plaques found at autopsy. The researchers noted that there was a greater amount of *Cp* infection in the shattered plaques, compared to the stable ones, implicating *Chlamydia pneumoniae* in the rupture of plaque and the development of acute heart attacks.[200] Two German studies released a year earlier concluded much the same—*Cp* was highly prevalent in rupturing plaque over stable plaque, indicating an active role in plaque destabilization.[201, 202] And this helps explain why…

Cp is associated with heart attacks and other acute coronary events

If *Chlamydia pneumoniae* germs take an active role in plaque rupture, you would expect to find a correlation between *Cp* infection and acute coronary events such as heart attacks and unstable angina. Both of these events are largely the result of rupturing plaque, and *Cp* has been associated with each of these types of problems, numerous times.

For example, in the year 2001 alone, many independent studies from around the world found a correlation between active infection with *Cp* and acute coronary events, including heart attacks and unstable angina. Here's a sampling of their conclusions:

"The detection of high titers of…antibodies to C. pneumonia in many patients with heart attacks, compared to control groups, suggests that chronic *Chlamydia pneumoniae* infection plays a role in the pathogenesis of atherosclerosis and acute ischemic events."[203]

...and...

"We found a strong association between high level seropositivity to *Cp* and acute coronary symptoms."[204]

...and...

"This study discovered that...antibody to *Chlamydia* was significantly associated with coronary artery disease, especially with heart attack, in Japanese men and the findings suggest that chronic infection of *Chlamydia* may be linked to the pathogenesis of heart attacks."[205]

...and so on. Since plaque rupture is also the cause of many strokes, it's not surprising to find that...

Cp is associated with cerebral vascular disease and strokes.

Many studies have established a link between cerebral vascular disease, including stroke, and infection with *Chlamydia pneumoniae*. In their own words, here are the conclusions of four separate studies published in a single year—2001:

"The results of this study demonstrate that patients with advanced atherosclerotic carotid disease have an increased incidence of *C. pneumoniae* infection. Recent infection could be responsible for instability of the carotid plaque, causing cerebral ischemic episodes."[206]

...and...

"The demonstration of *C. pneumoniae* in atherosclerotic middle cerebral arteries is consistent with the hypothesis that this bacterium is involved in acute and chronic cerebrovascular diseases."[207]

...and...

"This study confirmed that the observations of an association between antibody against *C. pneumoniae* and common carotid atherosclerosis in Western nations is also present in Japan. Our results suggest that *C. pneumoniae* infection is also an important risk factor for common carotid atherosclerosis."[208]

...and...

"CONCLUSION: We think that there is a relationship between chronic infection with *C. pneumoniae* and carotid atherosclerosis."[209]

Cp is associated with aortic aneurysms

Just as *Cp* germs are associated with the rupture of plaques, they are also implicated in the rupture of aortic aneurysms. Previous studies have suggested that active *Cp* infection can exacerbate inflammation in the aortic wall, accelerating the progression of the abdominal aortic disease, which can end in aneurysms.[210]

A study of the germ in a laboratory setting found that aortic tissue infected by *Cp* leads to the degradation of elastin in the aortic wall.[211] Recall that elastin is one of the extracellular matrix substances that holds the artery together. The study couldn't draw a hard and fast conclusion, but the fact the *Cp* helps disintegrate the aortic wall may partly explain the association between abdominal aortic aneurysms and *Cp* germs.

Additional evidence for the role of *Chlamydia pneumoniae* as a source of strokes and heart attacks will be presented in the following chapter. For now, however, let's move on to the other germs associated with cardiovascular disease, such as...

Herpes Simplex Virus

Most of the research of scientists around the world has focused on *Chlamydia pneumoniae* as a source of cardiovascular troubles. But several experiments point to the herpes simplex virus as a source of trouble, too.

A study published in 2000 found that people infected by HSV were twice as likely to have had a heart attack or to have died from heart disease.[212] A study from Finland at around the same time had similar results—chronic infection with the herpes simplex virus can significantly increase the risk of developing heart disease.[213]

It's believed that HSV increases cardiovascular risk in much the same manner as *Chlamydia pneumoniae*: by creating chronic inflammation in the arteries.

HSV can infect the cells of the artery, including endothelial cells and smooth muscle cells, and the virus itself has been found inside atherosclerotic lesions.[214] When endothelial cells are infected by HSV, they turn "sticky" by expressing adhesion molecules, an initial step of atherosclerosis which brings immune system cells to the site of infection.[215, 216] Infected cells also promote tissue factor and other procoagulant changes that enhance thrombosis—another early step which can lead to atherosclerosis in the artery.[217]

Cytomegalovirus

For more than a decade, scientists have conducted studies linking cytomegalovirus with cardiovascular disease. The evidence has been promising, although some studies failed to find an association.[218] But the positive studies follow the familiar outlines of other cardiovascular infections.

For example, a 2001 study demonstrated that atherosclerotic patients are more frequently infected with CMV compared to people without atherosclerosis.[219] And a year earlier, a study by the National Heart, Lung, and Blood Institute found that subjects with the highest levels of immune system antibodies to CMV (a sign of CMV infection) had a 76% greater chance of developing heart disease over five years, compared to those with the lowest levels (or none at all).[220]

Evidence of CMV infection been found in atherosclerotic arteries and two studies have linked CMV infection with the early stages of atherosclerosis.[221, 222]

One recent study associated CMV with premature heart attacks and a second study found that CMV infection was a strong predictor of death in patients with coronary artery disease, especially when combined with high CRP levels.[223, 224]

CMV is also associated with stroke. A 2001 study found that CMV infection played an important role in the disease process of atherosclerosis and subsequent strokes.[225]

But there exists another type of link between cytomegalovirus and cardiovascular trouble that is based on a different kind of evidence than we've been considering so far.

CMV infection has been connected to the failure of plaque-clearing surgery such as *atherectomy* and *balloon angioplasty*. And CMV has also been connected to accelerated hardening of the arteries in patients who receive heart transplants.

Atherectomy is a surgical procedure used to remove cholesterol plaque from inside arteries. A catheter is placed inside an artery and a clearing device—such as a laser beam or a rotating shaver—is used to clear the plaque away. After atherectomy a *balloon angioplasty* may also be performed. In this procedure, a balloon at the tip of the catheter is inflated. The balloon presses against the artery wall and widens the channel for blood to flow through, helping to restore circulation to the heart.

Often, however, within months after surgery the "cleared" artery becomes blocked again and the procedure will have to be repeated or a bypass operation performed.

Perhaps the most famous example of angioplasty failure in recent times happened to Vice President Dick Cheney. The vice president had his initial angioplasty in November of 2000. Within four months, the angioplasty had to be repeated when the vice president started experiencing chest pains. One of his "cleared" arteries had become blocked again, reducing circulation to his heart.

It's estimated that up to 50% of patients undergoing angioplasty will experience reblockage, or *restenosis*. This restenosis is caused primarily by the proliferation of smooth muscle cells.

Several studies have now linked cytomegalovirus infection to this type of restenosis from atherectomies and balloon angioplasties. A study published in the *New England Journal of Medicine* found that the risk of restenosis after atherectomy is five times higher than normal for people infected with CMV.[226] And a study in the *American Journal of Cardiology* reported that CMV infection was associated with restenosis following angioplasty.[227] It's suspected the CMV infection allows smooth muscle cells to proliferate, causing the artery to close up again.

You might think that patients who receive a heart transplant wouldn't need to worry about atherosclerosis, which generally takes many years of development before causing noticeable symptoms. But the fact is that half of all heart transplant patients suffer significant blockages in their new coronary arteries within five years of receiving their new heart.[228] Heart transplants are plagued by "accelerated atherosclerosis," a condition known as *transplant coronary artery disease*.

CMV has been associated with accelerated atherosclerosis in heart transplants. A 1996 Finnish study reported that CMV infection is associated with intense atherosclerosis in the coronary arteries of transplanted hearts. This accelerated atherosclerosis affects all the coronary branches soon after transplantation.[229] Additional studies from Germany and the USA reported similar findings, even associating CMV infection with a significantly increased risk of death.[230, 231]

In 1999, researchers from Stanford made a supplementary discovery when they analyzed data from heart transplant patients who had received *ganciclovir*, an anti-virus drug commonly given to heart transplant patients to prevent CMV infection. (CMV infection can increase the risk of the transplanted heart being rejected by the body.) The data showed that the patients who received the anti-CMV drug were nearly three times less likely to have coronary arteries blocked by atherosclerosis—an added indication that cytomegalovirus may very well be a factor in coronary artery disease.[232]

Helicobacter pylori

Many studies have associated *Helicobacter pylori* with coronary artery disease, stroke and an increased risk of heart attack.

A 1999 Italian study found that patients with acute heart attacks had a significantly higher prevalence of *Hp* infection compared to the control population.[233] Separate English and Polish studies from that same year found an association between coronary artery disease and *Hp* infection.[234, 235] And two later studies have linked both chronic and active *Hp* infection to patients who suffered acute heart attacks.[236, 237]

Other studies, however, have failed to find a significant association between *Hp* and cardiovascular disease.[238] One way to explain this discrepancy may be by taking into account the virulence of different strains of *Hp* bacteria. Three different experiments indicate that the link between *Helicobacter pylori* and heart disease depends on the infective strength of the germ.[239, 240, 241] In other words, some strains of *Hp* may be more damaging to the infected artery than other, milder strains, resulting in an increased risk of atherosclerosis.

Apart from heart disease, *Hp* is also implicated in strokes. A German study in 2001 identified *Hp* infection as an independent risk factor for stroke caused by atherosclerosis.[242] And the following year, researchers in Italy reported that *Hp* infection was significantly more frequent in middle-aged patients suffering from acute ischemic stroke.[243]

Finally, as you might expect, inflammation plays a key role in *Hp* research. Studies show an association between *Hp*-infected atherosclerotic lesions and inflammation.[244]

Total Pathogen Burden and the Risk of Coronary Artery Disease

Quite apart from this germ's link to cardiovascular disease, *H. pylori* has a lesson to teach us about infection as a hidden cause of disease.

Peptic ulcers can cause serious bleeding and pain in the digestive tract, requiring surgery. For most of the last century, peptic ulcers were thought to be caused by stress or spicy food. Not surprisingly, doctors prescribed bland food and rest as therapy for the disease. In the last decades, attention shifted to the gastric acids found in the stomach, so antacids and other acid suppressants became the preferred treatments. But while these medicines seemed to control the disease for a while, the ulcers almost always returned.

It wasn't until 1983 that Australian physicians isolated *H. pylori* bacteria in the stomach and identified it as a possible cause of ulcers. But there was great resistance to the idea; the medical establishment simply wasn't used to thinking of ulcers as the product of infective disease. It wasn't until more than a decade later, in 1996, when the FDA finally approved the first antibiotic treatment for eradicating *Helicobacter pylori* as a treatment for ulcers.[245] Antibiotic combined with acid suppressant therapy is so effective that 90% of patients are cured, with only rare cases of reinfection.

The lesson in this story is obvious.

After so many years thinking about cardiovascular disease as purely the result of non-infective risk factors, it's difficult for the medical community to accept the notion that strokes and heart attacks can be caused by an infective germ.

But it's a mistake to search for one single, infective cause of all atherosclerosis. As one researcher pointed out, "If common or widespread chronic infections are truly important risk factors for coronary heart disease, it is unlikely that a single infection will be shown to be causative. It is likely that the entire microbial burden of the patient from several simultaneous chronic infections is more important (e.g., *H.*

pylori-caused gastric ulcers+*C. pneumoniae*-caused bronchitis+periodontitis)."[246]

In other words, the more chronic infections you have—of all types—the more likely you are to have heart disease caused by atherosclerosis. A study released in 2000 supports this very idea.

Researchers from the Cardiovascular Research Institute in Washington, D.C. studied a group of patients for signs of infection by *Chlamydia pneumoniae*, cytomegalovirus, herpes simplex virus (type 1 and 2), and hepatitis A virus. They also tested for levels of C-reactive protein.

The amount of infectious germs a patient has is refereed to as his ***total pathogen burden***. It turned out that more than 75% of study subjects had been exposed to three or more of the five germs tested.

When the scientists ran the numbers, they found that, sure enough, an increasing pathogen burden was significantly associated with increasing risk for coronary artery disease. A similar association between increasing pathogen burden and levels of C-reactive protein was also found. Since C-reactive protein is suspected of actively promoting atherosclerosis, infections might contribute to coronary artery disease through systemic inflammatory response, as well.[247]

A second germ study in 2001 reached the same conclusion—infection plays an important role in heart attacks and death in patients with heart disease, and the risk posed by infection is related to the total amount of germs that the patient has.[248]

Another study in that same year had similar results: the number of infectious pathogens to which an individual has been exposed independently contributes to the long term prognosis—including a higher risk of future cardiac death—in patients with coronary artery disease.[249]

And, in their own words, here is the conclusion of researchers who studied the effects of infectious burden in 572 patients with cardiovascular disease in a 2002 study:

> "Our results support the hypothesis that infectious agents are involved in the development of atherosclerosis. We showed a significant association between infectious burden and the extent of ath-

erosclerosis. Moreover, the risk for future death was increased by the number of infectious pathogens, especially in patients with advanced atherosclerosis."[250]

As conclusions go, you can hardly get more conclusive: patients with the most chronic cardiovascular infections—such as *Chlamydia pneumoniae*, CMV, *Helicobacter pylori* and herpes simplex—have a greater extent of atherosclerosis and a higher risk of death.

But perhaps the most groundbreaking study yet was released in 2002 by the National Heart, Lung and Blood Institute in Bethesda, Maryland. It measured the infectious burden in people of all four germs that we've discussed in this chapter—*Cp*, *Hp*, CMV and HSV—plus one more, the hepatitis A virus. Not only did it find that multiple infections of these germs were an independent risk factor for coronary artery disease, it concluded that these germs were also a risk factor for endothelial dysfunction, a key concept we've discussed earlier in the book. Recall that endothelial dysfunction is the pathway toward the initiation and growth of atherosclerosis in arteries. This important study concluded that "Endothelial dysfunction provides the crucial link by which pathogens may contribute to atherogenesis (that is, the beginning of atherosclerosis)."[251]

All the studies above demonstrate the increased risk of being infected by many cardiovascular germs simultaneously. Of all the single pathogens we've talked about, however, the germ with the most evidence in its favor is *Chlamydia pneumoniae*. Despite the evidence presented in this chapter, it takes a special kind of argument to persuade scientists such as bacteriologists that *Cp* is a source of strokes and heart attacks. And that's just what we'll attempt to do in the next chapter called…

12

The Arguments for Chlamydia Pneumoniae as a Cause of Strokes and Heart Attacks

In the previous chapter, we outlined the many individual pieces of evidence that explains how *Cp*—the Heart Attack Germ—initiates and sustains inflammatory atherosclerosis and the creation of blood clots. But what about the big picture? How do you prove conclusively that the bacterium *Chlamydia pneumoniae* causes cardiovascular disease?

If you're a bacteriologist, you have a ready answer: Koch's Postulates.

German scientist and Nobel laureate Robert Koch is often called "The Father of Bacteriology," and with good reason. Along with the work of Pasteur, his experiments with anthrax and other microorganism in the 1800s established the validity of the germ theory of disease. Up until then, it was thought that disease was the product of imbalances in the four "humors" of the body (blood, phlegm, choler, and black bile) or even supernatural forces.

Koch's Postulates are criteria that Koch used to prove that a particular pathogen causes a particular disease.[252] Only four in number, the Postulates are easily summarized:

> **Koch's Postulates**
> 1. The pathogen must be present in nearly all cases of disease.
> 2. The pathogen must be isolated from the diseased host and grown in culture.
> 3. The disease must be reproduced when the culture is inoculated into the healthy host.
> 4. The organism must be recovered from the experimentally infected host.

The Postulates seem pretty commonsense today, but at the time they were developed they were a great advancement in medicine. Bacteriologists still use Koch's Postulates today as a guide when investigating the cause of disease.

One of Koch's great successes was his identification of a bacterium as the cause of tuberculosis (TB). TB is an infectious disease that attacks the lungs, causing coughing, weight loss and chest pain. If left untreated, TB can be fatal. Before Koch's experiments revealed the truth, there were many misconceptions about the cause and cure of tuberculosis.

For example, in the 1800s TB was though to be a consequence of a person's "lifestyle"—if a person contracted the disease, somehow his behavior was to blame.

The cure for TB was also thought to be a choice of lifestyle. In the late 1800s, American physician Edward Trudeau was stricken with TB. Believing that death was imminent, he decided to spend his last days in the Adirondack Mountains of New York. To his surprise, he recovered and Trudeau credited his recovery to the fresh air of the mountains. He built a resort for the convalescence of fellow TB victims and soon these "sanatoriums" were the preferred treatment for tuberculosis.

Koch, of course, demonstrated the fallacy of the "lifestyle" cause of tuberculosis. He proved that TB was caused by the bacterium *Mycobac-*

terium tuberculosis. When an infected person coughs or sneezes, the germ is released into the air and inhaled by the next victim. TB is a communicable disease, spread like the flu or a cold. Aside from living in crowded, unsanitary conditions, lifestyle has little to do with catching the disease.

The cure for TB is also independent of lifestyle. Long-term therapy with antibiotics kills the tuberculosis bacteria and prevents the onset of fatal symptoms.

Hmmm, wait a minute. Lifestyle…bacterium…coughing and sneezing…chronic infection…cured by antibiotics—does all this sound a little familiar?

It should. The shifting attitudes about the cause and cure of TB in the 1800s are very similar to the shifting attitudes about the cause and cure of cardiovascular disease today.

TB caused by "bad behavior?" That's what they say about cardiovascular disease. "Bad behavior"—such as eating the wrong foods, not exercising, etc.—is commonly held to be the ultimate cause of atherosclerosis. If someone suffers a stroke or heart attack, it's his lifestyle that is mostly to blame.

TB cured by a change in lifestyle, supervised by a medical facility? That's what they say about cardiovascular disease. By eating the right foods and exercising vigorously, people believe they will protect themselves from most strokes and heart attacks. Many doctors and hospitals encourage and profit from their sponsorship of "lifestyle remedies, supervised by a medical facility" as the numerous "Cardiac Rehabilitation Centers" attest to.

Koch showed that the origin of TB was not "bad behavior" and the cure was not "change of lifestyle, supervised by a medical facility." He proved that the cause and cure of TB was linked to bacterial infection, not behaviors, good or bad.

Today, researchers suspect much the same about cardiovascular disease. They realize that strokes and heart attacks cannot be fully explained by "bad behavior." There is an infective cause, as well—and they're using the Postulates as their investigative guide.

Just as Koch used his Postulates to uncover the infection behind tuberculosis, in this chapter we will use the Postulates to uncover the infection behind cardiovascular disease. However, these Postulates will have to be modified to fit the advances of medical knowledge, particularly as they relate to long-term infections, such as produced by *Chlamydia pneumoniae*.

Paul Ewald, a professor of biology at Amherst, discussed the problem of applying the Postulates to long-term infections in the *Atlantic Monthly*:

> "The health sciences are still grappling with the masking effects of long delays between the onset of infection and the onset of disease," Ewald says. "Any time you have hit-and-run infections, slow viruses, lingering or relapsing infections, or a time lag between infection and symptoms, the cause and effect is going to be very cryptic. You won't find these newly recognized infections by the methods we used to find old infectious diseases. We have to be ready to think of all sorts of new, clever ways to identify pathogens. We will have to abandon Koch's postulates in some cases."[253]

Or at least modify them, as we intend to do here.

For example, no one is arguing that *Chlamydia pneumoniae* infection is the *sole* cause of atherosclerosis. Anything that contributes to chronic inflammation in the artery is likely to contribute to atherosclerosis, including other types of germs. So *Cp* will never be identified in 100% of all atherosclerotic plaques, which is what you would demand from a strict adherence to the Postulates. And while a living germ may not be found in the artery, modern technology can reveal the antibodies to it, or pieces of its DNA, lodged in the plaque, indicating infection. So modifications of Koch's postulates are very common in today's medical science and shouldn't hinder our investigation.

We'll begin with the first requirement: "The pathogen must be present in nearly all cases of disease."

Scientists began their *Cp* investigations by demonstrating an association between *Chlamydia pneumoniae* and cardiovascular disease. If studies showed that people infected with *Chlamydia pneumoniae* have a higher risk of cardiovascular disease, that would be a good argument in *Chlamydia's* favor.

And, sure enough, that's…

Argument #1

Antibody evidence shows a strong association between chronic infection with *Chlamydia pneumoniae* and cardiovascular disease, including strokes and heart attacks.

To understand Argument #1 you need to know a few things about antibodies. So here goes.

Antibodies, a type of protein molecule, are a key component of your body's response to injury. The immune system creates antibodies when it detects a foreign substance in the blood, such as a germ. After antibodies are created, they float through the bloodstream and attach themselves to the surface of the invading germ. Once attached, the antibodies either destroy the germ directly or signal the body to send additional forces to destroy it.

Every type of germ creates its own type of antibody. So if a test shows that you have antibodies for *Cp*, it is certain that this particular germ has infected you.

All this talk about antibodies is necessary because testing for antibodies is how those Finnish researchers first discovered the link between *Cp* and cardiovascular disease. When they studied the antibodies of patients who had heart attacks or chronic coronary heart disease, they noticed that these patients were more likely to be infected with *Cp* than the general population. They also discovered that these same patients had a high level of the chronic type of *Cp* antibody, indicating long-term infections or reinfections.

Over the years, many antibody studies have consistently shown these same results: atherosclerosis, strokes and heart attacks are associated with *Chlamydia pneumoniae* infections. Here is a list of studies describing the association.

Early Studies Associating the Germ *Chlamydia Pneumoniae* with Cardiovascular Disease

Year	Institution	Study Results
1991	University of Washington	Higher levels of *Cp* antibodies meant a greater risk for plaques in the coronary arteries.
1992	Stanford University	Prior infections with *Cp* were associated with a greater risk of coronary artery disease.
1993	University of Minnesota	There was a significant cross-sectional association between past *Cp* infection and asymptomatic atherosclerosis.
1995	St George's Hospital Medical School, England	Higher levels of *Cp* antibody are more prevalent in subjects with coronary heart disease.
1995	Umea University Hospital, Sweden	Raised levels of *Cp* antibody were significantly more common in coronary artery disease patients than control subjects.
1995	St George's Hospital Medical School, England	*Cp* infections are associated with coronary heart disease.
1997	University of Milan, Italy	Heart attack patients had a significantly higher prevalence of *Cp* antibodies compared to blood donors. *Cp* reinfection may trigger heart attacks.
1997	St George's Hospital Medical School, England	In heart attack patients, increased levels of *Cp* antibodies predicted further adverse cardiovascular events.
1998	S.M. Annunziata Hospital, Italy	Heart attack patients had a higher prevalence of *Cp* infection and raised levels of *Cp* antibody compared to healthy control subjects.

As the chart demonstrates, different groups from around the world using different techniques of studying antibodies have all come to the same conclusion—there is a clear association between chronic infection with *Chlamydia pneumoniae* and an increased risk of atherosclerosis, heart attack and other cardiovascular troubles.[254, 255]

Once the association was made between *Cp* antibodies and heart attacks, scientists naturally wanted to know if there was also an association for stroke and other cerebrovascular diseases such as TIAs. Sure enough, that is exactly what they found.

In one experiment, researchers tracked the stroke rate of men who had high levels of antibody to *Cp*. After following the progress of these patients for six and a half years, they concluded that high antibody levels to *Cp* were associated with an increased risk for future stroke.[256] In a separate study, researchers found that *Cp* antibody is significantly associated with acute stroke and TIAs.[257] And a third study concluded that chronic *Cp* infection led to an increased risk of stroke and TIAs.[258]

All in all, if you want to prove that *Cp* infection leads to strokes and heart attacks, the antibody evidence makes a pretty good start.

But antibodies in the bloodstream are only one type of evidence. If *Cp* infection leads to atherosclerotic arteries, one would expect to find actual *Cp* germs or their cellular components, such as DNA, at the site of the disease. And that leads us to…

Argument #2

***Chlamydia pneumoniae* is detected in a high percentage of atherosclerotic plaques from different sites.**

It isn't easy to find *Cp* germs in the human body. Remember that *Cp* is a parasite—it hides within other cells, making *Cp* very difficult to see in a routine bacterial examination.[259] Sophisticated procedures, which require great skill to perform, are necessary. Fortunately, these tools, such as Polymerase Chain Reaction (PCR), immunocytochemistry and electron microscopy, can accurately identify the cellular traces of *Cp* germs when they find them.

With these new tools in hand, scientists searched for the germ at the sites of infection, in and around the plaque of diseased arteries. Their prime targets for testing were the coronary arteries and it's here that *Cp* was first detected.

In 1990, researchers in Johannesburg, South Africa discovered *Cp* in the coronary plaque of young black miners who had died from heart failure. Since then, *Cp* has been discovered nearly everywhere that arterial plaque has been discovered. Here is a listing of studies describing atherosclerotic arteries and cardiovascular tissue found to be infected by *Cp*.

Atherosclerotic Arteries and Cardiovascular Tissue Found to be Infected by *Cp*

Year	Institution	Tissue Infected by *Cp*
1992	National Centre for Occupational Health, SA	Coronary arteries
1993	University of Washington	Aorta
1995	University of Washington	Coronary arteries
1995	University of Washington	Coronary arteries
1995	University of Washington	Carotid arteries
1996	St Mary's Hospital Medical School, England	Aorta, iliac and femoral arteries
1996	University of Louisville	Coronary arteries
1996	University of Utah, LDS Hospital	Coronary arteries
1996	University of Milan, Italy	Abdominal aortic aneurysms
1997	Central Hospital of Kainuu, Finland	Abdominal aortic aneurysms
1997	University of Toronto	Carotid arteries
1997	University of Washington	Carotid arteries
1997	University of Washington	Peripheral arteries
1997	Uppsala University Hospital, Sweden	Aortic valves
1997	National Public Health Institute, Finland	Aortic valves
1998	Yamaguchi University, Japan	Carotid arteries
1998	Oulo University Hospital, Finland	Aortic valves

These studies prove that *Chlamydia pneumoniae* is found in atherosclerotic tissues throughout the body.

The significance of this is extremely important. As we've already discussed, aneurysms can rupture the abdominal portion of the aorta, heart attacks begin in the coronary arteries, and strokes often begin in the carotid arteries, the upper aorta and the aortic valves. Now we know that *Cp* germs are found in atherosclerotic tissue *in all five loca-*

tions, providing strong evidence of *Cp*'s association with these deadly events.

Moreover, the prevalence of *Cp* infection in atherosclerotic arteries is high. In 1998, one scientific paper examined all the available evidence from previous studies. Out of a total of 497 diseased tissue specimens, *Cp* was detected in 257 of them, for a rate of 52%—more than half.[260]

Keep in mind that *Chlamydia pneumoniae* is only one of the bugs suspected of causing atherosclerosis, so you shouldn't expect to find it in 100% of diseased arteries. For example, when one study looked for evidence of both *Chlamydia pneumoniae* and cytomegalovirus in the plaque of advanced carotid atherosclerotic lesions, they number of occurrences for either or both germs in the plaque rose to 71% of the arteries tested.[261]

To show that *Cp* germs are prevalent in diseased arteries is strong evidence, but that's only half of the story. It's possible that *Cp* germs could have the same rate of prevalence in normal, undiseased arteries. If that were the true, there would be no way to demonstrate that *Cp* infection correlates to a greater risk for cardiovascular disease.

So scientists set out to prove the second half of the story, which is…

Argument #3

***Chlamydia pneumoniae* is rarely found in normal arteries.**

When researches searched for *Cp* in diseased arteries, they also examined normal, healthy arteries. These normal arteries were used as "control groups" to match against the diseased tissue.

It was discovered that, although *Cp* germs were common in diseased arteries, they were *uncommon* in normal arteries. In one study, none of the normal arteries examined contained *Cp*, while diseased arteries harbored the germ.[262] A second study found the same—healthy arteries weren't infected by *Cp*, but diseased arteries were.[263] In other studies, the percentage of normal arteries showing traces of *Cp* was extremely low.[264]

A 1998 scientific paper summarized all the available evidence from a number of studies. Out of the total amount of normal arteries examined, only 5% were found to contain evidence of *Cp* germs. When compared to the rate of *Cp* found in diseased tissue, the researchers concluded it is much more likely that *Cp* germs will be found in diseased arteries than in normal arteries, showing a strong association between *Cp* infection and atherosclerosis.[265]

Let's review the arguments so far: 1) antibody evidence shows *Cp*'s strong association with cardiovascular disease 2) *Cp* is found in the majority of atherosclerotic lesions and 3) *Cp* is rarely found in normal arteries. These three arguments fulfill the first of Koch's Postulates: "The pathogen must be present in nearly all cases of disease."

At this point, you might think the case for *Chlamydia* is all sewn up. After all, if *Cp* is so strongly associated with cardiovascular disease it must certainly be the cause of the illness. But it's too early to make this conclusion, and here's why.

Establishing an association does not necessarily establish a cause. For example, there's a strong association between roosters crowing in the morning and the sun rising in the east. But it isn't the crowing that makes the sun come up.

With this in mind, some scientists theorized that *Chlamydia pneumoniae* might be nothing more than an "innocent bystander" in the whole process. As one researcher speculated, "It is possible that pre-existing atherosclerotic plaque within the vessel wall may simply serve as 'fertile ground' where the *Chlamydia* organism can grow as an 'innocent bystander,' in a manner unrelated to the development of the atherosclerotic plaque."[266]

To prove causation, we need to show that *Cp* is more than simply associated with cardiovascular disease. And the way to do that is to complete the rest of the criteria laid down by Koch.

So let's move on to his second Postulate: "The pathogen must be isolated from the diseased host and grown in culture."

To isolate a germ in culture means to grow and separate out a pure strain of a germ in a nutrient medium. A germ properly cultured from tissue is proof that a living germ came from the tissue.

Can *Cp* germs be isolated from a diseased host and grown in culture? The answer to that question brings us to...

Argument #4

***Chlamydia pneumoniae* germs have been cultured and isolated from atherosclerotic plaque.**

Two studies have successfully cultured and isolated *Cp* from atherosclerotic arteries. The very title of the first study, released in 1996, says it all: "Isolation of *Chlamydia pneumoniae* from the coronary artery of a patient with coronary atherosclerosis."[267] You can't get any more definitive than that...unless, of course, you consider this title from a second study, released in 1997: "Isolation of *Chlamydia pneumoniae* from a carotid endarterectomy specimen."[268]

Both of these studies fulfill the second of Koch's Postulates: "The pathogen must be isolated from the diseased host and grown in culture."

Well, that was quick! With two down and two to go, we can safely move on to the third Postulate: "The disease must be reproduced when the culture is inoculated into the healthy host."

Screeeech...Bang!

That's the sound of researchers crashing head-on into the third Postulate. (I guess it wasn't so safe to move on, after all.)

The third Postulate presents a bit of a problem. It requires that researchers infect a healthy subject with the germ and see if the subject gets the expected illness.

I can hear the researchers now—"OK, who's first? Hands in the air, all of you who'd like to volunteer for a stroke or heart attack!"

You see the problem? There aren't many healthy people willing to be infected with *Chlamydia pneumoniae* in the hopes they'll come down with cardiovascular disease. And chronic diseases pose a special problem—it might take four or five decades for disease to develop, a very long time for a single experiment. As you might expect, in any pathogenic investigation human research is often a sticking point when trying to fulfill Koch's Postulates.

Remember our discussion of *Helicobacter pylori* and peptic ulcers? The *H. pylori* researchers were faced with exactly the same dilemma. They needed to show that healthy people exposed to *Hp* would come down with peptic ulcers. But who would volunteer to let himself be exposed to a virulent bacterium in the hopes of contracting a potentially fatal disease?

The volunteer was Australian physician Barry J. Marshall, the scientist who, along with his research team, discovered *Helicobacter pylori's* association with ulcers. Unable to convince the medical community that *Hp* infection was the cause of ulcers, Marshall used himself as a guinea pig. In 1984 he drank a pure culture of *Helicobacter pylori* (no ice) and hoped for the best—which, in this case, was the worst.

Sure enough, a week later Marshall became ill with severe gastric infection and inflammation. His courageous self-experiment caught the attention of the medical world, and further experiments demonstrated conclusively that *Hp* infection is a cause of peptic ulcers. For his efforts, Dr. Marshall won the prestigious Lasker Award in 1995.[269]

Fortunately, not every researcher studying pathogenic disease has to go through self-experimentation or even experimentation on healthy human beings. Instead, researchers rely on animal studies. In fact, this was precisely the reason why Dr. Marshall took such dramatic action—he was unable to find a satisfactory animal model to study *Hp* infection and ulcers.

Cp researches have fared better. As luck would have it, rabbits make good substitutes for humans in the study of atherosclerosis. Like humans, rabbits develop atherosclerosis in their arteries. And, also like humans, they can catch pneumonia from *Cp* germs.[270]

In due course, studies with rabbits were begun by *Cp* investigators. The results from these studies lead us to...

Argument #5

***Chlamydia pneumoniae* induces the symptoms of atherosclerosis in animal studies.**

In a 1997 study, Canadian researchers infected a group of rabbits with a human strain of *Chlamydia pneumoniae*. The rabbits were infected by inhaling the germ, the same way that humans are infected. A separate control group of rabbits was not exposed to *Cp*.

The study was designed to answer a simple and direct question: does infection with *Cp* lead to atherosclerosis? By the end of a month, the researchers had their answer.

And the answer was, "Yes!"

Cp infection *does* lead to atherosclerosis. In the Canadian study, it turned out that the control group of rabbits remained healthy while several in the group infected with the *Cp* germ developed atherosclerotic lesions.[271]

Additional studies confirmed the results of the Canadian experiment. Researchers in Finland found that some of the rabbits that inhaled *Cp* germs developed the symptoms of atherosclerosis, while control rabbits did not.[272] Researchers at the University of Utah found the same:

within months of inhaling *Cp* germs, some infected rabbits showed signs of atherosclerosis, while uninfected rabbits stayed healthy.[273]

All three studies demonstrate that, after inhaling *Cp* germs, signs of atherosclerosis develop in the arterial walls of the experimental animals. As one of the University of Utah scientists stated about his own research, "These findings are best explained by assigning *a causative role to C. pneumoniae in the atherosclerotic process...*"[274]

With the data from these experiments, Koch's third Postulate is fulfilled. Only one more Postulate to go: "The organism must be recovered from the experimentally infected host."

This final Postulate follows logically from the others. If *Chlamydia pneumoniae* truly is the cause of an experimental rabbit's atherosclerosis, you would expect to find *Cp* in the rabbit's atherosclerotic lesions. And this, indeed, is...

Argument #6

Chlamydia pneumoniae can be recovered from experimentally infected hosts.

As part of the 1997 Canadian study, the researchers successfully cultured *Cp* from the atherosclerotic lesion of one of the infected rabbits, thus fulfilling the final criterion of Koch's Postulates.[275]

The chain of reasoning is complete—*Cp* is present in the majority of atherosclerotic cases, *Cp* can be isolated and cultured from diseased arteries, atherosclerosis begins when *Cp* infects a healthy host and it's subsequently found in the lesions of the infected host.

As Koch used the Postulates to argue that *Mycobacterium tuberculosis* infection leads to tuberculosis, we have used the modified Postulates to argue that *Chlamydia pneumoniae* infection leads to cardiovascular disease. As German researchers remarked after considering all the *Cp* evidence, "The Koch...criteria for the proof of the etiology are largely fulfilled...."[276]

Whew! In the course of only a few decades, *Chlamydia pneumoniae* went from being an accidental discovery, to recognition as one of the most ubiquitous pathogens known to man, to a key suspect in the leading cause of death in America.

The revolutionary nature of this discovery is still reverberating around the world, which is why the arguments for *Cp* don't end with Koch's Postulates. Numerous additional studies illuminate *Cp*'s role in atherosclerosis and, what is most important, suggest a cure.

These studies deserve a chapter of their own, so let's begin with the most encouraging research of all…

13

Antibiotics and the Prevention of Cardiovascular Disease

The more you know about the cause of a particular disease the more likely you are to find a successful treatment. And from the moment *Chlamydia pneumoniae* infections were suspected as a cause of atherosclerosis, researchers knew they were finally within sight of a possible cure for the majority of strokes and heart attacks.

The researchers were especially encouraged because medicine has a very potent weapon against bacterial infections like *Cp*...

Antibiotics

For the past 50 years *antibiotics* have been used very successfully to treat or prevent infections in the body. Antibiotic drugs destroy or limit the growth of microorganisms such as bacteria; and by killing bacteria, you eliminate the inflammation they produce. Since inflammation is the prime factor in the origin, growth and deadliness of atherosclerosis, you can see why researchers would be excited.

They reasoned that if a bacterial infection was a source of atherosclerotic inflammation, then antibiotics might be used to treat or prevent the disease. This, in turn, would lead to a reduction in the amount of strokes and heart attacks.

In fact, the researchers were quick to realize that antibiotic drugs might *already* be a secret benefit to people, quietly reducing strokes and heart attacks without anyone even being aware of it.

After all, many thousands of people use antibiotics every day. Perhaps patients using antibiotics to treat *Cp* respiratory diseases such as pneumonia or bronchitis were—as a happy coincidence—protecting themselves from inflammatory atherosclerosis, as well.

Since the 1960s, there's been a decline in the number of cases of atherosclerotic disease. Some researchers speculated that the reason for this decline was the growing use of steadily improving antibiotics.[277] It was only a matter of time before someone attempted to answer the question.

A recent study reviewed the records of 16,000 patients in Great Britain. Researchers wanted to compare the antibiotic use between patients who suffered heart attacks and those who did not. The researchers discovered that several groups of patients who received antibiotic treatments had a lower risk for a first-time heart attack than patients who did not receive the drugs. For example, patients who took the antibiotic *tetracycline* had a 30% lower risk for a first time heart attack. And for patients who used *quinolone*-type antibiotics the risk was even lower—55%.[278] The authors of the study noted that both tetracycline and quinolones are commonly prescribed by doctors to treat the respiratory diseases caused by *Chlamydia pneumoniae*.

Here was evidence that—quite by accident—doctors were already protecting their patients from cardiovascular disease by prescribing antibiotics. Although the researchers cautioned that this one study by itself does not prove that antibiotics were responsible for the reduction in heart attacks, they concluded that the study's findings "fit well with the hypothesis that respiratory tract infections with *C. pneumoniae* may play a role in the [cause] of ischemic heart disease."[279]

There were other compelling studies that also "fit well" with the hypothesis. Remember those rabbits infected with *Cp* in the last chapter? One team of researches wanted to know what would happen if the rabbits were given antibiotics after being infected with *Cp*.

It turned out that *Cp*-infected rabbits given a course of antibiotics showed a significantly lesser amount of atherosclerotic disease than infected rabbits given no antibiotics.[280] Again, more evidence that treating infection leads to a reduction in cardiovascular disease.

The rabbit researchers chose the drug ***azithromycin*** for their experiment. They chose this particular antibiotic for several important reasons.

As you know, *Cp* is a bacteria that acts as a parasite; it spends most of its life living inside host cells such as macrophages and endothelial cells. As a result, the immune system has a hard time finding the germ and mounting an attack against it. For instance, when *Cp* is holed up inside a cell, it is beyond the reach of immune system antibodies that could destroy it. Because of cunning ploys like this, most *Cp* infections last a long time. This results in the chronic inflammation that is the hallmark of *Cp* infections—and, of course, atherosclerosis.

The rabbit researchers knew this, which is why they chose azithromycin to use in their study. Azithromycin is part of the class of drugs called ***macrolide antibiotics***. These drugs are especially effective against bacteria that hide out inside cells. Macrolides are able to penetrate infected cells, concentrating the drug where it's needed most. Since *Cp* is a bacterium that spends most of its time inside cells, macrolides such as azithromycin would be the obvious antibiotic to use against the crafty pathogen. And studies showed that azithromycin was particularly effective against *Cp*.

In addition, azithromycin works fast. A single course over three days can do the trick, while similar drugs are prescribed for two weeks.[281] For these and other reasons, it's not surprising that many doctors use azithromycin as their drug of choice against the respiratory diseases caused by *Cp* germs.

And since *Cp* germs are also suspected of creating atherosclerosis, it's also not surprising that azithromycin would be the drug of choice in the first test of...

Antibiotics for the Prevention of Heart Disease

In 1997, British researchers released the results of an experiment that tested the effectiveness of antibiotics to prevent heart attacks and other cardiovascular troubles.

First, the researchers grouped together 213 male patients who had already suffered a heart attack. Each man was tested for evidence of *Chlamydia pneumoniae* infection by examining the amount of *Cp* antibodies in his blood serum. The researchers determined that—not surprisingly!—the patients with the highest levels of *Cp* antibodies were four times more likely to suffer death, a second heart attack or emergency coronary surgery. Clearly, the more *Cp* infection a heart patient was exposed to, the more likely the patient was to have additional serious cardiovascular trouble.[282]

Then the authors of the study treated the patients with the highest levels of *Cp* antibodies with either azithromycin or a placebo. The results after 18 months? As a group, the patients given azithromycin were four times less likely to suffer an additional cardiovascular event—such as death or heart attack—compared with patients who didn't receive antibiotic treatment.[283] A truly dramatic decrease.

Why would antibiotics be responsible for this reduction in heart troubles? Remember that the majority of serious coronary events are caused by inflamed, vulnerable plaque suddenly rupturing and producing blood clots. In their own words, the researchers reported that "azithromycin, by eradicating or suppressing infection, may have helped to 'stabilize' active plaque lesions, in part by dampening inflammation and hypercoagulation."[284]

In more familiar language, the researchers believed that killing *Cp* germs with azithromycin may have led to a decrease in the dangerous inflammation which makes plaque vulnerable and increases the likelihood of clots to form—the same ideas we've been discussing for the past several chapters.

In a second study with azithromycin, researchers worked with patients who had undergone surgery to clear a coronary artery clogged with atherosclerotic plaque. Typically, this surgery is performed to relieve angina. Arteries that are surgically cleared of plaque often become clogged again and the patient will have to repeat the surgery or undergo a coronary bypass operation.

In this coronary artery experiment, some of the heart patients were given azithromycin while others were given placebo pills. After six months, the patients who were given the azithromycin had lower frequencies of angina and reclogging of the artery.[285] Once again, it seems that antibiotics played a part in reducing cardiac troubles.

We know that antibiotics work effectively in typical human tissues. But can antibiotics kill or suppress the *Cp* germs that live specifically in cholesterol plaque?

Just such an experiment was carried out using the drug ***roxithromycin***, another type of macrolide. This 1999 study by Italian researchers examined the amount of *Cp* germs in diseased carotid arteries from two groups—those who were treated with roxithromycin and those who weren't. The scientists determined that taking roxithromycin appeared to effectively reduce the amount of *Cp* germs contained in the plaque.[286]

This discovery helps explain the results of another important test using antibiotics to prevent heart disease—the ROXIS study.

ROXIS stands for "Roxithromycin in Ischemic Syndromes." In this experiment, researchers studied patients from coronary care units in Argentina. Along with traditional therapy, the patients were given either placebo or a course of roxithromycin.

After 30 days, the researchers examined the rate of coronary events between the two groups. Taken together, the rate of severe recurrent angina, heart attack and cardiac death was significantly reduced in the patients who received the antibiotic therapy. The incidence of these events was 9% in the placebo patients and only 2% in those who received the antibiotic.

What accounts for the difference? As one of the researchers noted, "The antichlamydial activity of roxithromycin may have suppressed the reactivation of chronic infection within coronary plaque. In addition, the drug is known to have anti-inflammatory effects and this may have diminished a persistent inflammation within the plaque."[287] Again, the very subjects we've been discussing all along.

Summing up, the lead researcher of the ROXIS experiment commented that, "It may be that we are seeing the beginning of a new era in the treatment of symptomatic atherosclerosis. Looking ahead, this approach might lead to new ways of intervening earlier in the process of artery hardening, possibly even a preventive vaccine."[288]

Not every test of antibiotics has been strongly positive, however. In one trial, patients who had already suffered a heart attack were given azithromycin to see if a second attack could be prevented. After two years, patients who were given the azithromycin had a 7% reduction in the incidence of all-cause mortality, nonfatal heart attack, hospitalization for angina or coronary revascularization compared to patients on placebo. So, although the azithromycin patients had a reduction in risk, the amount of reduction was not considered to be significant.[289] A second study, performed by the University of Utah found that antibiotic therapy with azithromycin for patients with coronary artery disease was not associated with strong early reductions of ischemic events. However, the data did suggest that, in the long term, there might be worthwhile benefits to the therapy.[290]

The year 2002 saw more significantly positive azithromycin and other antibiotic studies, several of them focusing on cardiovascular patients infected with *Cp* germs.

In one experiment by British researchers, patients with coronary artery disease and who tested positive for *Chlamydia pneumoniae* infection were given either azithromycin or placebo for five weeks. Then a simple test was performed which measured the functioning of an artery. The patients who received placebo had no change, but the patients given the antibiotic showed a significant improvement in the functioning of the artery.[291]

In a second experiment, Finish researches studied 187 patients who were hospitalized for heart problems, treating them with either *clarithromycin* (another type of macrolide antibiotic) or a placebo for three months. The results? Patients treated with the antibiotic had a prolonged life and significantly reduced the risk of future heart attacks, unstable angina and stroke.[292]

In a statement released by the American Heart Association, Juha Sinisalo, a doctor at Helsinki University and the lead author of the Finish study, explained the beneficial results of the therapy in this test. "The most likely mechanism of action," said Dr. Sinisalo "is clarithromycin's antibacterial effect.... The action of clarithromycin seems to be long lasting."[293] According to the study, the patients who took the antibiotic had a 41% lower risk of heart attack and other cardiovascular troubles.

A third experiment performed in Switzerland assigned either roxithromycin or placebo to men infected with *Chlamydia pneumoniae* and suffering from peripheral artery disease. Previous studies had already established an association between *Cp* infection and atherosclerosis in the peripheral arteries.[294] In the Swiss study, the antibiotic was given for a one month period. At the end of nearly three years, the men were tested to see how much their illness had progressed. The study concluded that the antibiotic therapy was effective in preventing the progression of lower limb atherosclerosis for several years.

In addition, the amount of plaque in the carotid arteries of the men—a hot spot for strokes to develop—was monitored for six months. It was found that the amount of plaque in the arteries decreased in size for the antibiotic group, but remained constant for the placebo takers. Moreover, the regression of plaque size observed in roxithromycin-treated patients was significant for soft plaques, the most dangerous plaques in the body because of their tendency to rupture.[295]

Another experiment tried a different approach to antibiotic treatment for atherosclerotic arteries. In Chapter Eleven, I briefly mentioned that angioplasty procedures—where blocked arteries are surgically opened up with a catheter—are often plagued by reblockage within months after surgery. This reblockage—or restenosis—is caused primarily by the proliferation of smooth muscle cells caused by our old friend, inflammation. To keep the artery open, a small metal tube called a stent is inserted into the artery. But stents often fail because they don't stop inflammation and may actually become a source of inflammation, themselves. So even with a stent, the artery becomes blocked again, requiring more surgery.

Well, a team of doctors wondered what would happen if the stents were coated with a substance that would help stop inflammation. They chose an antibiotic called **rapamycin**, which is in the family of macrolide antibiotics we've been discussing throughout this chapter. The stents were designed to release tiny amounts of the antibiotic at a slow, steady rate, targeting the precise area where the stent was in place.

The team of doctors placed the antibiotic-impregnated stents in 45 patients in Brazil and the Netherlands. After two years in place, the doctors were astonished to find that the stents were 100% effective in preventing restenosis. Not a single stent became blocked.[296]

That startling 2001 study was replicated on a larger scale in 2002 when a second antibiotic stent test of 238 patients had the exact same results. Some patients received the antibiotic stents, while others didn't. After seven months, 100% of the rapamycin stents remained free from restenosis, a dramatic result. As an Associated Press article appearing in the New York Times reported, "to be 100 percent effective [is] almost unheard of in medicine...."[297]

Leaders in the medical community were astonished and elated by the success of the antibiotic stents. Dr. David Faxon, president of the American Heart Association, called the news "a major breakthrough" and Dr. Jesse Currier, associate director of the Adult Cardiac Catheterization Lab at the UCLA Medical Center, was quoted as saying "This is Neil Armstrong, one giant leap for interventional cardiology…this is a huge, huge quantum leap."[298, 299]

The chief benefit of the rapamycin stents may not be their antibiotic effect (that is, their ability to kill germs) but, rather, their anti-inflammatory effect. Remember that inflammation causes cells to proliferate, which is one of the reasons atherosclerotic lesions grow in size. And the proliferation of smooth muscle cells is the chief reason that stents become clogged and fail. Rapamycin is known to block inflammation and cell proliferation, and this may be the secret of its success.

And finally, in August of 2002, British researchers released the results of their study in which patients with heart disease were treated with either azithromycin or a second antibiotic, ***amoxycillin***. After a year follow-up, it was determined that the patients treated with the antibiotics were 36% less likely to suffer from unstable angina or to have had a heart attack, compared to those who were treated with placebo. Surprisingly, the researchers think that the antibiotics were targeting bacteria other than the two germs they were most interested in—*Chlamydia pneumoniae* and *Helicobacter pylori*.[300]

The studies above were most concerned with heart disease. But, as the Swiss study above suggests, since most strokes are the result of inflammatory atherosclerosis, there is every reason to suspect that antibiotic therapy will also be beneficial for the victims of cerebrovascular disease.

When I first explain to a patient that I intend to treat his heart disease with antibiotics, the patient often remarks that it's an unusual therapy and he worries if the treatment will be successful. As it happens, however, treating heart disease with antibiotics has *already* been incredibly successful. So successful, in fact, that antibiotics have all but eliminated one of the most common forms of cardiovascular illness in the United States—rheumatic heart disease.

The odds are, you don't know anyone currently suffering from rheumatic heart disease—in fact, I'll bet you're not really sure what it *is* exactly. Yet, within my lifetime, it was a major cause of illness and death in America. That should give you an idea of how effective antibiotics have been in controlling this disease. The story of treating rheumatic heart disease with antibiotics shares so many similarities with *Cp* infection that it's well worth exploring...

The Striking Parallels between Cp Infection and Rheumatic Heart Disease

When I first began medical school, my professors told me that most of my life as a general practitioner would be spent treating three diseases—syphilis, tuberculosis, and ***rheumatic fever***, an illness which often progresses to ***rheumatic heart disease.***

Back then, these three were among the most prevalent diseases in the United States and it certainly seemed that they'd be around for a long, long time. As it turned out, however, by the time I started my own practice, I hardly saw a single case of these three diseases.

The reason was antibiotics.

Each of these diseases is caused by germs that can be killed or controlled with antibiotics. The early antibiotic treatments such as ***penicillin*** and ***streptomycin*** were so effective that all three illnesses fell into rapid decline.

But, of the three, it's rheumatic heart disease that deserves our attention now because it illuminates much of what we know about *Cp* infection. So let's begin with a few facts about this illness.

Rheumatic heart disease is the direct result of ***rheumatic fever***, which, prior to 1960, was a leading cause of death in children. Although it can strike at any age, rheumatic fever typically occurs between the ages of five to fifteen years old.

The illness, which is caused by a streptococcus bacterium, is contagious. It can be passed from person to person simply by touching the same objects as an infected victim. Like other contagious diseases, rheumatic fever becomes more prevalent in crowded conditions and during the colder months when strep infections are most active.

The illness usually begins as a strep throat infection, then progresses to a fever that may last for two weeks. During an acute attack, the major joints of the body—knees, ankles, elbows and wrists—become hot, red, swollen, painful and lose much of their function.

Hmmm…where have we seen those five symptoms before?

They are—of course—the five familiar symptoms of inflammation. It turns out that much of the lasting damage done by rheumatic fever is caused, not by the strep germ itself, but by the body's inflammatory reaction to the germ. Rheumatic fever is considered to be an inflammatory disease of the connective tissues. In fact, anti-inflammatory drugs like aspirin are often used to control tissue inflammation during acute attacks. The streptococcus bacterium is most dangerous when it inflames the tissues of the heart, which is when rheumatic fever turns into **rheumatic heart disease**.

Inflammation, as you already know, is one of the body's chief defenses. It's thought that, because there is a similarity between streptococcus germs and heart muscle protein, the body mistakenly launches inflammation against the heart muscle as well as the invading germ.[301] Once again, here's an example of how inflammation can cause disease by attacking healthy tissue.

The inflammation of rheumatic heart disease commonly occurs in the **valves** of the heart. These valves regulate the flow of blood within the heart. When heart valves become inflamed, they do not open and close properly. They become leaky, making the heart work harder to keep up with the demand for adequate circulation to the body. These leaky valves produce **heart murmurs**, which are abnormal sounds of the heart. Using a stethoscope, a doctor hears the leaky valves as heart murmurs.

Because the valves don't open and close properly, the blood in the heart is pumped inefficiently to the rest of the body creating symptoms such as shortness of breath, chest pains and fatigue. Most of the time, the acute phase of rheumatic fever passes and the child recovers. But, as you know, inflammation often leads to lasting tissue stiffness and scarring and this has important consequences later in life.

Heart valves damaged by childhood attacks of inflammatory rheumatic heart disease may eventually lead to serious abnormalities in adulthood. As they years pass by, the leaky valves of the heart, stiffened and scarred by inflammation, put an added strain on the heart muscle, resulting in *congestive heart failure*. During congestive heart failure, the pumping action of the heart is so weak that it is unable to adequately supply blood to the rest of the body. Unless controlled by drugs or surgery, congestive heart failure can lead to disability and death. (I'll have much more to say about heart failure later in the book.)

Even in the days before antibiotics, not every child who developed rheumatic fever ended up with rheumatic heart disease; but many of them did. It is thought that some people may be genetically predisposed to develop rheumatic fever after infection with the streptococcus bacteria. By the time infected children reach the age of forty or forty-five, the consequences of valvular disease catches up with them and they become seriously ill.

Until a few decades ago, rheumatic heart disease was a major killer. But since the advent of antibiotics, the disease can be quickly extinguished at the first sign of illness. That's why penicillin is often used to treat strep throat in children. By killing the germ during the initial stage, you stop it from progressing to the heart.

One of the most frustrating things about the disease is that it can be surreptitious. It's not always possible to tell when a child has developed rheumatic fever. In mild cases, rheumatic fever produces no symptoms. There may be no outward evidence that the heart has become inflamed and injured. Yet, inflammation does its damage to the heart, waiting for decades to pass before finally revealing itself.

Moreover, once a patient develops rheumatic fever, he is prone to repeated episodes of reinfection. Streptococcal infection may rekindle itself several times in the victim's life, causing continuing rounds of inflammation in the heart, adding to the damage. Because of this, patients suffering from rheumatic heart disease may be given antibiotics on a long-term basis as a means of preventing reinfection.

Surprisingly, despite all we know about this disease, there is no definitive diagnostic test for rheumatic fever.[302] It is only by associating prior strep throat infection that the link was made between rheumatic fever and a particular germ. To this day, making a diagnosis depends largely on a description of symptoms. The fact the rheumatic fever is extinguished with antibiotics strongly supports the conclusion that it's an infective disease.

Now that you know the basics, it's easy to see the many parallels between rheumatic heart disease and heart disease created by *Cp* infection.

For both diseases:

- The cause is a contagious bacterium that follows seasonal patterns.
- The initial illness is a respiratory disease.
- The initial illness can be mild, producing no symptoms.
- Infection can begin during childhood.
- The susceptibility of the victim to the bacterium is though to be related to genetic factors.
- The heart damage is caused, not by the bacterium itself, but by inflammation, a response to injury by the immune system.
- Inflammation leads to stiffness and scarring in the heart.
- The heart may suffer from reinfection.
- Heart damage can happen slowly, over the course of decades.
- The damage can happen secretly with no symptoms before being discovered in adulthood.

- Anti-inflammatory drugs, such as aspirin, are used to treat inflammation.
- The use of antibiotics is indicated to treat the disease.

For most people, the notion that a germ can lead to heart disease—which can then be successfully treated with antibiotics—initially sounds like an unlikely, far-fetched idea.

But, as rheumatic heart disease illustrates, *there's nothing new* about infective bacteria causing heart disease, about inflammation damaging the heart, or about successfully treating heart disease with antibiotics. All of these facts are well established. The only thing new is the identification of *Chlamydia pneumoniae* and other pathogens as additional sources of infection and inflammation, which cause their own, unique damage to the heart.

There is every reason to suspect that the success of antibiotics against rheumatic heart disease will be repeated with *Cp*-induced atherosclerosis. The studies above are just the first indications of what's to come.

Many physicians have already drawn their own conclusions. A recent report reveals that, on the basis of the present studies, 14% of the cardiologists surveyed were already treating their patients suffering from heart attacks, bypass surgery, angioplasty, and angina with antibiotics to stop infection and inflammation and thus reduce the risk of cardiovascular events.[303] As with rheumatic heart disease, antibiotics are used both to treat on-going *Cp* infection (which leads to vulnerable plaque and blood clots) and to extinguish *Cp* infection early on before it even has a chance to create atherosclerosis.

It's been more than half a century since I attended medical school. No doubt, the professors in med school today are telling their students that a great deal of their time as general practitioners will be spent treating cardiovascular disease. I believe that—in the near future—antibiotics and other therapies that treat infection and inflammation will make strokes and heart attacks as rare as rheumatic heart disease is today.

14

Cardiovascular Germs and the Symptoms of Alzheimer's Disease

A Few Facts about Alzheimer's

Alzheimer's disease, an irreversible brain disorder, is the leading cause of dementia in the elderly. The symptoms of Alzheimer's include the deterioration of intellectual faculties, such as memory and reasoning ability, accompanied by emotional and personality changes. It is estimated that four million Americans suffer from Alzheimer's and it's the third largest cause of death in the nation, behind cardiovascular disease and cancer.

The loss of mental capacity from Alzheimer's is gradual, and the progression of the disease varies in each individual. In general, however, patients live for seven to ten years from the time of diagnosis. With the passage of time, the victims of Alzheimer's can no longer care for themselves and they become bedridden, making them susceptible to a disease, such as pneumonia, which will end their life.

For the brain to function properly, the nerve cells in the brain (called *neurons*) must be able to communicate with each other. The neurons in Alzheimer's patients, however, deteriorate and die, losing their ability to communicate and creating the patient's loss of mental functions.

Scientists have uncovered two types of neuron degeneration that are the hallmarks of Alzheimer's—amyloid plaques and neurofibrillary tangles.

Amyloid plaque, a hard, waxy substance composed in large part by protein, forms outside the neuron as a result of degeneration. *Neurofibrillary tangles* are twisted, silk-like fibers the build up inside nerve cells. The areas of the brain that are related to memory are the most likely to show plaques and tangles. I mention these twin hallmarks because they play an important part in the following discussion.

At the present time, no one is really sure of the cause of Alzheimer's, although people with a family history of the disease seem more likely to develop it. Much of the present research is focused on environmental factors—such as the ingestion of aluminum or lead—and genetic factors.

The most promising genetic factor is the ***APOE gene***, which is responsible for the creation of proteins that interact with amyloid plaques. Studies show that people with variations in this gene are at an increased risk for developing Alzheimer's. Depending on the variation, the risk can increase anywhere from two-to ten-fold, but only if the gene works in combination with other risk factors. By itself, the gene cannot create Alzheimer's.[304]

In the past few years, however, researchers have uncovered a promising new factor that is of particular interest to the study of the Heart Attack Germ…

The Surprising Link between Atherosclerosis, Strokes and the Symptoms of Alzheimer's Disease

As doctors and researchers studied the problem of mental decline in the elderly, they noticed a relationship between Alzheimer's disease and cardiovascular disease. Hypertension, diabetes, smoking, coronary artery disease, atrial fibrillation and atherosclerosis in general are all known to significantly increase the risk of developing Alzheimer's.[305, 306] And people with severe atherosclerosis are three times more likely to get Alzheimer's disease.[307]

Of course, both cardiovascular disease and Alzheimer's are diseases of the elderly, so you would expect some overlap between the two. In fact, the second highest cause of dementia in the elderly is strokes in the brain caused largely by atherosclerosis, a condition known as *vascular dementia*. Modern medicine has always made a clear distinction between Alzheimer's disease and the strokes that cause vascular dementia but, as one scientific paper pointed out, "In recent years, evidence is increasing that the two may be more closely linked than just by chance."[308]

The most compelling evidence for the link between strokes and Alzheimer's was discovered in 1997 by a team of researchers from the University of Kentucky. They used data from the "Nun Study," a long-term study of aging and Alzheimer's disease funded by the National Institute on Aging. This study tracks the mental impairment of nuns from the School Sisters of Notre Dame religious congregation. In this particular case, the researchers studied 102 sisters who were between 76 and 100 years of age. The sisters were examined every year and, upon their death, each sister agreed to donate her brain for autopsy.

The researchers found that the sisters whose brains exhibited the twin hallmarks of Alzheimer's disease—amyloid plaques and neurofibrillary tangles—didn't always suffer memory loss or dementia. In other words, even though their brains had Alzheimer's disease, the sisters didn't *act* as if they had Alzheimer's.

However, if an autopsy showed the presence of strokes in the brain *in addition* to Alzheimer's, then the sisters were much more likely to suffer from memory loss or dementia. The researchers found that if strokes happened in certain areas of the brains affected by Alzheimer's, the nuns were 20 times more likely to develop the actual symptoms of Alzheimer's disease.

This was an amazing finding. It seems that not all people with Alzheimer's suffer from a decline in mental ability. For many, mental problems occur only when their Alzheimer's is combined with strokes. The researchers concluded that as little as one or two small strokes increased the risk for symptoms to appear. And once the symptoms appeared, one or two small strokes made the symptoms much more severe.[309]

Researchers point to the example of Sister Mary as a case in point for their findings. A member of the Nun Study, Sister Mary passed away three months short of her 102nd birthday. On autopsy, her brain was discovered to be severely devastated by the ravages of Alzheimer's—many areas were withered away by plaques and tangles, leaving holes in the structure of the brain. And yet, despite the severity of her disease, she displayed none of the symptoms of Alzheimer's. To the end, she lived with clarity of mind and an enthusiasm for living. The researchers found it incredible that she was able to function so well with so much Alzheimer's damage.[310]

And Sister Mary was not alone. Out of 61 deceased nuns found to have Alzheimer's in the brain, 19 showed none of the mental symptoms associated with the disease.

What was their secret? None of the 19 had suffered from strokes. The combination of stroke with Alzheimer's, it seemed, made all the difference.

Other studies have found supporting evidence. Strokes often result from atherosclerosis in the carotid arteries, the arteries that supply blood to the brain. Dutch researchers found that as atherosclerosis in the carotids increases, so does the risk of dementia from both strokes and Alzheimer's disease.[311]

The lead author of the Nun Study research, David Snowden, summed up his investigation this way:

> "Our findings indicate that stroke may be a critical factor in determining whether Alzheimer's symptoms appear and if they appear, how severe they will be....Preventing strokes may reduce your risk of developing the symptoms of Alzheimer's, and once the symp-

toms appear, preventing stroke may result in less severe symptoms."[312]

And, of course, preventing strokes is a key subject of *The Heart Attack Germ*.

So the good news of this book is that, by preventing stroke, you may very well prevent or reduce the severity of the symptoms of Alzheimer's—an unexpected bonus from the treatment of cardiovascular disease.

A key reason why the link between stroke and Alzheimer's remained unknown for so long is the hidden nature of...

Silent Strokes

Silent strokes are strokes that take place in the smallest arteries of the brain. Typically, a piece of cholesterol plaque will break off from a larger artery and travel through the bloodstream until it becomes snagged in a smaller blood vessel. Because the resulting occlusion affects a tiny area of brain cells, the amount of damage is most likely not critical to the function of the brain. The occlusion may cause no symptoms at all, or symptoms so slight that they are mistaken as something else, such as a fainting spell. So a small stroke may go unnoticed by the patient or the people around him, which is why they're given the name "silent."

It's fair to say that silent strokes are a hidden epidemic. A study of brain scans by the National Heart, Lung and Blood Institute estimates that 11% of the American population between the ages of 55–70 have suffered a silent stroke, which translates into millions of people. It's also believed that between 10 and 40% of people who've had Transient ischemic Attacks have also suffered a silent stroke.[313]

Although any one silent stroke may not produce symptoms, the cumulative effect of many silent strokes can lead to the symptoms of vascular dementia. But Alzheimer's makes a significant change in this equation. In patients with Alzheimer's, just a few silent strokes can have grave consequences: *only one or two silent strokes in an Alzheimer's brain are enough to produce the symptoms of memory loss and dementia.*

So stopping strokes—even the smallest of them—becomes critical for people at risk for Alzheimer's.

Until now, many people assumed that mental impairment was an unavoidable consequence of old age. But this new research on Alzheimer's and silent strokes reveals that aging, by itself, is not responsible for mental changes. In the absence of disease, it is normal for people to retain the full function of their mind well into their 9th and 10th decades of life.

It's only when disease is present that memory loss and confusion take place. And since many elderly suffer from silent strokes, the effects of cardiovascular disease were not taken into account as a cause for their mental impairment.

At this point, we need to stress an important distinction. The evidence we've considered so far has been restricted to the effect that stroke has on the *symptoms* of Alzheimer's. No one is quite sure yet what causes Alzheimer's to appear in the brain in the first place. But there is some startling new evidence that the cause of Alzheimer's *and* atherosclerosis might arise from the same basic source. The evidence begins with the recent discovery of an old friend…

Inflammation and Alzheimer's

If you remember, one of the earliest clues that atherosclerosis was tied to infection and inflammation was the fact that people who received antibiotics for non-cardiovascular diseases—such as pneumonia—were less likely to develop heart problems. Quite by accident, the antibiotics they were taking for other illnesses secretly protected them from heart troubles, as well.

Much the same thing happened in the world of Alzheimer's. Population studies reveal that arthritis sufferers have a much lower rate of Alzheimer's disease.

Arthritis, of course, is a chronic, inflammatory disease, and patients are often given anti-inflammatory drugs to control their illness. As it happened, the reduction in Alzheimer's disease was traced back to the regular use by arthritis patients of anti-inflammatory drugs.[314] Studies estimate that the prevalence of Alzheimer's disease is reduced by 40—50% in patients using anti-inflammatory drugs.[315] And, as one paper reported, "Twenty…studies that have been published to date indicate that populations taking anti-inflammatory drugs have a significantly reduced prevalence of Alzheimer's disease or a slower mental decline."[316]

Clearly, inflammation has something to do with the progression of Alzheimer's.

This anti-inflammatory evidence fit well with an emerging theory about Alzheimer's. New research was suggesting that the regions of the brain affected by Alzheimer's disease are also affected by chronic inflammation. In fact, evidence seemed to indicate that inflammation plays a key role in the development of Alzheimer's.

Many scientists hypothesize that the amyloid plaques and tangles that are the hallmarks of Alzheimer's are themselves the products of inflammation and act to keep the inflammatory process going. Much of the recent data points to chronic inflammation as the reason why nerve cells degenerate and die in the brain of Alzheimer's victims.[317, 318] In animal studies, the use of ibuprofen—an over-the-counter pain reliever that is also an anti-inflammatory drug—reduced by half the amount of amyloid plaques in Alzheimer's-like brains, underlining the connection between inflammation and the disease.

Once the connection was made between inflammation and Alzheimer's, of course, scientists set about searching for the cause of the inflammation. Since inflammation is the immune system's response to injury, they looked for a possible source of injury to the brain. It didn't take them long to find…

Herpes Simplex Infection and Alzheimer's

As we've discovered, infectious germs are often a source of inflammation—and the brain can harbor infection just like any other part of the body. Since the link between atherosclerosis, strokes and Alzheimer's was just coming into focus, researchers wondered if the pathogens of cardiovascular disease might have something to do with Alzheimer's.

As mentioned in Chapter Ten, the cold sore virus, herpes simplex, is associated with cardiovascular disease. Now, recent studies suggest that it is *also* associated with Alzheimer's.

To begin with, herpes simplex is known to infect the brain and create inflammation in the same areas that Alzheimer's does. With this as a starting point, studies have determined that a herpes simplex infection, combined with the APOE genetic cofactor, creates a strong likelihood for the development of Alzheimer's.[319, 320]

And a team of researchers from the University of California reported that a protein found in the herpes simplex virus mimics beta-amyloid, a protein that forms the amyloid plaques that are a hallmark of Alzheimer's. Further, they found that the herpes simplex protein killed brain cells and formed amyloid plaque in lab experiments.[321]

It's too soon to draw any hard and fast conclusions from these findings, but one explanation is that herpes simplex infection helps creates inflammation in the brain that leads to the build-up of the amyloid plaques, resulting in Alzheimer's.

But herpes simplex is not the only infectious germ linked to Alzheimer's disease...

Chlamydia Pneumoniae and Alzheimer's

Chlamydia pneumoniae—that ever-present germ that seems to be associated with so many ills—is now associated with Alzheimer's.

Let's begin by remembering that *Cp* is already implicitly associated with strokes in the brain. Studies have connected *Cp* infection to the presence of atherosclerosis in the carotid arteries, well known as a source of strokes.[322] Additional studies have specifically linked *Cp* infection to a significant increase in the risk of stroke.[323, 324] And since stroke is associated with an increased risk of Alzheimer's symptoms, there already exists a known link between *Cp* and Alzheimer's.

With this knowledge and the new association of inflammation with Alzheimer's disease, researchers wondered if *Chlamydia pneumoniae* germs could be a source of inflammation in Alzheimer's.

Up to this point, no one was even sure if *Cp* existed in the brain. So researchers from several Universities began a three-year study and, for the first time, discovered *Cp* living in brain cells. Moreover, their research revealed a strong association between *Cp* infection and Alzheimer's.

Out of the 19 Alzheimer's brains that they studied, 17 were found to contain *Cp* infection. That means that nearly 90% of the Alzheimer's brains had *Chlamydia pneumoniae* in them! Just as importantly, *Cp* showed up in the brain of only one of 19 control patients who had died of other diseases, further demonstrating *Cp*'s association with Alzheimer's.

The germ was found in the part of the brain that usually sustains the most damage in Alzheimer's disease. And the parts of the brain not affected by Alzheimer's showed little evidence of *Cp* infection. The *Cp* germs were alive and active in the brain and the scientists were able to grow the *Cp* from brain tissue samples in the lab.[325]

As one of the researchers explained, "What we have here is an organism that can get inside (brain) cells and can potentially trigger them to cause inflammation."[326]

And as we've seen, inflammation is one of the chief suspects for the plaques and tangles associated with Alzheimer's. But the *Cp* germs don't infect the neurons of the brain, which are the cells that become imbedded with plaques and tangles. Instead, *Cp* infects the brain's **glial cells**, a network of cells and branches that support the tissues of the brain. It's thought that the inflammatory cells and chemicals responding to the *Cp* in the glial cells attack the neighboring healthy neurons, damaging them, as well—an old, familiar story of inflammation. "We think it's the inflammation that's really doing the damage," said a member of the research team.[327]

It should be noted that other studies have failed to find *Cp* in Alzheimer's brains,[328] but the tests for *Chlamydia pneumoniae* are very sophisticated and difficult to perform, so mistakes can be made.

For example, in a paper presented at a meeting of the Canadian Association for Clinical Microbiology and Infectious Diseases, researchers found that testing for *Cp* in Alzheimer's brains had to be performed multiple times to ensure that the germ was detected. The results of their careful testing confirmed the positive results of the first study. None of the normal brains contained *Cp*, but 85% of the Alzheimer's brains were infected by the germ.[329]

Clearly, there are many threads that link the germs of cardiovascular infection, inflammation, atherosclerosis and Alzheimer's. The research is so promising that doctors are already preparing trials to test the effectiveness of antibiotics as a treatment for Alzheimer's.[330]

PART 2:
Preventing Strokes, Heart Attacks and the Symptoms of Alzheimer's Disease with WIN/WIN Therapy

1

A Philosophy of Healing

All diseases harm you in the same manner—they interfere with the process of renewal in your body.

The human body is in a state of constant renewal; it employs thousands of mechanisms to repair or replace the parts that become injured by things such as age, trauma or infection. Your body already knows what needs to be done to repair any damage. Disease is a hindrance to this process.

As a physician, my job is to assist your body as it attempts to heal itself. Every treatment I give, every drug I prescribe, every course of action I urge my patients to adopt is based on this simple philosophy.

WIN/WIN Therapy is consistent with this view of medicine. WIN/WIN stands for "***Whip Infection/Reduce Inflammation.***"

Chronic inflammation interferes with the renewal process of the arteries of the heart and brain after they've become injured. WIN/WIN Therapy stops this chronic inflammation and allows the arteries of the heart and brain to repair and restore themselves to health, as they naturally want to do.

Taking control of the usual risk factors—cholesterol, hypertension, smoking, etc.—is a part of WIN/WIN Therapy because these factors contribute to artery injury and chronic inflammation. But WIN/WIN Therapy goes beyond the traditional risk factors by also controlling cardiovascular infections, a major source of injury and chronic inflammation. WIN/WIN Therapy recognizes that *nothing* is more important to cardiovascular health than the early diagnosis and treatment of chronically infected and/or inflamed arteries because this is what leads to atherosclerosis, strokes and heart attacks.

This breakthrough discovery was important to me both professionally and personally. Let me tell you about...

My Experiences with Cardiovascular Disease—Past and Present

Both of my brothers died from heart attacks more than 25 years ago.

My brother William was the Chief of Staff at the hospital where we both worked as surgeons and general practitioners. Until the moment he was stricken, he was performing surgery and caring for his patients with his usual attentiveness and dedication. His attack came suddenly and was a great shock to me. As closely as I and his fellow doctors worked by his side, we saw no indication he was suffering from cardiovascular disease.

My brother Frederick, on the other hand, did have some indications of cardiovascular problems. As a child he suffered from Bright's disease, an illness which damaged his kidneys and led to hypertension. Despite occasional symptoms of advancing atherosclerosis, he held a demanding series of jobs as the musical director for many Broadway musicals. One day at work, like my other brother, he suffered a major attack and quickly succumbed.

When I saw both of my brothers die of cardiovascular disease, I decided to make some major changes in my life. In the mid-1970s, I moved my home and practice from Chicago to the beautiful town of Naples near the southern tip of Florida. I replaced the harsh winters and hectic pace of Chicago for the tropical breezes and relaxing beaches of the Gulf Coast.

I tried to limit the hours I spent at the office and in the hospital. I hoped that a change in location and work habits might afford some protection from the stresses associated with cardiovascular problems. I had already stopped smoking back in the 60s when the Surgeon General made his first report on the hazards of cigarettes. But I knew that my family history indicated I was a prime candidate for an early heart attack, just like my brothers.

Like much of Florida, Naples had a large retirement population. As a consequence, my practice shifted from general practice to a focus on the problems of the elderly, especially the prevention of strokes and heart attacks.

By the early 80s, the traditional risk factors were well established and a new generation of drugs was developed for the treatment of cardiovascular problems such as hypertension and arrhythmias.

But I felt as if medicine was up against a stone wall in preventing strokes and heart attacks. I encouraged my patients to stop smoking, watch their cholesterol, exercise, eat a proper diet and all the rest, but cardiovascular disease was still a major problem for people, even when all the rules were being followed.

Every treatment and suggestion helped, but all these little "helps" seemed to get us down to the same spot—about a 30% less chance of stroke or heart attack. Most people never got below that, to 50, 60, or 70% lower risk. It was very frustrating to me.

Flash forward to the present. It's been more than 25 years since I moved my practice to Florida. Certainly, cardiovascular medicine has changed dramatically during the past two and a half decades. But how far have we really advanced in our ultimate objective—preventing strokes and heart attacks?

Here's a story that might serve as an example—a typical case history of the way modern medicine treats cardiovascular disease in the new millennium.

A new patient named James arrived in my office, referred to me by a local druggist. James is 50 years old and in excellent shape. He runs four miles a day, maintains his weight, doesn't smoke and drinks red wine every day for his heart. On examination, his cholesterol levels were right where they should be. He had slightly elevated blood pressure, but not enough to be of concern. His family history was good and he had no obvious disease such as diabetes that would contribute to the development of cardiovascular problems. In sum, James had no significant risk factors and felt completely healthy.

That is, until about a month before he saw me. That's when he noticed that, during his daily run, he would start having back pains. When he stopped running, the back pains would disappear. James visited his doctor, who told James that his back pain might actually be angina, a symptom of reduced blood flow through the arteries of the heart. Alarmed, James decided to travel to a major clinic in Ohio that specializes in cardiac care.

At the clinic, they performed *angiography* on James, a special kind of X-ray examination that is used to visualize blood vessels of the heart. The angiogram revealed a 90% blockage of his right coronary artery.

They performed a standard operation for restoring blood flow—a balloon angioplasty. In this procedure, the surgeon inserts a balloon-tipped catheter into the clogged artery. As the balloon is inflated, the cholesterol plaque is pushed aside, enlarging the diameter of the artery. Afterward, the surgeon installed a *stent*—a small metal tube—designed to keep the artery open. Within a day or two, James was sent home with a prescription for a statin drug to lower his cholesterol levels.

After I heard his story about the clinic, I asked James, "How long do you think you've had this 90% blockage in the right artery?"

"I don't know. I never thought about it."

"You've probably been running with this thing for a long time," I said. "Did the doctors at the clinic say when you developed this disease?"

"No."

"Did they tell you what was the cause of your atherosclerosis?"

"No."

"How did they explain the fact that the rest of your arteries were clean, except this one area that was blocked?"

James shrugged. "Well, they didn't."

"Why did they give you a drug to lower your cholesterol when it's already low?"

"I don't know. They just told me it was a good thing to do."

"Did they say what the future would hold for you?"

"No. They just said to come back in a while and they'd look at it again."

Now, James just came from one of the most prestigious clinics in America, a clinic with modern, up-to-date facilities and modern, up-to-date doctors. After all this first-rate care, why would he come to see me simply on the recommendation of a druggist? Frankly, I don't think it was me in particular he wanted to see. He just needed to talk to somebody because there was a nagging doubt in his mind.

The nagging doubt was this: James didn't really understand what was making him ill.

Even worse—he felt that the doctors in the clinic didn't really understand what was making him ill, either. And if they didn't know that, how could they make him well?

He was right.

The doctors in the clinic performed the angioplasty, they gave him the stent, they gave him the cholesterol-lowering drug (even though his cholesterol was already low), and they sent him on his way. They did all the things that the protocols told them to do, without once stopping to ask themselves, "How does a man with no risk factors develop atherosclerosis?" All the physicians knew was that doing a balloon angioplasty with a stent was better than doing nothing—after all, an artery that was closed would be opened by the surgery. So that's what they did, then turned their scalpels to the next patient in line.

But because the physicians blindly repeated the same procedures based on statistics without any regard as to what was making him ill, James had absolutely no confidence that his problem was solved.

That is why he came to me. He had tried hard to follow all the rules for cardiovascular health, and he ended up with advanced atherosclerosis and a metal tube in his heart. If he was doing all that he should, then why did he have atherosclerosis?

If you've read Part I of The Heart Attack Germ, you already know the answer. James' story reveals…

The Major Flaw of Conventional Therapy

No matter how carefully I examine my patients, I never see their disease.

It's not because I'm unobservant. Quite the contrary; I pride myself on my ability to identify illnesses that may have slipped the attention of other physicians. But the fact is, when a patient comes to see me in my office, I never see any disease at all.

What I see instead is *the body's response to injury*—a key concept from earlier in the book.

Most medical symptoms are responses to injury. If you come to me with a cold, your sneezing and runny nose are not the disease, but your body's response to the injury caused by a cold virus. If you come to me with pneumonia, your fever and congested lungs are not the disease, but your body's response to an injury caused by multiplying pneumonia germs.

Why is this distinction so important? Because if I only treat your symptoms—that is, your response to injury—I am not treating the injury itself. And that leads to big trouble.

For example, if you come to my office suffering from a strep throat, I could treat you with pain relievers that will ease your suffering. But the underlying illness—tissue injury caused by streptococcal germs—remains unaffected by this treatment. The germs will continue to damage your body, with potentially fatal results. To cure you, I must always look beyond your symptoms and discover the true cause of your injury; only then can I hope to make you well.

Which brings us to strokes and heart attacks.

In a very real sense, atherosclerosis—the build-up of cholesterol plaque—is a *symptom*. It is the body's response to arterial injury. No amount of effort to remove, reduce or go around the plaque will actually cure the underlying injury that created the plaque. It's like trying to cure your strep throat with an aspirin: you might ease the painful throat for a while, but the underlying cause of the sore throat remains, growing more dangerous with each passing moment.

This is what happened to James at the clinic. The doctors treated the cholesterol plaque by pushing it aside and creating a tunnel through it for blood to flow. By doing so, an artery that once was closed was now open, which eased the pain of his angina. But the underlying illness that created the plaque was left untreated.

It's no wonder that James was still worried. The doctors were only concerned with relieving the immediate problem of an artery narrowed by cholesterol plaque. But his underlying problem is arterial injury and inflammation, which the doctors did little about. James had no risk factors so "reducing risk factors" was not an option. Under the clinic's care, his atherosclerosis will continue to progress and spread, creating more problems for him in the future. (Although by giving James statins, his physicians are unwittingly reducing inflammation. The latest research indicates that even people with low cholesterol can benefit from cholesterol-lowering drugs, most likely because of reduced levels of inflammation.)

Every day, this same scenario is repeated hundreds of times in clinics and hospitals throughout the country. This is the major flaw of conventional cardiovascular therapy. Correcting this flaw is…

The Advantage of WIN/WIN Therapy

Whip Infection/Weaken Inflammation Therapy—or *WIN/WIN Therapy*—is the first cardiovascular therapy that actively targets the underlying source of strokes and heart attacks, i.e., arterial injury and the resulting chronic inflammation in the arteries of the heart and brain. Not only is injury and inflammation responsible for the creation of cholesterol plaque, it is also responsible for weakening the plaque and making it vulnerable to rupturing and producing blood clots.

Chronic inflammation is provoked by diseases and conditions such as diabetes, hypertension, oxidized LDL-cholesterol and other risk factors that injure the artery wall. That's why taking control of risk factors is an important part of WIN/WIN Therapy.

But as we discovered in Part I, a previously unknown source of arterial injury is infection by cardiovascular germs such as *Chlamydia pneumoniae*. Using antibiotics and antiviral drugs, WIN/WIN Therapy kills or controls these germs to reduce inflammation in the artery. In this way, patients who suffer from advanced atherosclerosis can significantly reduce the risk of stroke, heart attack and other cardiovascular troubles, and patients with early atherosclerosis can slow or stabilize the progression of disease.

Let me tell you about it.

2

The Five Steps of WIN/WIN Therapy

Whip Infection/Weaken Inflammation Therapy—or *WIN/WIN Therapy*—is a safe, painless, non-invasive and inexpensive treatment for atherosclerotic disease that significantly reduces the risk of stroke, heart attack and the symptoms of Alzheimer's disease.

Despite the fact that WIN/WIN Therapy is a new and innovative therapy, every part of WIN/WIN Therapy is well known and time-tested. It uses the same medicines and treatments found in doctors' offices, health clinics and hospitals across the nation.

WIN/WIN Therapy aids in the prevention of strokes, heart attacks and the symptoms of Alzheimer's because it targets chronic infection and inflammation, the root cause of atherosclerosis, plaque rupture and the creation of blood clots.

WIN/WIN Therapy uses antibiotic and antiviral drugs to control the newly discovered cardiovascular germs that keep chronic inflammation smoldering inside infected arteries. These drugs have been around for many years and their safety and efficacy is well established.

Studies suggest that antibiotic therapy can significantly reduce the risk of serious cardiovascular events in patients who are already suffering from heart disease. And by starting antibiotic therapy early, it may be possible to slow the advancement of plaque before it gets to a dangerous stage of development, creating a preventive cure.

WIN/WIN Therapy has five basic steps:
1. Receive a thorough cardiovascular examination.
2. In addition to a standard blood test and cholesterol screening, test for inflammatory risk factors—such as C-reactive protein and fibrinogen levels—and for infectious risk factors, such as *Chlamydia pneumoniae* and the other germs of cardiovascular disease.
3. Use conventional therapy to treat the diseases and conditions that contribute to strokes and heart attacks.
4. Use antibiotic, antiviral and anti-inflammatory drugs to control cardiovascular infection and inflammation.
5. Control personal risk factors that contribute to arterial injury and inflammation.

Aside from reducing cardiovascular events, WIN/WIN Therapy also protects the patient by reducing the risks associated with cardiovascular surgery, such as angioplasty and coronary artery bypass. I'll have more to say about this important point in a later chapter.

Taking the First Step

Do you feel well? Do you follow the risk factor guidelines for a healthy heart by the American Heart Association (AHA)? Are you a young adult and feel that heart disease is a problem only for the elderly?

Then maybe you feel that WIN/WIN Therapy is not for you.

It's only natural that people who feel well believe they are not at risk. But according to the AHA, an estimated 48% of men and 63% of women who die suddenly of heart attack **had no previous symptoms.**

It's only natural that people who follow the AHA guidelines believe they are not at risk. But researchers say that up to half of all patients with cardiovascular disease have **none of the traditional risk factors.**

It's only natural that people who are young adults believe that, since they are not at high risk, they shouldn't worry about cardiovascular disease. But **atherosclerosis can begin in the teenage years,** growing worse as time passes. The heart attack that strikes at age 50 may have been set into motion while you were still in high school.

No matter if you're young, feeling well and following all the rules, the hidden processes of infection and inflammation that will lead to a stroke or heart attack can be simmering away inside you, unnoticed until disaster strikes. That's why you must make the commitment to begin WIN/WIN Therapy *now*, and not wait until the damage is done.

It requires a shift in thinking beyond the traditional risk factors and lifestyle changes promoted in so many cardiovascular health books. There are limits that "healthy living" and "self-help" can do for preventing strokes and heart attacks.

The reasons are infection and inflammation.

People readily accept the fact that there is no self-cure for infectious diseases like pneumonia or polio. Patients know that no amount of dieting, exercise or vitamins will stop the infection of a pneumonia germ or polio virus. They understand that only going to their doctor and getting antibiotics or a vaccine shot will assist in stopping these infections.

The same holds true for the infections and inflammation of cardiovascular disease. Simply controlling risk factors is often not enough to prevent the strokes and heart attacks that are caused by infection and inflammation. Only going to a doctor and getting the appropriate drugs to kill or control germs and limit inflammation in the arteries will stop the progression toward a stroke or heart attack.

Moreover, self-diagnosis is impossible for the individual to accomplish on his own. Arterial infection and inflammation happen on a microscopic scale, hidden from view. Even dangerously advanced atherosclerosis may not provoke symptoms until a fatal attack happens.

That's why it's worth repeating this simple point: atherosclerosis is an inflammatory, and often infectious, disease. Therefore, treating atherosclerosis—and cardiovascular disease in general—always requires the care of a physician. Always consult your physician before starting or changing any medical treatment.

The detection of cardiovascular disease requires that a physician conduct a complete cardiovascular examination, which leads us to…

Step 1
Receive a thorough cardiovascular examination.

Without question, the first step of WIN/WIN Therapy is critical. Every adult needs to have a complete cardiovascular examination—the earlier, the better, even if you look or feel healthy. If nothing else, you'll establish a set of measurements that will indicate how your health has changed over the years. You'll find this an invaluable aid in future examinations.

Because examinations are so critical, I've devoted a large section of the book to the topic. It's a subject I've been eager to share with you.

As a doctor, I've performed surgery, delivered babies, worked in the ER—done just about everything a general practitioner can do. But for me, the most challenging—and satisfying—moments in medicine are when I examine my patients and make the diagnosis that leads to recovery.

I'd like to share that experience with you…from the doctor's point of view.

I'm sure you've had quite enough of it from the *patient's* point of view; a trip to the doctor is by turns tedious and nerve-wracking.

Part of the problem is that, despite all the probing and poking you've endured over the years, the common instruments, tests and procedures in a medical office are still fairly mysterious to most people. Doctors rarely take the time to explain what they're looking for or how they judge the significance of their findings.

So I'd like to give a step-by-step account of how I conduct a cardiovascular examination—not only what I do physically, but what's going on inside my mind as I do it.

There's one bit of good news I can share with those of you who are nervous about medical examinations in general. Aside from the blood test, which requires the use of a small needle to draw blood, every test that I advise you to have for a thorough cardiovascular exam is completely safe, painless and non-invasive—not to mention, relatively inexpensive. And the treatments I most often recommend are also safe, painless, non-invasive and inexpensive.

All in all, taking a cardiovascular exam is a breeze: *not* taking one is the scary part. Aside from taking some of the mystery and anxiety out of your next doctor's appointment, I hope this chapter will be the standard by which you judge your next cardiovascular examination.

The very phrase "cardiovascular examination," however, is a little misleading. It sounds as if the only things being examined by the doctor are the patient's heart and arteries. But there are literally thousands of medical factors that influence the health of the cardiovascular system—everything from alcoholism to zoster—and the doctor must be alert to all of them.

While it would be impossible to touch upon every subject in a single chapter, I can point to the chief factors that weigh on my mind as I examine my patients. And often what's uppermost in my mind are...

The Causes and Symptoms of Heart Failure

The focus of this book has been atherosclerosis and its influence on cardiovascular health, specifically strokes and heart attacks. Very often, *heart failure*—a disorder in which the heart fails to pump blood at an adequate rate throughout the body—is the end result of atherosclerotic disease.

Since patients rarely come to see me when they're feeling well, a symptom of heart failure may be the first worrisome event that finally brings them to my office. Because the examination process so often points to heart failure, it's important to understand what it is, why it occurs and how the doctor can recognize it.

Heart failure is often referred to as ***congestive heart failure*** because, when the pumping action of the heart begins to weaken, many parts of the body become congested with fluid. This congestion is caused by blood pooling in the veins and organs in the body. The blood slows and stagnates because a weak, failing heart isn't strong enough to pump it forcefully through the body's many blood vessels.

Heart failure can be categorized by its location: ***right-sided heart failure*** and ***left-sided heart failure***.

When discussing the heart, it's natural to think of this organ as a single pump. It's more precise, however, to regard the heart as a *pair* of pumps—side by side, beating in unison. The right side of the heart is one pump—it pulls blood from the body and sends it to the lungs to pick up oxygen. The left side of the heart acts as a second pump—it pulls the oxygen-rich blood from the lungs and sends it out to the rest of the body.

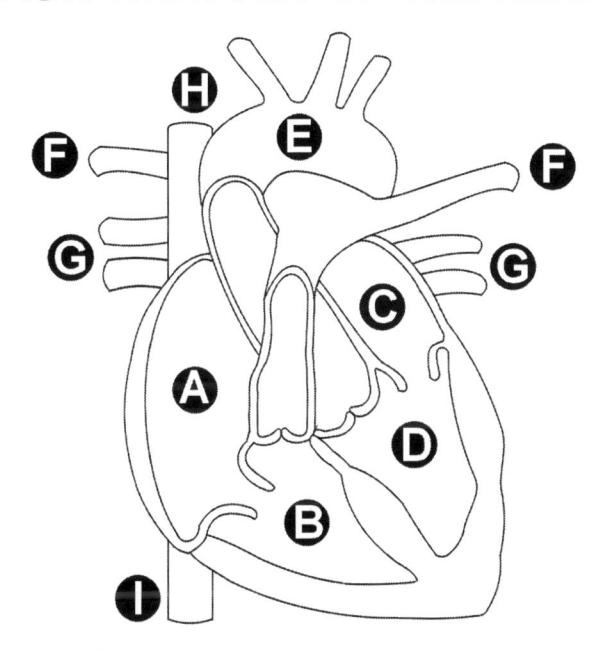

BASIC ANATOMY OF THE HEART

A - Right Atrium   } Right side of heart pumps oxygen-poor
B - Right Ventricle } blood to the lungs

C - Left Atrium   } Left side of heart pumps oxygen-rich
D - Left Ventricle } blood to the body

E - Aorta (blood to the body)
F - Pulmonary Arteries (blood to the lungs)

G - Pulmonary Veins (blood from the lungs)
H - Superior Vena Cava (blood from the head and arms)
I - Inferior Vena Cava (blood from the trunk and legs)

VALVES OF THE HEART

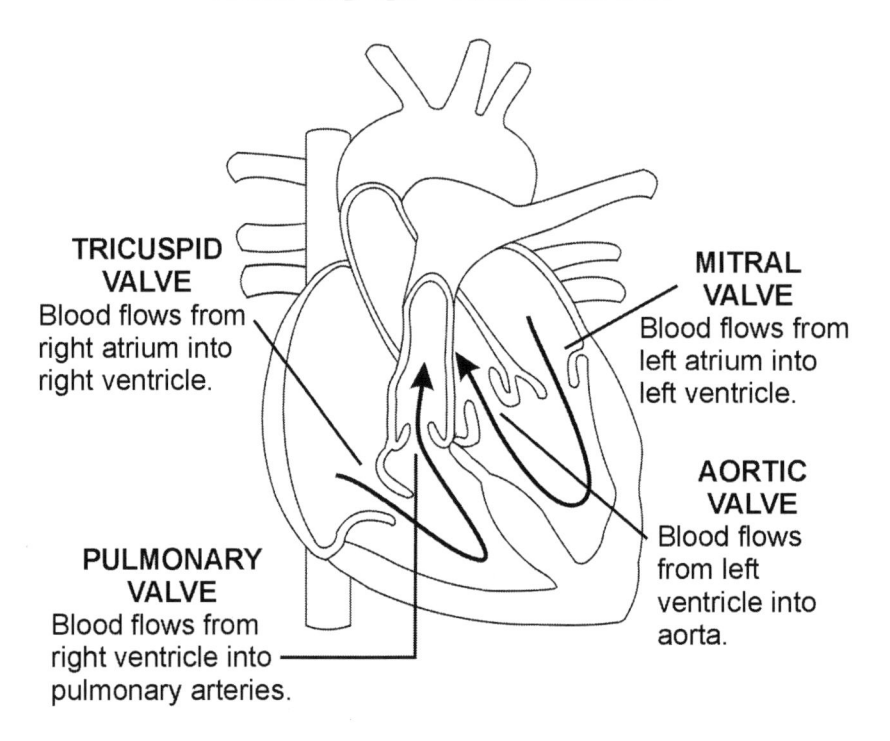

TRICUSPID VALVE
Blood flows from right atrium into right ventricle.

MITRAL VALVE
Blood flows from left atrium into left ventricle.

AORTIC VALVE
Blood flows from left ventricle into aorta.

PULMONARY VALVE
Blood flows from right ventricle into pulmonary arteries.

The valves of the heart are small openings that allow blood to flow between the chambers of the heart or between the chambers and their associated blood vessels. Heart valves are designed as one-way gates, allowing blood to flow in one direction only. When valves become damaged by disease, they fail to seal properly and blood flows in both directions, reducing the efficiency of the heart.

PUMPING ACTION OF THE HEART
Part I - Contraction

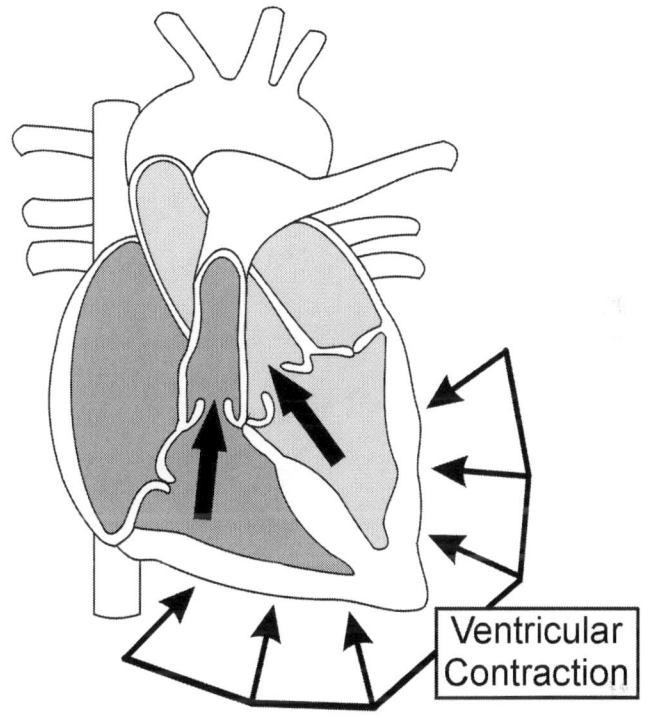

Ventricular Contraction

The pumping action of the heart begins with a weak contraction of the upper part of the heart, which forces blood into the lower chambers. There's a short pause, then a strong contraction of the bottom part of the heart. This powerful ventricular contraction squeezes blood out of the lower chambers and forces the fluid through the open valves of the aortic and pulmonary arteries, away from the heart.

PUMPING ACTION OF THE HEART
Part II - Relaxation

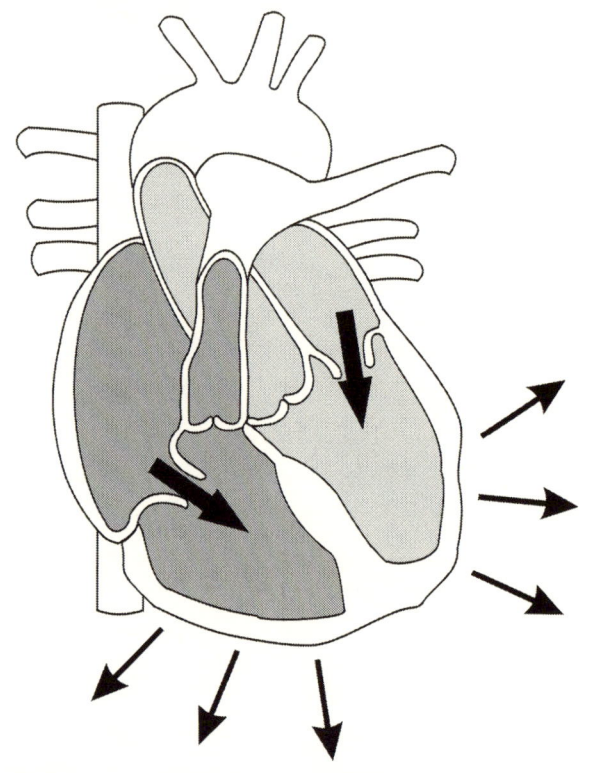

After the contraction of heart muscle that squeezes blood out of the heart, the lower chambers of the heart relax, creating a partial vacuum. This helps blood to flow from the top of the heart into the bottom, setting the stage for another cycle of contraction and relaxation that pumps blood throughout the body.

Either side of the heart can weaken and suffer heart failure, leaving the other side strong and functioning normally—at least for a while. Often, however, weakness in one side of the heart leads to weakness in both. You can often tell which side of the heart is failing—right or left—by the location of congestive symptoms.

For example, during *right-sided heart failure*, blood tends to pool in the lower extremities causing swelling in the legs, feet and ankles. During *left-sided heart failure*, blood pools in the blood vessels of the lungs which, in turn, creates fluid in the lungs.

The accumulation of fluid in the lungs causes coughing and shortness of breath. Since the word *pulmonary* refers to the lungs and *edema* means "an excessive accumulation of fluid," this condition is called *pulmonary edema*, a common consequence of heart failure.

As heart failure runs its course, the patient suffers from general weakness and fatigue because the body simply isn't getting enough circulation to function properly. In severe cases, heart failure leads to death.

Strictly speaking, heart failure is not a disease but the result of some underlying illness that is damaging the heart. Diagnosing heart failure is only the beginning step—the real trick for the physician is uncovering the reason *why* the heart is failing.

Often, a specific cause of heart failure can't be determined. But, without doubt, atherosclerosis in the coronary arteries and old heart attacks are prime causes of heart failure. Both conditions damage the heart muscle, which weakens the pumping action of the heart.

But there are many other problems besides atherosclerosis and heart attacks that can lead to heart failure:

- abnormalities in the heart, such as tumors or damaged heart valves
- infections of the heart, which weaken the heart muscle
- disturbances in heart rhythm
- heart defects present at birth

- alcoholism
- smoking
- obesity

In sum, anything that damages or hinders the pumping action of the heart can lead to heart failure.

Heart failure is often associated with an ***enlarged heart.*** A normal heart is typically the size of a clenched fist. But when heart muscle is damaged, it can turn thin and flabby. When it does, the heart takes on an engorged shape. The weakened muscles lose all their tone and dilate outwards, allowing the blood-filled chambers of the heart to expand like an over-inflated balloon. A normal-sized heart now becomes an enlarged heart, a sure sign that the pumping action of the heart is compromised.

But there is second type of heart enlargement that is usually associated with ***high blood pressure***, or ***hypertension.*** (See our discussion of hypertension in Chapter Nine.) Diseases such as atherosclerosis and diabetes narrow the diameter of blood vessels throughout the body. This causes an increased resistance to the flow of blood through the arteries. To overcome the resistance, the heart pumps harder, which raises the body's blood pressure.

So a rise in blood pressure may indicate an increased strain on the heart, which is laboring mightily to force blood through narrowed blood vessels. This means that—day-in, day-out—the heart is working harder than it should. Eventually, this extra effort leads to a common consequence of high blood pressure—***hypertrophy,*** a condition where the muscle of the heart become over-developed.

Why does extra effort lead to this type of heart enlargement? Because the heart is made of muscle, and muscles typically become larger when they are forced to work hard. You might think that a larger heart would mean a *stronger* heart, creating a vigorous circulation. But just the opposite is true.

Hearts enlarged by hypertrophy are, in a sense, "muscle-bound." The thickened muscle reduces the size of the heart chambers that hold the blood, so less blood is pumped with every heartbeat. Hindered by overdevelopment, the heart muscle is also unable to pump blood the way it should. As a result, circulation to the body is reduced, resulting in the symptoms of heart failure—dizziness, shortness of breath, fatigue, swelling, etc.

So anything that makes the heart work harder than it should can lead to trouble. Long-term lung diseases—such as *emphysema* (a disease marked by the destruction of lung tissue, often associated with smoking) or *chronic bronchitis* (long-term infection of the airways of the lungs, leading to excess fluid)—are often linked to heart failure because of the extra burden they place on the heart. In order to get enough oxygen from diseased lungs, the heart has to strain with effort, producing hypertrophy and, ultimately, heart failure.

Another lung problem that leads to cardiac trouble is *pulmonary emboli*, or blood clots in the lungs. Typically, these clots begin in the large, deep veins of the legs, travel through the bloodstream, and then become lodged in the lungs. Many small clots—or one very big one—can reduce the circulation in the lungs. To pull sufficient oxygen from the lungs the heart has to work harder, leading, once again, to hypertrophy and heart failure.

By now it should be apparent that a cardiovascular examination involves much more than just an assessment of the heart and arteries. There are scores of diseases and conditions that affect the health of the heart, and the doctor has to consider them all.

It may seem like an overwhelming task, but in this chapter I hope to capture the method I use in narrowing down the cause of symptoms and making the diagnosis. Knowing where to focus the examination is key, and the focusing process begins with…

The Written History

For obvious reasons, before I see the patient, I'd like to review his previous medical history, analyzing earlier diagnoses and the success—or failure—of treatments.

But I'm never content to rely on the conclusions of other doctors. It's always necessary to re-diagnose the patient, so I'm sure of what I'm dealing with.

As it happens, many of the cardiovascular patients that come to see me are misdiagnosed. They've been receiving treatment for a seemingly minor problem that turns out, upon examination, to be a serious cardiovascular illness.

For example, it's common to find that a nagging backache—assumed to be caused by muscle strain, neurological disease or arthritis—is in reality a serious aneurysm of the aorta. It only feels like a backache because the aorta happens to travel along the back of the body. If the cause of the backache is misdiagnosed, it's likely that the patient will be given aspirin or aspirin-like drugs, which may make the aneurysm bleed and rupture.

On the other hand, there are several non-threatening conditions that can mimic acute cardiovascular symptoms such as heart attacks and angina. In this case, the patient is spending time and money for treatments that will do him no good.

A very common error in diagnosis is the presence of *gallstones*, small, hard pebbles of cholesterol and calcium salts, which appear in the gallbladder or in a bile duct. A *gallbladder attack* can present the same set of physical signs as a heart attack. The *vagus nerve* runs through the abdomen, near the heart. When the gallbladder goes into spasm from gallstones, the vagus nerve can be stimulated, creating the identical symptoms of angina or a heart attack. It's not unusual to find that patients being treated for heart disease will have their heart symptoms suddenly vanish once their gallbladders are removed by surgery.

Other common causes of misdiagnosis are *acid reflux* (when acid produced by the stomach travels back into the throat), *panic attacks* (an intensely felt but inappropriate "fight or flight" response from the body) and *costochondritis* (a painful inflammation and swelling of the cartilage of the ribs).

There are many other difficulties to arriving at a correct diagnosis. A patient may have more than one illness at a time—and both illnesses may cause the same symptoms.

Say, for example, a patient comes in complaining of chest pains and, upon examination, it turns out that his coronary arteries are narrowed. It's tempting to conclude that the narrowed arteries are the cause of his pain, but it may very well be that the pain is generated by some completely separate and potentially more serious illness, such as a tumor. So just because a physician finds evidence of disease in a patient, it doesn't mean that the patient has received an adequate diagnosis of his problem.

Another reason why patients come to me misdiagnosed is because the tests they've received are too general in nature or they are performed by a technician, rather than a doctor familiar with the patient.

When a technician performs a test such as echocardiography, he performs it the same way on everybody. He's not looking for anything in particular, just a general overview of the heart.

When I perform echocardiography, however, I've already made several findings in the examination that will make me take a hard look at particular problems. I've had many people come to me with aortic valve disease that was missed in previous tests. A technician may not see valve disease until it's severe. But a doctor familiar with the patient and performing his own examination is much more likely to detect valve disease at its earliest stages.

Typically, when a patient walks into the doctor's office for the first time, the office nurse hands him a sheaf of insurance papers and a medical history questionnaire to fill out, right then and there. In the space of a few minutes—with nothing to refer to but his own memory—the patient is expected to remember a lifetime of symptoms, illnesses, surgeries and medications.

I find it's much better to mail a medical history questionnaire to the patient's home a few days before he comes in. With access to records and undistracted by time pressure, he's much more likely to fill out the form completely and accurately, which gets the examination off to a good start.

Here are the most important things I look for in the patient's medical history:

Age

To make a diagnosis of cardiovascular disease, age is a significant factor to keep in mind. I'm always considering age as it relates to *prevalence*, that is, the total number of cases of a disease (or condition) in a given population at a specific time.

Here's an obvious illustration of how prevalence influences diagnosis. After World War II, I served in the Army Medical Corps and spent most of my time stationed in the U.S. Canal Zone in Panama. When officers and enlisted men came to me complaining of fever, I would always consider the diseases prevalent in tropical Panama that would cause such a fever, such as malaria.

In later years, when I practiced in snowy Chicago, I would rule out malaria as a cause of fever almost a hundred percent; it simply wasn't prevalent in the Windy City.

So prevalence is a valuable tool for narrowing down a diagnosis. In cardiovascular disease, prevalence has a great deal to do with the age of the patient.

For example, both adults and children can experience chest pain. It's very possible that the adult may be suffering from coronary artery disease and I would focus on that during examination. Most likely, however, a child with chest pain is suffering from some other illness, so I wouldn't consider coronary artery disease a likely cause when forming a diagnosis.

When examining a patient for the source of their cardiovascular problems, I mentally place them in the following age groupings, based on prevalence:

Less than 16 years of age

In this age range, I would be looking mostly for evidence of uncorrected anatomy problems, such as physical flaws in the heart and arteries. These defects might be due to some drug the patient is taking that doesn't let the heart develop as it should. Or the flaws might be created by disease, such as German measles, which can cause defects in the walls of the heart.

Between 16 and 35 years of age

Again, I'd be looking at the patient's cardiovascular anatomy. There are several diseases that assert themselves around this age that can influence the heart and cardiovascular system. For example, *Marfan syndrome*—a genetic disorder largely affecting connective tissue—can lead to a degeneration of the aorta, creating an aneurysm. I would also be on the lookout for evidence of chronic infection, such as severe or repeated herpes, and serious lipid abnormalities in the bloodstream. These are the types of things that—at this age—lead to trouble down the road. And while it's quite likely that the patient has atherosclerosis at this young age, the noticeable symptoms of disease usually don't show up until later in life.

Between 35 and 45 years of age

In this decade of life, the chronic processes that lead to cardiovascular trouble are surreptitiously moving forward. The patient may have the beginnings of hypertension, coronary artery disease, cerebrovascular disease and so on, but most people are doing pretty well. They have no disabling symptoms. It is only by careful examination that the presence of cardiovascular disease is revealed.

Between 45 and 55 years of age

At this age we see a real blossoming of chronic disease states, such as infection by the cardiovascular germs, which lead to cardiovascular illness. The results of bad health habits such as smoking, an unbalanced diet and limited physical activity are also beginning to manifest themselves. Health problems such as diabetes, high blood pressure and obesity become factors. This is the age when hardening of the arteries really seems to accelerate for most people. The presence of cardiovascular symptoms are easily recognized—angina, TIAs, heart attack and so on. This is the decade when most people realize they are in serious trouble.

Between 55 and 65 years of age

Good news! In my experience, people who make it to age 55 without evidence of serious cardiovascular disease will probably do okay—atherosclerotic diseases will not be their main problem later in life. On the other hand, whatever was diagnosed at age 45 is now more apparent…and more dangerous. The beginning signs of heart failure are common here.

Between 65 and 75 years of age—and beyond

This is when chronic disease states—such as valvular disease and diabetes—become really prominent, influencing longevity and health. After age 65, there is a limiting of the body's ability to repair itself after sickness. The aging process really starts to make itself apparent as part of the diagnosis. You get slower, your body gets stiffer and your mind isn't as alert as it once was.

Weight and Height

We've already discussed obesity as a significant risk factor for the development of heart disease, especially when accompanied by diabetes or hypertension. But determining whether someone is significantly overweight is not simply a matter of counting pounds—it requires comparing the patient's weight relative to his height. Although the patient provides me with his weight and height in the written history, I'll always check his figures with my own office weight scale and height rod.

I'll use these figures in a mathematical formula called the **Body Mass Index** or **BMI**, which results in a number that compares the patient's weight to his height. Experience has shown the BMI number to be a useful guideline for determining if the patient is over–or underweight.

The formula for calculating your BMI number is:

$$BMI = (\text{weight in pounds} \times 703)/(\text{height in inches})^2$$

For example, if your weight is 170 lbs. and your height is 70 inches (5'10") the calculation would be:

$$BMI = (170 \times 703)/70^2$$

$$BMI = 119{,}510/4900$$

$$BMI = 24 \text{ (rounded off)}$$

Ideally, I'd like to see a BMI number in the low 20s. A patient is considered overweight when the BMI number reaches 25 and obesity begins at around 30. In practice, when a patient's BMI starts to approach 28 is when I really start to worry that weight will play an important factor in cardiac illness.

Sex

When it comes to cardiovascular disease, there's no great difference in the way I approach the examination process of male or female patients. Statistically, hardening of the arteries seems to strike men more than women. And from my own experiences, I'd say that women do not have as many clinical symptoms as men do. But by the age of 75, the differences level out.

There's another small difference I've noted. As mentioned above, there is an age range where hardening of the arteries seems to be accelerated, typically from age 45 to 55. Among women, I've found that menopause seems to produce accelerated changes in the course of cardiovascular disease. Since menopause can go from age 39 to 55, there is an increased range of years where menopause may enhance the development of cardiovascular disease in women.

Menopause occurs when a woman stops making enough of the female hormone *estrogen.* For the past several years, **Hormone Replacement Therapy (HRT)** for postmenopausal women has been promoted as a way to decrease the risk of heart attack for women with heart disease. HRT was thought to be beneficial because it reduced cholesterol levels in the bloodstream of older women.

Although my female patients often inquire about this type of therapy, I've never been convinced of its effectiveness. The latest studies suggest that hormone replacement therapy is not beneficial for women with heart disease, and may even increase the risk of heart attack for some women during the first year of treatment.[331]

In fact, a major new study has radically changed the conventional wisdom of Hormone Replacement Therapy. A study conducted by the National Heart, Lung, and Blood Institute called the **Women's Health Initiative** tested the effectiveness of long-term estrogen plus progestin hormone replacement therapy in the fight against cardiovascular disease in postmenopausal women.

Rather than prevent trouble, however, the HRT therapy seemed to provoke it. In July of 2002, the researchers revealed that patients receiving the therapy showed a significant increase in heart attacks, strokes and breast cancer. The study also showed a significant increase in blood clots in the lungs and legs of patients receiving HRT therapy. The statistics were so alarming, that the long-term, government-sponsored study was ended three years early because of the increased risks.[332] It appeared that the HRT therapy was doing more harm than good.

Family and Personal Medical History

Next, I am interested in the family and personal medical history of certain cardiovascular troubles and risk factors. For obvious reasons, I'd like to know how recently the patient or any close family member—including mother, father, sister, brother or grandparents—had any of the following:

- High blood pressure
- Stroke
- Heart attack or other heart trouble
- Diabetes
- Aneurysm of the aorta or brain artery
- Any type of vascular surgery such as bypass operations, balloon angioplasty, or surgery of the neck arteries
- Poor circulation in the lower extremities
- Eye problems
- Obesity
- Shingles and other important conditions or diseases

Before examining a new patient, I'll review his written history and note the areas that seem to need attention. If someone has already had cardiovascular surgery such as a bypass operation, it's important to know how long ago this was done. If it was done ten years ago and they're still symptom-free, then their disease process is not very serious. But if they had it done six months ago and they're still having symptoms, then it's likely to be very serious.

If there is a family history of cardiovascular disease, the physician should make a diligent search for the problems associated with the disease, even if the patient has no symptoms whatsoever.

"Family history" is not limited merely to genetic factors. Infections can run in families—husbands pass germs on to their wives, mothers pass germs on to their children, and so on. If I discover that a patient is infected with one of the cardiovascular germs, I may need to treat the patient's spouse as well, to prevent reinfection. Even gum disease, which is implicated in cardiovascular illness, can be passed between husband and wife through kissing.

The next important step prior to hands-on examination is the…

First Impression of the Patient

Most of my patients aren't aware of it, but their physical exam begins the moment they walk into my office.

My first impression of the patient's cardiovascular health is formed simply by watching him enter the room. How does he walk? How firm is his handshake? Is his hand cold or warm? Is his skin flushed or gray? How does he sit? How does he get up?

Simple observations such as these can reveal much about the patient's cardiovascular status and alert me to possible problems. Even something as simple as the condition of the patient's teeth tells me whether he pays attention to his personal care or not, which has implications for my success in getting him well.

For many years, my patients had to undergo a rather rigorous heart test before they even got to my office door.

My first practice was located on the second story of a business building. The building was built in the 1920s—a time when elevators were still an uncommon luxury. The only way to reach my office was by a long, narrow staircase—19 steps in all. I soon learned that if my patients could make it easily to the top of the stairs, the odds are they were in pretty good cardiovascular shape! If they arrived at my door huffing and puffing, however, I knew it was quite likely their vascular system had already been damaged.

During the course of our initial conversation, I'll ask the patient to tell me about the specific health problem that brought him to my office. The response is usually straightforward, but sometimes—for various reasons—the patient doesn't reveal the full story.

Why? It's not that he wants to purposefully mislead me, but he's already got his mind set on what the problem is. Without knowing it, he shapes his responses to fit what he already suspects.

Perhaps this sounds familiar: you take your car to the repair shop, certain that the knocking noise you hear is transmission trouble, only to find out from the mechanic that the knocking noise is made by something shifting around in the trunk.

Doctors face this same problem. Patients will diagnose their own illness and—often unconsciously—want the doctor to confirm the diagnosis. To that end, the patient will only mention the symptoms that fit the self-diagnosis. The patient doesn't realize he's not telling the whole truth, so it's up to the physician to ask the kinds of questions that will tease out as much information as possible.

Visual Inspection

Before physically examining the patient, it's important that he disrobe completely, if only for a few moments, so that I can inspect every inch of his body. The appearance of the skin and body structure provides important clues to his cardiovascular health.

One of the chief things I'm looking for is evidence of the viral infections that have been implicated in cardiovascular disease. I'll scan the entire body searching for the blisters, pimples and cold sores of herpes infections. Often the patient isn't aware that he has a herpetic eruption on his back or his buttocks. When he takes his clothes off and I notice the sore, he'll mention that he scratches the area every once in a while, but he never thought to look at what it was. So I can't rely on the patient to be fully aware of the state of his skin—only by having him disrobe and looking for myself can I be sure.

It's important to recall, however, that the infections of cardiovascular disease are usually well hidden. They are chronic, low-level micro-infections of the arteries that produce no symptoms. The only clue to their existence might be the occasional, acute flare-up of the virus in the form of a skin lesion. So just because I don't see evidence of infection on the skin, it's no guarantee that the patient doesn't harbor the virus.

In fact, I believe it's appropriate to say that the presence of atherosclerosis is an indication that the patient *is* infected by one or more of the germs of cardiovascular disease. By the time of middle age, nearly everybody becomes infected by one or more of these germs. And the studies suggest it's a pretty safe bet that the atherosclerosis I see is associated with these types of infection.

One virus we haven't talked about is the ***varicella-zoster virus***, another type of herpes virus, which is responsible for childhood chicken pox. Like other herpes viruses, varicella-zoster is ubiquitous—nearly everyone gets infected by it at some point in life. And once the initial acute infection fades, the virus can surreptitiously stay alive in the body, creating a chronic infection.

At any time, the virus can flare up again. The germ travels along nerve fibers, so any tissue that contains nerve fibers can be attacked by the virus. Since every organ has nerves that go to it, the virus can go just about anyplace in the body.

In later life, the varicella-zoster comes out of hiding and causes ***shingles***, a painful skin rash I often seen in my elderly patients. The virus goes all the way to the nerve tip, which is why it produces this often excruciatingly painful rash on the skin. It's amazing to think that a childhood infection like chickenpox can lay low for up to 60 or 70 years, then suddenly spark to life again and cause an entirely new kind of acute skin disease.

The varicella-zoster can also reappear again in a facial condition known as **Ramsay Hunt syndrome**, a form of paralysis of one side of face. The paralysis indicates that the varicella-zoster virus is active in the nerve cells in the brain, which is certainly one place you don't like to see it. The varicella-zoster virus is known to inflame blood vessels in the brain, causing strokes. So, although varicella-zoster has yet to be associated with atherosclerosis, this virus has serious cerebrovascular consequences and I'm always on the lookout for it.

Examining the skin also means examining the inside of the mouth and throat as well, using the tongue depressor to obtain a better view. The herpetic lesions of the skin often show up in the membranes that line the mouth and throat.

Cerebrovascular Disease and Nerve Function

Because cholesterol plaque and blood clots are the chief cause of occlusive strokes, atherosclerosis has a profound effect on brain function.

"Brain function" is not merely limited to conscious processes, such as the ability to think or remember. It also encompasses the many physical abilities that depend upon the proper functioning of the brain and nervous system. Difficulty in swallowing or weakness in a limb may have nothing to do with muscle damage and everything to do with brain cell injury from atherosclerosis.

It's very common for Transient Ischemic Attacks (TIAs) to result in numbness or tingling in the arms or legs. It's a minor complaint and people won't visit the doctor because of it, believing that it's just because of the way they happened to be lying on the bed or sitting in a chair.

Symptoms such as these are not recognized by the victim as originating from strokes—specifically, "silent strokes." A patient may simply think that he is "getting old" and these types of problems are the normal, unavoidable consequence of aging. In fact, however, they are *not* normal—they are symptoms of a specific disease process. With treatment, the disease process can be controlled; without treatment, the patient is at risk for significant damage to his health.

Certainly, if the patient tells me that his family has a history of stroke or diabetes or other risk factors, I would pay special attention to this potential problem. But since "silent strokes" are undetected by the victim (or by his friends and family), I always have to be alert for the subtle symptoms of stroke during my examination. Often, the patient unknowingly tips me off to the problem during our conversation. I'm always suspicious when the patient uses phrases such as...

- I must be getting old
- I'm not as sharp as I used to be
- I can't wait to retire
- I don't read as much as I used to
- I'm not making new friends anymore
- it's not as easy to think
- my memory is not as good as it was
- it's harder to make up my mind
- my balance is not as good as it was
- I get light headed easily

...and so on. It makes me think that "growing old" is not the problem, but a particular illness—namely, cerebrovascular disease—that can, and should, be treated.

As part of the cerebrovascular examination, I'll ask the patient to perform a number of simple tasks, such as doing arithmetic problems in his head. These mental acuity tests are designed to reveal the concealed presence of atherosclerotic disease affecting the brain.

Dizziness is also a tip-off of cerebrovascular disease. There are four blood supplies to the brain: two carotid arteries and two vertebral arteries. Circulation to the brain is critical, which is why nature gives us four separate blood supplies for backup. But when atherosclerosis becomes severe, the accumulation of cholesterol plaque becomes too much for the backup mechanisms to handle. The loss of blood flow results in dizziness, a common symptom of cerebrovascular disease.

Apart from the brain, atherosclerosis can also affect nerve function in different spots of the body. One of the most revealing tests for nerve damage is a balance test, which checks for *ataxia*.

Ataxia is a failure of muscular coordination. The ataxia exam is similar to the test for drunk driving. I have people stand on one leg, and then close their eyes, and see if they can stand on that one leg for a reasonable length of time.

When you close your eyes, all the information to control your balance comes through your spinal cord. So if you close your eyes and fail to keep your balance, it may be because the spinal cord has been injured.

Atherosclerosis can injure the brain through stroke, of course. But not many people realize that atherosclerosis can also cause spinal injury.

When the body suffers atherosclerotic disease, it can affect the arteries that go from the aorta to the spinal cord. Cholesterol plaque can occlude these arteries, cutting off circulation to the spinal cord, causing nerve damage.

Often this damage is hidden from the patient because his vision compensates, aiding his sense of balance. But with the eyes closed, vision can no longer help out. The result is walking and balancing problems, possibly caused by atherosclerosis. I make a point of asking all my elderly patients if they lose their balance in the dark, for the same reason.

I'll also have the patient close his eyes and attempt to touch his nose with his index finger. This might reveal some atherosclerotic damage to the upper part of the spine, around the neck. Or I might have him walk down the hall and study him to see if he leans to one side or the other when he walks.

In advanced cases of mental impairment, the caregiver or spouse comes in with the patient and explains the problem. Often, the problem is Alzheimer's.

In this book, we've learned of the association between Alzheimer's disease and stroke. Preventing or limiting stroke is extremely important in reducing the symptoms of Alzheimer's patients. So every Alzheimer's patient needs a thorough cardiovascular examination to evaluate his risk and take appropriate action.

Blood Pressure

The *sphygmomanometer*, or *blood pressure cuff*, was introduced more than 100 years ago, yet it remains one of the most useful tools in the doctor's office and is usually the first instrument I use to examine the patient. Here's a short description of how I use it and what I'm looking for.

The dangers of atherosclerosis increase dramatically when the body suffers from hypertension. So I'm very interested in knowing the status of your blood pressure. If it's too high, I'll need to bring it under control with medication to reduce your risk of a stroke or heart attack.

Typically, patients will wait for 10 to 15 minutes in the waiting room before I see them. This short wait provides at least one benefit—it gives time for their blood pressure to settle down. Many activities—such as smoking a cigarette or physical exercise—can influence blood pressure. So sitting in the waiting room, doing nothing more strenuous that reading a magazine, allows the blood pressure to return to normal. And that's really what I'm after—establishing a baseline number for the patient.

Using the blood pressure cuff, I can quickly determine the systolic and diastolic numbers. The first reading is taken while the patient is sitting in an upright position. But one set of numbers is never enough to get a true understanding of the patient's vascular condition.

A few minutes after the first reading, I'll lay the patient down flat on the examination table and check their blood pressure again to see if the reading has changed in any way or not. I'll also check their pulse at that time and note if the heart is going slower or faster.

Then I stand them up and take the pressure again. I take it right away, as soon as they stand, in order to see what the effect of gravity has on their vascular system. It's a way of determining the "tone" of their heart and arteries. Sometimes people react strongly to suddenly getting upright—their blood pressure might drop for 10 or 15 seconds, or it might rise for a few moments.

These different postures let me know if the patient has a highly reactive vascular system. I need to know this because, if they have a problem, it might have an adverse effect on the way a medicine might work on them. If a person is highly reactive, you wouldn't want to give medicine that can lower the blood pressure—they might faint on you. Or if pressure goes up too high and the pulse goes very rapid, they might faint again, because the heart goes too fast. So examining them under different conditions establishes a kind of base level for that particular patient.

Once I establish that the patient has high blood pressure, I'll try and find the cause of the hypertension during the course of the examination. This is often a difficult task. As we've already discussed, 90% of all hypertension is called *essential hypertension*, which means a cause can't be determined. But there are a few things that are known to cause a rise in blood pressure and those can be found by examination and blood tests.

For example, the kidneys play an important role in maintaining proper blood pressure by regulating the volume of blood in the body and by producing *renin*, a hormone that influences blood pressure. So as part of a cardiovascular examination I'll check the kidneys for tumors, kidney stones, infections…anything that might prevent them from functioning properly.

As it happens, the kidneys are often damaged by atherosclerosis itself. When cholesterol plaque clogs the arteries that lead to the kidneys, the loss of circulation impairs the kidneys, which, in turn, leads to a rise in blood pressure. So determining why your blood pressure numbers are too high can be a complicated business.

But exactly what numbers are considered "too high?" Most often, doctors use 140/90 as the cutoff point—higher than that and you start getting into trouble. In my own experience, however, I feel the numbers should be a set lower at 130/85.

Why? Well, after following some of my patients for 20 years or more, I've noticed that patients at 140/90 have a tendency, later in life, to go higher. In contrast, people at 130/85 generally stay the same, unless they develop a specific disease which influences blood pressure. I wouldn't rule anything out, but I'd feel very comfortable saying to a patient with 130/85 and no outstanding cardiovascular problems, "Hey, you're doing pretty good and maybe I'll see you in a year or two."

With a baseline blood pressure established, the next task is a…

Peripheral Examination

Generally, the next thing I do is check the pulses of the peripheral arteries. The feel of the pulses in the wrists, arms, legs, feet and neck can reveal quite a bit about the health of the patient.

The pulse is related to how well the heart muscle pumps out a wave of blood during the heartbeat. With practice, doctors can associate the quality of the pulse with specific problems.

Different names are often attached to the feel of the pulse, such as *"thready"* which would indicate that the heart is not beating very strongly. A thready pulse is often associated with shock, where the blood pressure is lowered and the heart is beating very rapidly but not filling up well, so it can't get the blood out.

If the pulse seems overly strong, it's referred to as a *"bounding" pulse*. Most people have experienced this type of pulse during moments of intense effort, such as running or lifting weights. The pulse will be so strong you can feel it rushing through your head.

That kind of intensity is similar to the bounding pulse found in people suffering from heart failure. When the body senses that it isn't getting enough circulation from a failing heart, it sends a signal to the heart to beat harder. If I notice a bounding pulse when the patient is at rest, it's a likely sign that something is amiss.

The speed of the pulse is also important but, because it varies so much in healthy people, there's plenty of room for a "normal" heart rate. Typically, I would be concerned if the speed were less than sixty beats a minute or more than a hundred. If the patient is athletic, however, it wouldn't be unusual for a healthy heart to dip down to fifty-five or even fifty beats per minute.

But a rapid pulse may also indicate the presence of several kinds of disease, not the least of which is heart failure; beating faster to increase circulation is one way the body tries to compensate for heart failure.

The pulse rate is part of a simple but helpful test I use to diagnose problems such as heart failure in the office. First I take the patient's pulse and blood pressure, then ask them to walk a few times up and down the office hallway. Afterwards, I sit them down and check the pulse and pressure again to see how long it takes the heart to recover. Normally, the heart should take between thirty seconds and a minute to recover. If it takes longer to resume a normal, rhythmic state, then I'll suspect a problem with the heart.

There's a similar pulse test I use quite often. Most hearts should be able to handle the stress of walking at the rate of a thousand feet in six minutes. If the patient doesn't have other limiting factors—such as asthma or arthritis—I'll ask them to walk the prescribed distance around my office building. If the patient can complete the test in time without becoming uncomfortable, it's likely they don't have clinically significant heart disease. This low-tech, inexpensive test has proven to be a pretty accurate estimation of the heart's *cardiac reserve*, a measure of the heart's ability to respond to demands that exceed ordinary circumstances. A low cardiac reserve may indicate some form of heart trouble, such as coronary artery disease.

I take the pulse in many different spots of the body because each location tells me something different about the patient.

First I feel for the pulse in the arteries of the wrists and feet. The pulses here are usually pretty easy to locate so if I have difficulty finding them my suspicions are aroused—somewhere the circulation to the extremity is being impaired. Naturally, I'd like to know where—and why.

Often this can be accomplished simply by checking the pulse further up the limb. Starting at the ankle, for example, I'd feel for the strength of the pulse at the back of the knee, then further up the leg at the femoral artery. In this way I may be able to determine where the problem lies. Generally, if people have poor pulses in their wrists or feet, it's usually associated with considerable hardening of the arteries, which means I'd have to be especially vigilant for signs of coronary artery disease.

Occasionally I'll find an obstruction in a leg artery that the patient isn't even aware of. The leg looks good and the patient feels pretty normal, but checking the ankle I'll find practically no pulse at all. In a case like this, there is collateral circulation supplying an adequate supply of blood to the leg—at least for a while. But ongoing atherosclerosis may eventually close off this circulation, as well.

Poor pulses in the feet are particularly worrisome if the patient smokes or has diabetes. These things seem to accelerate the occlusive effect of the lower arteries—one of the many reasons why the patient's history is a critical part of the examination.

While I'm checking the pulses in the extremities, I also pay attention to the warmth or coldness of the limbs. Warmth usually indicates a good blood supply while coldness is associated with impaired circulation. If the patient complains of a weakness in a limb, a lack of circulation is certainly high on the list of possible causes.

Warm sweats are usually associated with fevers, but a cold sweat generally means a collapse of blood pressure. When something feels cold, generally it means that a lot of sweat is evaporating quickly which cools the body. If I see a patient in a cold sweat, I'm pretty sure that there is some kind of cardiovascular problem that I need to pay attention to.

Color is also a good indication of circulation in the extremities. Over the years I've seen a number of patients with *blue toe syndrome*, a condition where the toes of a foot take on a bluish color. It's usually an indication of serious atherosclerosis in a larger artery. Particles of plaque flake off from the artery and lodge in the circulation of the lower extremities, especially in the toes. The reason the toes turn blue is not completely understood, but we think it's because of pooling blood.

Lack of peripheral circulation from atherosclerosis, especially to the feet and legs, can create or aggravate many kinds of health problems, such as leg ulcers. Poor circulation makes it much more difficult to treat infections in the leg and, if an occlusion is bad enough, it can even lead to gangrene, a major cause of amputation.

After examining the limbs, I'd feel the patient's abdomen for several reasons. First, I'd check the pulse of the aorta in the abdomen to see if there's an *abdominal aortic aneurysm*. An aneurysm, if you remember, is the enlargement of a blood vessel due to disease or weakness in the vessel wall. Normally, you'd just barely be able to feel the aorta in the lower abdomen. But an *abdominal aortic aneurysm* can be large enough that its pulse is strongly felt through the skin.

As it happens, the pulse of the heart is part of the problem with an aneurysm. When a large vessel like the aorta balloons outward, the pressure in the distended part is almost identical to the pressure in the artery. As a result, the weakened walls of the aneurysm are under constant pressure. In addition, the shape of the aneurysm creates turbulence within it. The churning action contributes to the forces acting against the integrity of the artery wall.

Pulsation only adds to the strain. The weakened artery wall tries to contain the pulses from the heart, but the pulse constantly stretches the artery, putting it under stress. Eventually, the things that hold the artery together are slowly broken down, creating *aortic dissection*, the peeling away of the artery wall from inside, which leads to rupture.

Thoracic aneurysms occur in the part of the aorta that runs through the patient's chest. Its position makes it difficult to diagnose in the doctor's office, but there's one trick I use that may reveal it: I check the pulses in both wrists at the same time. If there is a delay in the pulse from one wrist to the other, it's a good indication than an advanced thoracic aneurysm is present.

Also in the abdomen, I'd check to see whether the liver is enlarged, which is often an indication of disease. The liver can be an important factor in cardiovascular troubles. Among the many functions of the liver is the production of cholesterol. If the patient has high cholesterol levels, it may be because the liver isn't functioning properly. Several medicines commonly used for cardiovascular disease can damage the liver. So it's important to know if the patient is starting with a healthy liver or not.

Below the abdomen, I'd feel for the pulse of the femoral arteries, which supply blood to the legs. Once again, the strength of the pulse can reveal a blockage somewhere upstream.

While taking the pulse throughout the body, I'll note any irregularities in the pulse's rhythm, a sure sign of cardiac arrhythmias. These arrhythmias may be of no great importance, or they may indicate a problem. At this stage, it's impossible to tell. To really understand their significance, I need to examine the patient with the electrocardiograph machine. But right now it's time to move on to…

Auscultation of the Lungs and Heart

The next step would be to listen to the heart and lungs using the stethoscope. The medical name for this procedure is called *auscultation*, a word you are unlikely to hear again except as a Jeopardy question.

Often you'll see that a stethoscope has two types of listening devices at the end. The bell-shaped part is better for picking up low-frequency sounds while the round diaphragm device is better at the higher frequencies.

As I've mentioned, the lungs play an important part in cardiovascular fitness, which is why they're always included in the examination.

Lung problems such as emphysema and chronic bronchitis limit the amount of airflow through the lungs, either through the destruction of tissue or the build-up of fluid in the lungs. These diseases are commonly referred to as either **Chronic Obstructive Lung Disease (COLD)** or **Chronic Obstructive Pulmonary Disease (COPD)** because they obstruct the airflow over a long period of time. The heart is under continual strain to compensate for this loss, which, of course, leads to heart failure.

Listening to the lungs can tell me a lot about their health and, consequently, the health of your heart. What kinds of sounds am I listening for when I put the stethoscope to your chest ask you to breathe deep?

Ideally, I'm hoping to hear...not much at all.

The sound of air rushing through healthy lungs should make no more noise than you'd expect to hear when breathing through your mouth. An unhealthy lung, however, can make a number of different sounds. Through experience, the doctor can associate the type of sound—and whether it occurs during inhalation or exhalation—with a particular problem.

"Crackles," "wheezes" and *"rhonchi"* may sound like the names of sugary breakfast cereals, but in fact they're the common classifications of sounds within the lungs. These noises come from various locations of turbulent airflow in the lungs.

"Crackles" sound like someone wrinkling cellophane inside the chest wall. Fluid in the lungs is a common source for this type of noise. Since the build-up of fluid in the lungs is one of the symptoms of congestive heart failure, a crackling noise would certainly arouse my suspicions in that direction.

"Wheezes" sound like moaning gusts of wind as they rush through a grove of trees. Wheezing sounds seem to be especially prominent when the patient exhales. Fluid in the lungs can cause this type of sound as well, so heart failure must also be considered when wheezing is present.

"Rhonchi" is a kind of bubbling, gurgling noise. It's often found in patients who suffer from diseases that constrict the airways in the lungs—such as asthma—or in patients who are bedridden and experience a build-up of fluids in the chest.

Many times you'll notice your doctor thumping on your chest or back with his fingertips. It's another way of checking for fluid in the lungs. I expect to hear a particular kind of sound from the tapping. It's hard to put into words the quality of sound I'm listening for, but I know it when I hear it. It's the difference in the sound that you hear when you tap on a hollow pipe compared to a pipe filled with fluid—a certain resonance that tells you whether the lungs are clear or congested.

After checking the lungs, the next stop for the stethoscope is the heart itself. But first, I need to look and feel for the heart with reference to certain landmarks of the body. Just noticing the location of the heart is often enough to clue me in to possible trouble.

The *clavicles* or *collarbones* sit atop the rib cage. If I locate the middle of the clavicle on the left side of the body, and go straight down I should find a key cardiac landmark called the **Point of Maximum Intensity** or **PMI**. Located along this mid-clavicular line, the PMI is the point where the heartbeat feels the strongest, at the base of the heart called the *apex*. I can judge the exact location of the point by feeling for the heartbeat with my hands. Occasionally, when feeling for the apex beat, I'll feel a trill or buzzing in the heart, in which case I might suspect a heart problem such as rheumatic heart disease.

The actual location of the PMI can, by itself, be a pretty good diagnostic tool, especially in older patients. I can tell if the heart is enlarged by how far the PMI is to the left of the mid-clavicular line.

I listen to the patient's heart with the stethoscope while he's both sitting and standing to see what difference it makes to the heart sounds. Ideally, I should only hear two distinctive heart sounds with the stethoscope; extra sounds in the heart are classified as *heart murmurs*. Typically, murmurs are described as clicking, knocking or fluttering noises.

The sounds are caused by an abnormal turbulent flow of blood through the heart or perhaps by the opening and closing mechanics of the heart valves.

The valves, you'll remember, regulate the flow of blood through the heart, just like the valves in a faucet regulate the flow of water through a pipe. These valves are designed to allow the flow of blood in one direction only. When valves are damaged by trauma or disease, they tend to leak, allowing blood to backwash through the valve in the wrong direction. This is the kind of abnormal, turbulent flow that creates heart murmurs.

A normal heartbeat has a distinctive sound to it, often characterized as "LUB-dub." The first sound—"LUB"—is associated with the mitral and tricuspid valves, and the second—"dub"—with the aortic and pulmonary valves.

Trouble might be brewing when I hear a third heart sound appearing before the normal heartbeat. This third sound is often characterized as "duh-LUB-dub." Typically, this sound is associated with aortic valve disease.

And then there is a fourth heart sound—"duh-LUB-dub-boom." When I hear that final "boom," it's a tip-off that the bottom part of the heart is beginning to fail.

And then again, it may not. The trouble with listening to heart murmurs is that—by themselves—they are only indications that heart disease *may* be present. It's risky to diagnose any specific ailment from murmurs alone. At this point, listening to heart murmurs merely suggests the direction I should take for further examination.

Finally, I will place the stethoscope over the carotid arteries in the neck. If the carotids are severely clogged with atherosclerosis, the turbulent flow of blood through the arteries makes a distinctive sound called a ***bruit*** (pronounced broot). The word comes from an Old French term *bruire*, which means "to roar," which is a pretty good approximation of the sound. The sound of a bruit puts me on notice that the patient may be at risk for stroke.

Eye Examination

Patients are often surprised when I pick up an *ophthalmoscope*—that small, hand-held instrument that illuminates and magnifies the interior of the eye—as part of the cardiovascular examination. As I approach them with the device in hand and its bright, halogen light floods their vision, I can sense their puzzlement that I would bother to study a part of their body which has no apparent connection to heart disease.

But the eyes are—quite literally—an open window onto the arteries of the body. It is one of the few places a doctor can observe a blood vessel as it actually appears.

Nearly everywhere else in the body, the blood vessels are covered by skin and tissues; it's impossible to view them directly. Therefore, everything we know about them can only be inferred. But in the interior of the eye, on the retina, the blood vessels lie completely open and exposed for observation. With the help of the ophthalmoscope, there is simply no better place to study the condition of a patient's blood vessels with such clarity and accuracy.

This unobstructed vision allows for a good evaluation of what is happening in these vessels. I can witness—first-hand—the quality of circulation through the vessels, noting obstructions, bleeding or even the death of arteries. Often, I can see particular spots where circulation is impaired from atherosclerotic occlusions. Instead of the vessels being nice and thick, they turn white and shriveled, or perhaps bumpy. I might even see that the arteries have a kind of golden cast to them because they are full of cholesterol. Sometimes I can pick up a hint of high blood pressure from a narrowing of the blood vessels in the eye.

The benefits of these observations are not limited to the eye itself. What I discover in the arteries of your eyes has important cardiovascular implications for the rest of the body.

For example, looking at the eye helps me evaluate the health of the carotid artery. It happens that the first artery that comes off the carotid is called the ophthalmic artery, which feeds circulation to the eye. If a piece of cholesterol plaque breaks off from the carotid, the first place it's likely to enter is the smaller ophthalmic artery. This piece of cholesterol can temporarily occlude the vessel, resulting is a loss of vision in one eye for a few minutes.

This condition is called *amaurosis fugax*, and patients often describe its symptoms as someone pulling the shade down on a window. Blood clots and debris breaking off from the aorta or valves of the heart and traveling to the eye can also lead to this condition. So if someone comes to me complaining of occasional loss of vision and the arteries in his eyes appear damaged, it's a tip-off that the patient's heart and carotid arteries need to be thoroughly examined for evidence of atherosclerosis.

But the sense of vision is not located exclusively in the eyes. Atherosclerosis can affect your eyesight in another spot entirely. The *occipital lobes*, located in the back of the brain, process the images from the eyes in an area called the *visual cortex*. The blood supply for this part of the brain comes from the vertebral arteries. Any reduction in circulation in these arteries can cause vision problems.

Often when people wake up in the morning with a crick in their neck, they might not see too well for a minute or two. This is because the position of their head while sleeping reduced the flow of blood through the vertebral arteries, which are located in the neck. Their vision will be temporarily impaired until the blood starts flowing normally through the arteries to the back of the brain. Broken pieces of cholesterol plaque inside the vertebral arteries can also cause the same kind of vision problem by reducing the flow of blood to the visual cortex.

Usually, vision problems such as the above don't appear until atherosclerotic disease is well advanced. So changes in a person's vision are very important and make me extremely suspicious of disease elsewhere in the cardiovascular system. Surprisingly, patients may neglect to mention loss of vision during a cardiovascular examination, believing only their eye doctor would be interested in such a symptom. So I always make it a point to examine the eyes myself and ask the patient point-blank whether he suffers any vision problems, especially if he's suffering from aggravating diseases such as diabetes or hypertension.

At this point, we come to the "heart" of the cardiovascular examination…

The Resting Electrocardiograph

All muscle—including heart muscle—moves in response to electrical stimulation from nerve fibers. Electrical currents travel down the nerve fibers of the heart in a systematic progression, stimulating the heart to contract in an orderly way. This well-organized contraction of heart muscle creates the rhythmic pumping action of the heartbeat.

An *electrocardiograph*, or *ECG*, is a machine that measures the electrical currents of the heart as it beats. An *electrocardiogram* is the graphic representation of these currents—the familiar up-and-down tracings of an inked needle across a moving roll of paper. The actual tracing itself is called a *waveform*. By studying the waveform on the electrocardiogram, I can follow the movement of electricity through the heart muscle, and this gives me a wealth of information about the physical condition of the heart.

If the electrical impulses through the heart are irregular, then the beating of the heart will be irregular. An irregularity in the normal rhythm of the heartbeat is called *arrhythmia* or *dysrhythmia*. Arrhythmias are often a sign that the heart has been damaged by disease. This damage impairs the present function of the heart and can create serious health problems in the future.

When the heartbeat suffers a serious arrhythmia, the pumping action of the heart becomes weakened. Which means that the volume of blood pumped through the body will be reduced, and that always means trouble.

When I examine your electrocardiogram, I'm basically looking for two things: abnormalities in the conduction of electricity through the heart muscle and abnormalities in the heart rhythm. Both of these irregularities are associated with a host of heart problems.

The Limitations—and Necessity—of ECG Examination

As a diagnostic test, the ECG has limitations. For one thing, it only records electrical impulses in the heart that manage to travel up through the chest to the electrodes on the skin. There are many electrical subtleties that the standard ECG doesn't record. As a result, the ECG is just a summary of electrical activity—it doesn't always tell me everything I'd like to know. For patients who really need a detailed analysis, hospitals provide a surgical test called *electrophysiology*, which attaches electrodes to the heart itself.

Also, the ECG records heart activity during a small window of time, typically only a matter of a few minutes. This snapshot in time may not be sufficient to pick up arrhythmias that only occur at irregular intervals.

And the heart performs differently under different conditions. The *Resting ECG* records the heart at rest, as the patient lies on a table. But when the patient is up and moving around, the heart can change its electrical character, causing arrhythmias that will be missed by the Resting ECG.

Despite its limitations, however, it's very important that everyone gets an ECG examination early in their adult life, even if they are healthy. One of the best ways to diagnose cardiovascular disease is to examine a previous ECG and compare it to a new one, to see what the changes are. But, quite often, people walk into my office who have never had an ECG before. It makes diagnosis very difficult because there's no baseline study available—and everyone's heart is as individual as they are.

The organs in our bodies are rarely perfect instruments. They may be flawed at birth or develop flaws later in life. An obvious example is the eye and eyesight: many people are either born with poor eyesight or develop problems such as *presbyopia* (an inability to clearly see nearby objects) later in life as the eye ages.

The heart is often not a perfect instrument, either. The electrical connections which transmit current through the heart can be flawed at birth or develop flaws later in life, as the heart ages or suffers damage from disease. The ECG can detect these electrical flaws, but it doesn't necessarily tell me why they are occurring.

It's a dilemma I'm faced with often. A patient may come to me with chest pains and I may see something suspicious on the ECG, but I can't assume that what I see is the cause of the chest pains. When I analyze an abnormal ECG, I always have to ask myself, "Is this disturbance just an insignificant characteristic of the patient's heart or is it an irregularity caused by damage to the heart?"

It's always easier to answer this question if I have a previous ECG for comparison. If a patient has no history at all of irregular heartbeats, then suddenly starts to show arrhythmias, that's a tip-off to a current disease process at work. That is why I advise everyone to obtain a copy of their earliest ECG, which can be carried around to any doctor who needs to see it.

Although it's no guarantee of cardiovascular health, a normal ECG is a very favorable sign. Certainly, having a normal one is better than having an abnormal one!

Reading the Electrocardiogram

The ECG exam begins with the bare-chested patient lying on his back on the examination table. A series of electrodes are attached to various spots on the upper body. The movement of small electrical currents in the heart is transmitted through the skin to the electrodes. The ECG machine amplifies the currents and reproduces them on the graph paper.

Below are some simplified illustrations of the typical electrocardiograms I find during office examinations.

NORMAL SINUS RHYTHM

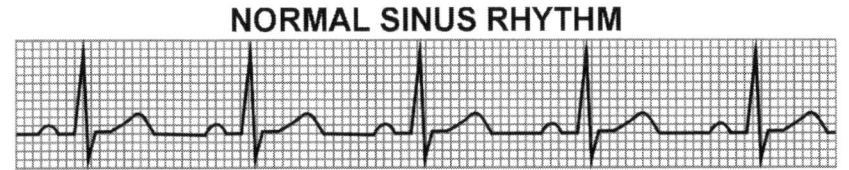

An electrocardiogram is often referred to as a "rhythm strip" because it's a graphic representation of the rhythm of the heartbeat. In this simplified example, the heart beats with a regular rhythm at a normal speed.

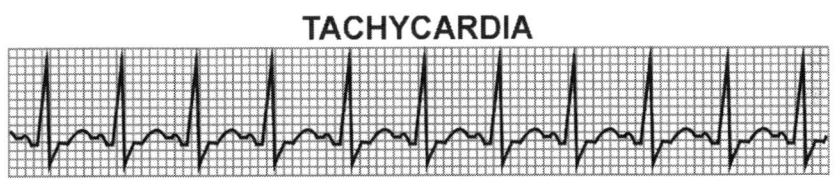

TACHYCARDIA

In this example of tachycardia the beats are still uniform in their rhythm, but there are many more beats in the same amount of time, indicating a rapid heartbeat.

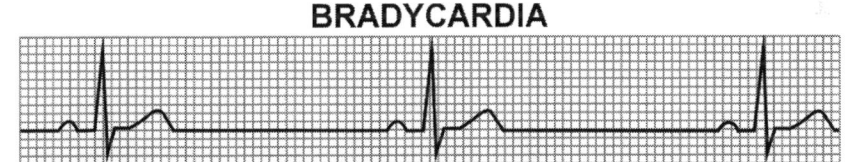

BRADYCARDIA

During bradycardia, the beats are regular but their number has decreased, indicating a slowed heartbeat.

ARRHYTHMIA

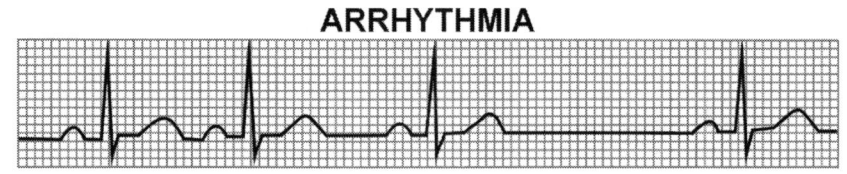

And in this example of arrhythmia there are varying times between the start of one beat and the next, indicating that the heartbeat has become irregular.

The heart is divided into four chambers for holding blood: two upper chambers called the left and right *atria* and two bottom chambers called the left and right *ventricles*. Different types of arrhythmias generally get their name by referring to the site of origin of the electrical impulse and the part of the heart involved in the conduction of the current, which is why the terms *atrial* and *ventricular* keep popping up in the names of arrhythmias.

A normal heartbeat cycle starts with an electrical impulse from the *sinus node*, a small mass of specialized cells near the top of the heart (actually located in the right atrium) that acts as a "pacemaker," generating impulses at regular intervals. Like a pebble dropped in water, the impulse spreads out in concentric waves throughout the heart muscle. The top of the heart contracts first, then the wave travels down specific pathways to the bottom part of the heart, which contracts in response to the impulse a split-second later.

These waves from the sinus node follow one another, creating the rhythm of the heartbeat. But as the waves radiate out, they may not be transmitted smoothly through the heart muscle. By studying the electrocardiogram, I can often tell where—and why—the electrical connections in the heart have gone awry.

The smooth progression of the current through the heart can be hampered by several problems. A chief reason is nerve and muscle damage caused by old heart attacks. When you have a dead part of the muscle, no electricity is transmitted through it, so the current that powers the heartbeat has to go a roundabout way. Or, just the opposite, the current may be short-circuited and never arrive at where it should. This abnormal timing of currents is easily seen on the ECG, which is why the electrocardiograph is very good at diagnosing past heart attacks.

Once the conduction of current is impaired by heart damage, the heartbeat loses its ability for uniform, rhythmic contractions. These disturbances in rhythm can profoundly affect the pumping ability of the heart, leading to all kinds of cardiovascular troubles.

Arrhythmias can be categorized many different ways, but to keep things simple let's just classify them by the risks the pose—*minor arrhythmias* and *significant arrhythmias*. The following list is by no means exhaustive, but it reflects the broad categories of what I typically see in my practice. First up are...

Minor Arrhythmias

Minor arrhythmias are rarely a real health threat. Often they are not even noticed by the patient. Occasionally, however, harmless arrhythmias are strongly felt by the patient and, because they are noticed, become a cause for concern. Eventually, most patients become accustomed to their presence and they fade into the background of everyday living.

The most common minor arrhythmias have to do with the speed of the heartbeat. *Tachycardia* is defined as a fast heartbeat, usually above 100 beats per minute. *Bradycardia* is a slow heartbeat, usually below 60 beats per minute.

The heart, of course, is specifically designed to accommodate a wide range of heartbeat speeds. When exercising, the heart needs to beat faster to increase circulation to the skeletal muscles. When resting, the heart allows itself to beat slower, conserving energy. So variations in heartbeat rate are common throughout the day.

Unlike the muscles of our arms and legs—which move when we tell them to—the heart muscle is not under our direct, conscious control. We can't order the heart to beat or not to beat the same way we order a hand to wave or a knee to bend. Instead, the heart (and all other organs) is controlled by the ***autonomic nervous system***, autonomic meaning "self-controlling."

Left by itself, the heart will beat at a basic rate of 25 beats per minute. But nerve impulses generated by the autonomic nervous system, which is responding to the needs of the body, tells the heart how fast—or how slow—to beat. As previously noted, a normal heart rate falls within a range of values, but the average is about 72 beats per minute.

Normal changes above and below the basic heart rates are often called ***sinus tachycardia*** and ***sinus bradycardia***, "sinus" referring to the origin of the heartbeat, the sinus node. Generally, it means that the heart is responding appropriately to the influences that control the heart, so these changes in heart rhythm are not much to worry about.

Occasionally, however, sinus tachycardia is a symptom of an underlying problem. We've already talked about heart failure as a cause of rapid heartbeats. But conditions such as anxiety, emotional stress, fever and anemia can also cause sinus tachycardia, and these issues, of course, need to be addressed. Most things that stimulate the autonomic nervous system end up stimulating the heart, as well.

Premature beats are also usually harmless arrhythmias, but they account for most of the symptoms that patients complain—and worry—about. They are often felt as "skipped beats"—a strongly felt pause in the usual rhythm of the heart. These palpitations can also be experienced as a fluttering or thumping in the chest, and can be accompanied by dizziness or weakness.

Although it feels as if the heart has "skipped a beat," quite the opposite is true. Instead, the heart has taken the beat *earlier* than usual, which is why the beat is called premature. This early beat has no effect on the timing of the next natural heartbeat but, to the patient, the perceived delay makes it seem as if the beat has been dropped altogether.

Usually, of course, it's the sinus node that originates the heartbeat. But premature beats can originate from other locations in the heart. If the beat begins at the top of the heart, it's called a *premature atrial contraction (PAC)*. If it begins at the bottom of the heart, it's called a *premature ventricle contraction (PVC)*.

Why would the heartbeat start anyplace else but the sinus node? Well, nature has wisely designed the heart with a lot of redundancy built into it. After all, it's truly a matter of life and death if the heart should fail to beat! So the heart has several fail-safe mechanisms that can kick in if parts of the heart begin to falter.

As part of this redundancy, nearly every part of the heart muscle is capable of originating a heartbeat. That way, in case the sinus node fails, some other location in the heart will take over.

PACs and PVCs are still a bit of a mystery. No one is really sure why they occur in a healthy heart, but it appears they can be aggravated by smoking, alcohol and caffeine. Also, we think that premature beats may be due to some irregular nervous influence to the heart, such as being anxious or emotionally upset. Some people are simply born with a delicately balanced heart—even minor disturbances make it beat irregularly. Premature beats may be isolated, occurring once or twice a minute for a limited time, or they occur with much greater frequency, lasting for the life of the patient, but still causing no great problems.

Occasionally, premature beats may be a symptom of some type of heart disease. One way to grade the significance of a premature beat is to ask the patient when it occurs. Most often, he'll reply that the "skipped beat" occurs when resting or sitting down, but disappears when he walks around or engages in activity such as playing tennis. Under these conditions, I feel that most premature beats are not clinically significant—that type of arrhythmia is not going to bother him very much.

When PACs and PVCs are combined with other cardiovascular symptoms, however, it may be a marker for an abnormality in the heart, such as coronary artery disease. If this were the case, I'd definitely look into it more as the examination progresses.

Supraventricular tachycardia is a general term to describe several types of arrhythmias where the top of the heart beats more rapidly than normal. I know the name is a mouthful, but if you consider each term individually, the meaning becomes clear: a fast heartbeat that's located above (supra–) the ventricles.

This type of arrhythmia is caused by a short-circuiting of the normal currents through the heart. The current keeps traveling around the top of the heart, forcing it to beat rapidly. Most episodes last a short time—a few seconds to a few minutes—but if they last longer they may cause symptoms such as palpitations, light headedness, anxiety and chest pain. Smoking, caffeine and alcohol may contribute to this usually benign arrhythmia. However, if the arrhythmia lasts a long time, it may indicate a more serious problem.

First degree Heart Block (or ***First degree AV Block***) is a type of bradycardia that is caused by a slowing down of the electrical current from the upper part of the heart to the lower part. "First Degree" indicates that all the current eventually gets through, it just takes longer than usual. This condition is often a consequence of aging and usually produces no symptoms.

Significant Arrhythmias

Arrhythmias such as premature beats are often referred to as "*regular irregularities*" because the hiccup in rhythm of the heart happens the same way each time. Conversely, there is second type of arrhythmia called an "*irregular irregularity*," where the heartbeat becomes chaotic. This presents a new level of risk to the patient and may indicate an underlying disease process.

One of the most common "irregular irregularities" is ***atrial fibrillation****,* a specific kind of Supraventricular tachycardia. The electrical currents coursing through the atrium are so disorganized that top of the heart begins to shake and quiver, producing more than 350 heartbeats per minute. Under these conditions the top part of the heart can't pump blood efficiently to the lower part.

Many people have no symptoms, but others will feel the typical complaints of significant arrhythmias—weakness, lightheadedness, fainting, confusion, shortness of breath, chest pain and low blood pressure.

It's possible to live a long life with this type of arrhythmia—episodes of atrial fibrillation can last from a few seconds to forty years. But, in the long-term, it can be quite a problem. It's often associated with an increased risk of stroke because blood clots can form inside the quivering atrium, then travel to the brain.

When I see atrial fibrillation in a person who is 40 to 45, I think of thyroid disease because this type of arrhythmia is strongly linked to an overactive thyroid. In a person who is older, the sudden appearance of atrial fibrillation usually indicates the presence of cardiovascular disease such as hypertension, coronary artery disease or heart failure.

A famous episode of atrial fibrillation happened in 1991 to George Bush, Sr. While jogging, he suffered an irregular heartbeat and, after spending two days in a hospital, he was diagnosed with *Graves' disease*, a condition caused by overproduction of thyroid hormone. Despite his arrhythmia, the former President made cardiovascular headlines again in 1997 by parachuting from an airplane at age 72, recreating a wartime exploit. As his example shows, with proper therapy patients with atrial fibrillation can keep it under control and lead a long, active life.

Sick Sinus Syndrome is another example of an "irregular irregularity." Normal heartbeats get their cue from the rhythmic firing of the sinus node, the pacemaker of the heart. Sometimes the sinus node becomes irregular in its stimulation—sometimes too fast, sometimes too slow. This fluctuation influences the rate of the heartbeat, causing the typical symptoms of significant arrhythmias—weakness, fainting, etc. The sinus node becomes less reliable as people age, or it can become damaged as a result of a particular injury, such as ischemia or scarring. In extreme cases, an artificial *pacemaker* will have to be surgically implanted in the patient to return the heart to normal beating.

As mentioned above, in first degree Heart Block, the electrical impulses from the top of the heart are slow in reaching the bottom of the heart. A potentially more serious matter is **second degree Heart Block**, where some of the impulses fail to reach the bottom, and the ventricle isn't stimulated to beat, creating an arrhythmia. In **third degree Heart Block** none of the impulses make it through at all and the ventricles have to beat without guidance from the top of the heart, resulting in bradycardia. It causes the typical symptoms of significant arrhythmias, but may also include sudden death. Third Degree AV Block is usually the result of heart damage such as coronary artery disease, heart attacks or rheumatic fever.

Ventricular tachycardia is always a very serious matter. As the name implies, it's a rapid heartbeat whose origin is in the ventricles, the bottom part of the heart. The rate of heartbeat can go as high as 300 beats per minute.

Because the heart fails to pump adequately, the usual symptoms appear—lightheadedness, faintness, shortness of breath, and so on. If the attack is sustained, emergency treatment may be required.

Ventricular tachycardia is associated with some kind of underlying disease, such as coronary artery disease or heart failure. So the ultimate cause of the arrhythmia will always have to be diagnosed to assure the proper treatment.

The chief worry of ventricular tachycardia is that is will slip into **ventricular fibrillation**, the disorganized, rapid quivering of the ventricles that is the chief cause of cardiac arrest. Without immediate intervention, the patient will die.

If I notice something unusual during the ECG or if the patient has a particular kind of complaint such as a pounding heart or dizzy spells that the resting ECG doesn't catch, I may continue examining the heart with an…

Ambulatory Electrocardiograph

As we discussed in Chapter Eight, daily living can provoke the sympathetic nervous system into triggering episodes of cardiac arrhythmias and heart troubles. Physical exercise, emotions, stress, even sleep can induce changes in the heart's electrical behavior that would probably be missed during a five-minute examination in the doctor's office.

These limitations of the resting electrocardiograph can be overcome by using an *ambulatory electrocardiograph*—a portable, battery-powered electronic device for continuous, 24-hour monitoring of the heart.

The electrodes of the ambulatory electrocardiograph machine, often called a *Holter monitor*, can be hooked up to the patient in a matter of minutes in my office. The small recording unit is then attached to the patient's belt or carried around by a strap.

After the machine is attached, I'll instruct the patient to wear the monitor continuously for 24 hours while performing his daily routine. The machine is unobtrusive enough that the patient can walk, eat, work at his office, do chores around the house and even sleep with the unit attached.

The next day I'll remove the machine and download the recorded electrocardiogram, which will document any unusual changes to the heart's electrical behavior that occurred during the past 24 hours. I also have the patient keep a timed diary of his activities and symptoms so I can match changes in his electrocardiogram to possible triggering events. In this way, the ambulatory ECG can catch troubling arrhythmias that the five-minute resting ECG would miss.

The Holter Monitor also becomes useful in another critical area...

Mental Stress Testing

As we discussed in Chapter Eight, the heart and blood vessels can undergo tremendous changes when the sympathetic nervous system is stimulated by stress. Physical and mental stress can increase the heart rate, raise blood pressure and generate spasm in the coronary arteries, which reduces the supply of blood to the heart, creating ischemia, and possibly triggering a heart attack.

Everyone reacts differently to moments of stress. The cardiovascular system of some patients is able to shrug off stress without too much difficulty—their heart rate and blood pressure don't overreact and their coronary arteries stay open. Other patients are highly reactive to stress—their heart rate and blood pressure rise more than required, and ischemia quickly begins.

In Chapter Eight I showed how an individual's cardiovascular response to stress can predict future heart trouble. That's why physicians often have their patients perform an *exercise treadmill test* while connected to an electrocardiograph machine or other heart monitoring device. The purpose of the test is to see whether the heart suffers ischemia or other difficulties during the stress of physical exercise, which gives the physician insight into the patient's future risk.

The treadmill stress test was originally designed to solve a business problem. A major corporation found that when they promoted middle-aged men to high positions—after spending a lot of time and money on their training—the executives would often end up with a heart attack, even though they seemed perfectly healthy. So the corporation asked their doctors to devise a medical test that would answer the question, "Who can we promote and feel reasonably certain that they'll stay alive?"

The doctors devised the physical stress test, which they felt could identify the people most likely to have heart attacks in the future. They believed that when you place someone under physical stress and they respond with changes in their ECG, it's more likely that they'll suffer a heart attack.

There are many problems with the treadmill method. First of all, not all people are equipped to handle the physical requirements of the test. They may have arthritis, or trouble walking, or diminished lung capacity, etc. So you don't get the same results as you would with a person without those difficulties.

Even more troubling, the test can be dangerous. You might be stressing a heart that is already damaged, and the heart cannot take the added physical stress. That's why a physician always has to be present during the taking of the test—the patient might actually suffer a heart attack while taking it.

In my opinion, however, the biggest flaw with the treadmill test is that it is not a *stress* test as much as it's a test of the physical capacity of the heart. Most heart attacks don't happen as the result of physical strain—they happen during moments when the body is at rest. As we've seen, a good percentage of heart attacks happen when the patient is asleep and not undergoing any physical stress at all.

It's more important to test for the patient's reaction to *mental* stress, which is more likely to trigger an acute cardiovascular episode.

One of the reasons mental stress is often overlooked by physicians is that, unlike moments of physical stress, where ischemia often results in painful angina, the effects of mental stress are mostly "silent" in nature—there's no outward sign of coronary spasm and ischemia. Which means neither the doctor nor his patient is aware of the effect that mental stress is having on the victim.

However, hidden episodes of silent ischemia *can* be captured on an electrocardiogram.

When you decrease circulation in any part of the heart muscle, it alters the heart's electrical pathways. This alteration of current shows up on the electrocardiogram, specifically a certain segment of the waveform called the **ST segment**. When the electrocardiogram records changes in the ST segment, I can infer the presence of ischemia and spasm in the coronary arteries.

Occasionally, moments of ischemia caused by mental stress can be picked up by the portable Holter machine during the course of a 24-hour monitoring period. In fact, the Holter can be programmed to automatically detect episodes of silent ischemia, alerting the doctor to their presence. But catching them is purely a matter of luck—there's no guarantee that the patient will suffer a stressful ischemic episode during the examination period, even if he wears the Holter for 24 hours straight.

What's needed is a dependable method of provoking mental stress in a patient while he's actually in the doctor's office. (Although some would argue that simply going to the doctor—and paying the bill—is mental stress enough!) Fortunately, there are standard procedures for *mental stress testing*, which in some ways is superior to physical stress testing as a method of predicting future heart trouble.

Provoking mental stress in a patient it isn't nearly as grim as it sounds. The mild frustration of word games or mental arithmetic is usually enough to separate the "hot responders" from patients who are not easily stressed. By having the patient perform simple mental tasks while connected to the Holter monitor in my office, I can uncover hidden episodes of ischemia, which aid me in predicting the patient's risk for cardiovascular troubles.

Here's an example of the value of mental stress testing. A 1996 study from Duke University followed 126 volunteers with coronary artery disease. The members of the group were given mental stress tests which included counting backwards, giving a short speech, public reading of a text and so on. Each volunteer was hooked up to monitors to record heart abnormalities during the test.

After following the subsequent health of the group for five years, the researchers discovered that the people who had ischemia during the mental stress test had a two to three times higher risk of death, heart attack, progressive chest pain or pain requiring an operation such as angioplasty or bypass surgery.[333] Clearly, mental stress testing was effective in singling out the patients most at risk for further cardiac events.

One of the methods that the researchers used in this study to provoke mental stress is a common technique known as *mirror tracing*, one of several methods I use for my own patients during the simple, safe and painless *Sit-Down Stress Test*.

During the Sit-Down Stress Test the patient is hooked up to the Holter monitor and asked to trace a series of images in a mirror using his finger. It sounds simple enough, but the mirror image is maddeningly difficult to trace correctly, provoking mental stress in the patient and—depending on his reaction—moments of ischemia in his heart, which the Holter electrocardiograph will record. Several other mental challenges are used, and then the patient is allowed to relax to see how long it takes for his cardiovascular system to return to normal.

Following are some typical examples of a Sit-Down Stress Test.

THE SIT-DOWN STRESS TEST
NORMAL STRESS TEST RESULT

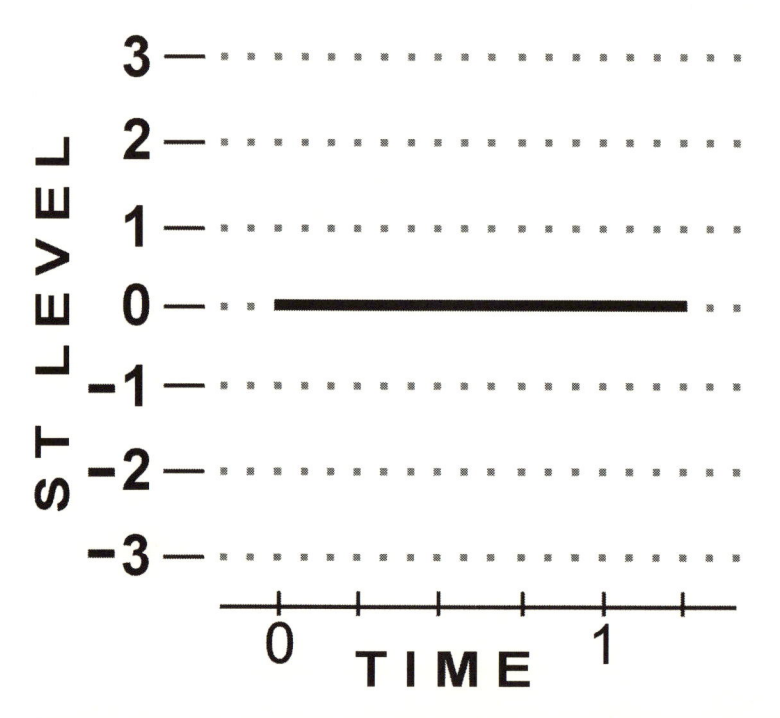

The graph above is the result I expect to see from the Sit-Down Stress Test of a healthy patient. The "ST LEVEL" numbers are an indirect way of detecting ischemia in the heart. The "TIME" numbers indicate the length of the test - in this case, one hour. Throughout the test, the patient's level of blood flow remained constant, indicating no arterial spasm. The patient's risk of death, heart attack, angina, or heart surgery in the near future is low.

The Five Steps of WIN/WIN Therapy 291

THE SIT-DOWN STRESS TEST
ABNORMAL STRESS TEST RESULT

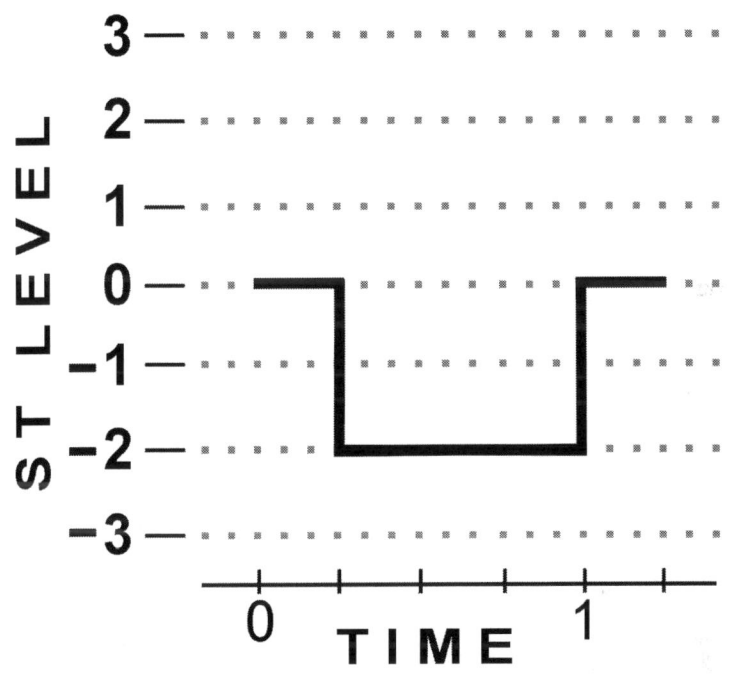

The graph above indicates a serious loss of blood flow to the heart. At the beginning of the test, the patient has a normal reading. But 15 minutes later his level of blood flow has dropped. It stays low throughout the test, and only returns to normal when the test is over and the patient relaxes. This indicates that, for this patient, mental stress has a significant impact on heart ischemia. If this patient has other risk factors, then the likelihood of him having heart troubles in the near future is high.

Ultrasonic Examination

Ultrasound technology has been the most important advance for the diagnosis of cardiovascular disease during my lifetime as a physician. There are three types of ultrasonic examination that I perform on my patients. First up is…

Echocardiography

Echocardiography is a diagnostic test that uses ultrasonic waves to create images of the heart. Although the electronic wizardry of the ultrasound machine is complex, this safe, painless and completely non-invasive examination is easy to perform, right in the doctor's office. The doctor simply places a small hand-held probe (it looks like a microphone) against the surface of the patient's chest, directing the beam of ultrasound at different angles to view particular areas of the heart.

Similar to the way the sonar on a ship works, the ultrasound probe generates harmless sound waves that travel through the skin to the heart. The waves reflect back to the probe, the electronics do their magic, and a moving image of the heart appears on a television screen.

It takes a trained eye to interpret the picture, called an *echocardiogram*, but with enough practice the walls, chambers and valves of the heart are easily detected. For example, below are two echocardiograms I took of the aortic valves of one of my patients.

ECHOCARDIOGRAM

CLOSED AORTIC VALVES

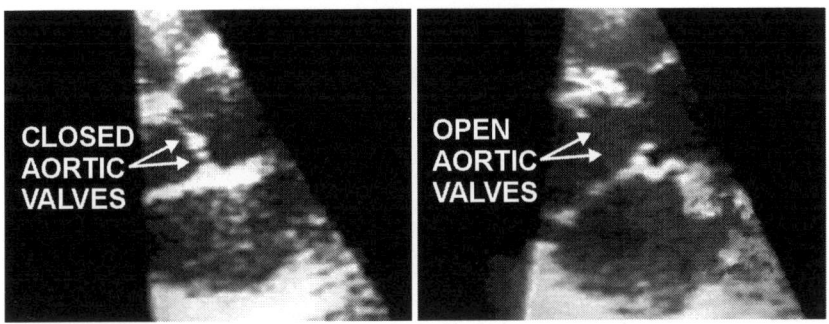

OPEN AORTIC VALVES

The first echocardiogram shows the valves in the closed position, as blood fills the heart. A moment later, the second echocardiogram shows the same valves swept open as blood is pumped out of the heart and funneled into the aorta by a contraction of heart muscle.

The ability to see "real-time" motion such as this reveals crucial information about the condition of the heart. An experienced doctor can spot trouble simply by watching the many elements of the heart move in response to the contractions of the heartbeat.

Depending on the patient's history or what I've uncovered through examination, I'll pay special attention to specific parts of the heart. Did the patient have rheumatic fever as a child? Then the heart valves will need close examination. Is the patient coughing from congestion in the lungs? Ultrasound will show if the patient is suffering from heart enlargement and possible heart failure.

During examination, there's a mental checklist I use to make sure I've covered everything.

The first thing I look for with the ultrasound probe is whether the heart is situated normally in the body. There are several medical conditions in which key structures of the heart—or the general position of the heart in the chest—are abnormal. There's even a rare condition called *dextrocardia* in which the heart—normally located in the left side of the chest—is flipped completely and sits in the right side.

Once I'm satisfied that the anatomy looks as it should, I'll examine the valves of the heart. The health of the valves—which regulates the flow of blood through the heart—is a critical factor in many kinds of heart disease.

The valves are made of a strong, flexible membrane, like the webbed foot of a duck. This flexibility allows the valve to spread wide when opened yet form a tight, leak-proof seal when the valve is closed.

The trouble comes when a valve and its membrane begin to lose flexibility. Any kind of damage to the valve—such as infection during rheumatic fever—can lead to stiff, inflexible scar tissue and a narrowing of the valve opening.

Once valves lose their flexibility, they can no longer open and close properly. The valves leak and regurgitate blood with every heartbeat, creating a backflow. This condition decreases the normal flow of blood through the organ. And if the valve opening is narrowed, it further decreases the volume of blood pumped by the heart. In order to make up for the lost blood flow, the body signals the heart to work harder, which—as you know—can lead to hypertrophy and heart failure.

Stiff and scarred valves also increase turbulence in the blood within the heart. Instead of being pumped out, blood slows down and pools in the heart chambers, allowing blood clots to form. Once created, these blood clots can leave the heart and wander to other areas of the body. That's why valve damage increases the risk for strokes—clots created by leaky valves travel from the heart and become lodged in the arteries of the brain, creating the occlusions that lead to stroke.

How can I tell if the valve is damaged? First, by the way it looks. A damaged valve may appear thicker than usual on the echocardiogram, thanks to scar tissue (fibrosis) and the build-up of calcium deposits on the valve (both conditions caused by our old friend, inflammation). Valve openings narrowed by disease can also be picked up by ultrasound.

Second, I can tell a damaged valve by the way it opens and closes during the course of the heartbeat. Instead of looking flexible, the valve moves stiffly or it hardly moves at all, nearly frozen in place. The valve may be so stiff and brittle that it becomes partially broken and a hinged flap flutters wildly in the bloodstream.

Occasionally, a patient's valve is *too* elastic, looking floppy and fluttering on the echocardiograph screen. A "floppy valve" fails to seal tightly, once again creating backflows of blood that reduces the efficiency of the heart. This condition, called **valve prolapse**, is typically present at birth or develops in childhood. Valve prolapse usually causes only mild symptoms or no symptoms at all. Occasionally, however, the symptoms become acute and the patient develops **prolapse syndrome**, which is marked by fatigue, arrhythmia and other problems.

Next, I look at the upper and lower chambers of the heart and see whether they're normal-looking or distorted in some way, either too big or too small. The left ventricle is the heart's main pumping chamber; if the heart is going to suffer from hypertrophy, this is the most likely place for enlargement to happen.

Then I look for abnormalities in the motion of the heart. As the heart pumps, the outside walls of the heart should expand and contract with the undulating fluidity of a jellyfish gliding through the sea. Once you know what to look for, it's easy to pick out irregularities in heart motion using ultrasound.

Sometimes portions of the heart muscle move stiffly, with restricted action. Or perhaps sections of the heart bulge outwards during the heartbeat. And occasionally I'll notice that an area of the heart appears to beat out of sync with the rest of the heart. These kinds of abnormalities in wall motion would indicate damage to the heart muscle, either through trauma, infection or lack of circulation, such as an old heart attack.

Next, I would look at the condition of the aorta, the large artery that carries blood from the heart to the rest of the body. Normally, the walls of the artery should look smooth on the echocardiogram. But when the artery is diseased by atherosclerosis or calcium deposits, the walls of the aorta take on a bumpy, almost shaggy, appearance.

As blood surges into the aorta with every heartbeat, the walls of a healthy aorta should expand and contract smoothly, with every pulse. The movement of an artery coated by cholesterol plaque, however, looks stiff and inflexible. Under these conditions, I'd be concerned that showers of cholesterol plaque might break off from the diseased aorta and travel to the brain, causing a stroke. If the aorta here seems abnormally large, it may indicate an aortic aneurysm, which is prone to rupture.

Naturally, patients are anxious to know if their ultrasound examination reveals actual coronary artery disease. On rare occasions, it's possible to pick up evidence of atherosclerosis in the coronary arteries. Usually, however, the echocardiogram is not detailed enough to make out plaque in the small arteries of the heart so I'd be reluctant to make any firm diagnosis simply from an echocardiogram.

But there's another type of ultrasonic examination that can tell me the likelihood for both coronary artery disease and the patient's risk for a stroke or heart attack…

Cerebrovascular Ultrasound

I've already described how important the carotid arteries are for cardiovascular health: atherosclerosis in the carotids greatly increases the risk of stroke, the symptoms of Alzheimer's and other cerebrovascular problems. But what's not commonly known is that the very presence of disease in the carotid arteries *also* indicates the presence of heart disease.

Studies have shown that, in the vast majority of cases, if a patient's carotids have atherosclerosis, his coronary arteries are likely to have atherosclerosis, as well. Similarly, if the carotids are normal, the coronary arteries of his heart are likely to be normal, too.

In fact, the health of the carotids can also predict the patient's risk for a heart attack. One study of elderly subjects found that those patients with the most amount of carotid artery disease were nearly four times more likely to suffer a heart attack or stroke compared to those with the least amount of carotid disease.[334]

In sum, the health of the carotids is an accurate bellwether for the health of the heart. I'm able to predict coronary artery disease with 90 to 95% accuracy simply by knowing the health of the carotid arteries. This holds true even if the patient looks and feels healthy, with no signs of cardiovascular troubles.

At this point in the examination, however, I've only been able to infer the presence of atherosclerosis in the carotids by listening for bruits or noticing signs of mental impairment from stroke. Fortunately, because of their large size and shallow location, the carotids can be imaged by the echocardiograph machine and it's easy to detect the presence of disease within them. Not only does ultrasound remove much of the guesswork from diagnosis, but ultrasound can also reveal the earliest stages of plaque build-up that no amount of hands-on examination could ever reveal.

The left and right carotids, located on either side of the neck, lie close enough to the skin that the pulse can often be seen. After a few adjustments to the echocardiograph machine, I'll apply the ultrasound probe to the neck, sliding it up and down the length of each artery to view as much of it as possible.

From the base of the neck, I can follow a carotid up to the head where, right below the jaw line, each carotid splits into two separate arteries: the *internal carotid* and the *external carotid*. The external carotids supply blood to the face and scalp. The internal carotids supply blood to the brain. The point where the internal and external arteries split off from one another is called the *bifurcation*. Naturally, after the branching off point, the internal carotid is the one I'm most interested in since it leads directly to the brain.

But the bifurcation presents its own special problems. Because of the way the bifurcation is constructed and how blood flows around it, it's the point most likely to collect cholesterol plaque. Since most blockages occur right here, I'm especially curious to see how the bifurcation looks.

What sorts of things am I looking for? First and foremost is the presence of cholesterol plaque. Following is an illustration of where I place the ultrasound probe to examine the right carotid artery before it reaches the bifurcation point. Right below the illustration is a photo of what the probe sees in this position.

The Five Steps of WIN/WIN Therapy 299

VASCULAR ULTRASOUND OF A CAROTID ARTERY

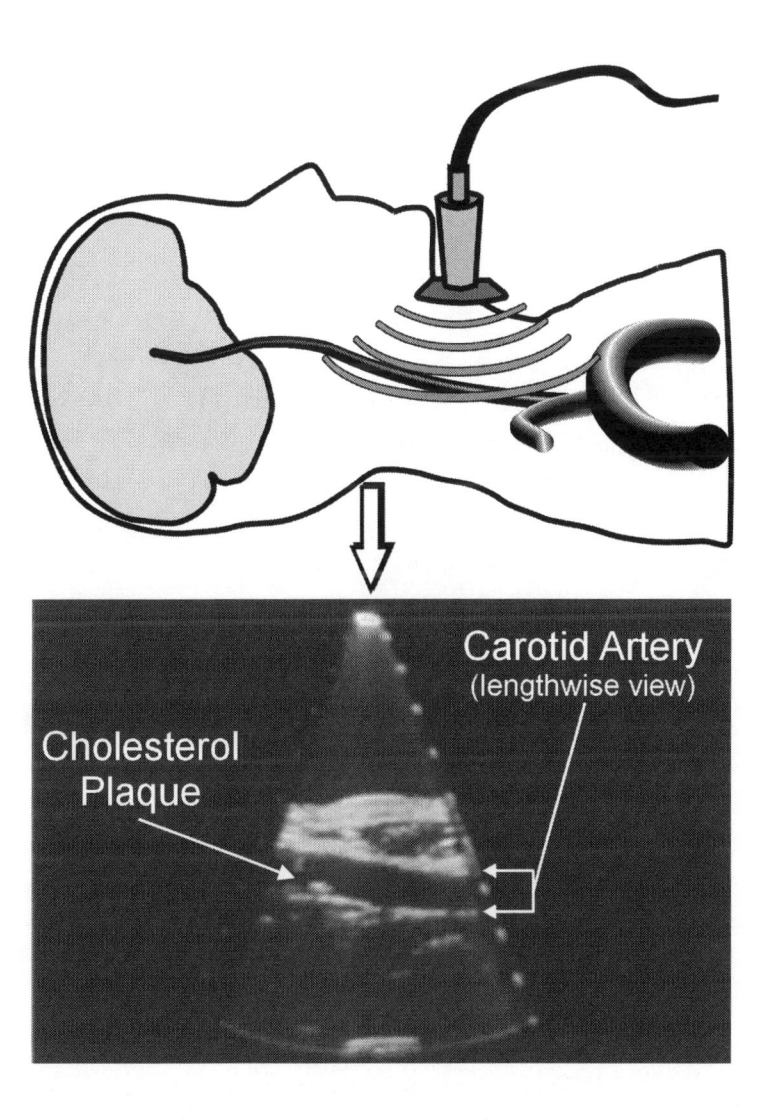

Carotid Artery
(lengthwise view)

Cholesterol Plaque

In the ultrasound photo, the carotid artery looks like a long, hollow tube running through the middle of the picture. The arrow at the left end of the tube points to an unmistakable deposit of cholesterol plaque within the artery.

This mound of cholesterol obstructs the artery by nearly 30%. Yet, it's quite likely that the patient has no idea that he's suffering from atherosclerotic disease, which is putting him at an increased risk for stroke and the symptoms of Alzheimer's—not to mention the associated risk of heart disease. Typically, it takes a 75% obstruction before symptoms start to appear, which is exactly why ultrasonic examination is so important: early detection means an early start to WIN/WIN Therapy.

Aside from the presence of plaque, there are other things to look for in the carotids. Typically, diseased arteries become stiffened by atherosclerosis, so I look to see whether the artery expands and contracts easily with each pulse. I might press down with the probe slightly to test whether the artery is compressible, as it should be.

Hardening of the arteries is often the result of calcification and ultrasound can indirectly reveal it. Since calcium is a mineral and not soft tissue, ultrasonic waves can't penetrate it. As a result, the artery image will have dark shadows in certain spots, an indication that deposits of calcium are blocking the view.

Also significant is the shape of the artery itself. I can tell if the artery is relaxed, in which case it has a round, open look. Or I can tell if it's experiencing spasm, which gives it a flattened or squared-off shape. Witnessing actual spasm first-hand will certainly influence my assessment of the patient's risk for cardiovascular problems down the road.

Atherosclerosis has a habit of thickening the walls of the arteries that it inhabits. So checking the thickness of the artery wall in the ultrasound image is a further indication of disease.

Just as the health of the carotids corresponds to the health of the heart, there is another great indicator of cardiac trouble: *peripheral artery disease (PAD)*.

As mentioned earlier, people who suffer from peripheral artery disease have a higher risk of death from stroke. But it's also true that patients with PAD have a significantly higher risk of heart attacks and cardiovascular death, as well, even if the patient shows no symptoms of disease.[335]

Therefore, knowing the health of the arteries throughout your body is a big help in predicting heart trouble ahead. There's one more ultrasonic examination I can perform in the office that's perfectly suited to detecting PAD, even at its earliest stages…

Doppler Ultrasound

Doppler ultrasound works on a different principle than ultrasonic echocardiography. If you remember your high school science, the *Doppler effect* is an apparent variation in the frequency, or pitch, of a sound. When an object is moving toward you, the pitch of the sound appears to rise. When the object moves away from you, the pitch appears to fall.

When the Doppler probe is placed on the patient's skin, blood cells rushing through a nearby artery will reflect the sound waves back to the probe. By analyzing the shifting frequencies of the rushing blood, the Doppler machine can determine how much and how quickly blood is traveling through an artery.

That—of course—is the key to discovering peripheral artery disease. In healthy arteries, the flow of blood is fast and plentiful. In arteries diseased by atherosclerotic plaque, however, the flow of blood is slow and trickling. The Doppler probe can be placed at the many different locations where PAD reveals itself—ankle, knee, leg, wrist, arm and neck arteries. The further away you are from the heart, the more likely you are to have impaired circulation.

Instead of an echocardiographic picture, however, the Doppler machine creates two different types of data—sounds transmitted to an audio speaker and wave-like tracings on a moving strip of chart paper.

The sound from a Doppler machine is really just an aid to making sure that the ultrasound probe is in the right position. When the probe is placed correctly over an artery, the audio speaker rumbles to life with the swooshing sound of blood pulsing through the vessel. Through experience, the volume and tone of the sound can give you a broad hint whether the blood flow through the artery is adequate or not. If the sound is diminished or—even worse—not present at all, it's likely that circulation is very low at that spot. The rumble of turbulent blood flow within the artery, a consequence of cholesterol plaque, can also be heard with the probe.

But for a definitive analysis, you have to study the waveform tracings that the Doppler machine creates on paper. Illustrated below is a typical tracing of four pulses through a normal artery.

DOPPLER ULTRASOUND TRACINGS

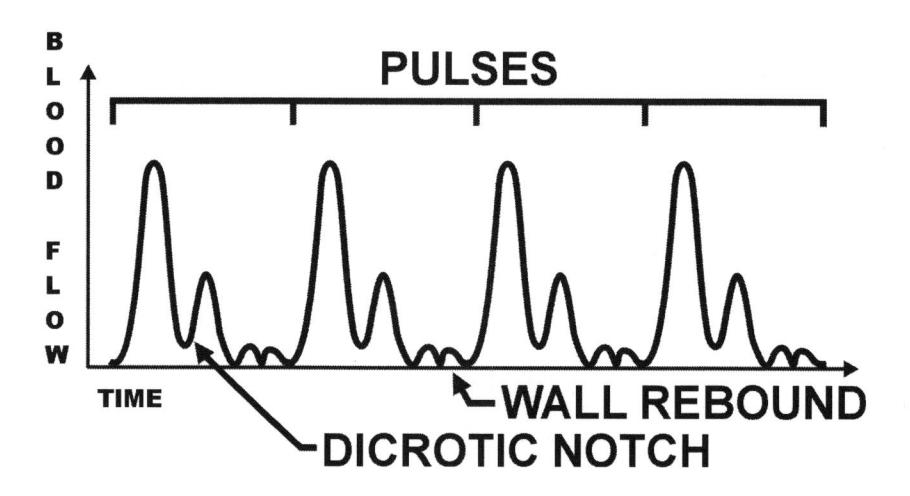

As the sample tracing shows, each pulse begins with a large, upward curve showing the rush of blood through the artery as the heart muscle contracts. As the heart relaxes, the curve drops, indicating that the volume and velocity of the blood is lessening. But the downward slope is interrupted by a smaller, secondary upstroke called the *dicrotic notch.* This brief upturn corresponds to the abrupt closure of the aortic valves in the heart, which the blood flow responds to. Then the curve continues its downward course, punctuated by even smaller bumps caused by the *rebounding of the artery wall* from the currents of blood.

The towering height of each pulse indicates a plentiful blood flow. The clearly seen dicrotic notches and wall rebounds are indications that the artery is elastic and not stiffened by hardening of the arteries. When these telltale signs of a healthy artery begin to disappear, it's likely that the artery is becoming clogged with atherosclerosis. If there is a circulatory problem, inflexibility of the blood vessels caused by scarring, cholesterol and calcium deposits is one of the first signs of disease. The shape of the Doppler tracings lets me judge the severity of disease, from mild to severe. Following are some graphs that chart the decline in circulation that the Doppler ultrasound can reveal.

DOPPLER ULTRASOUND TRACINGS OF DECLINING CIRCULATION IN A PERIPHERAL ARTERY

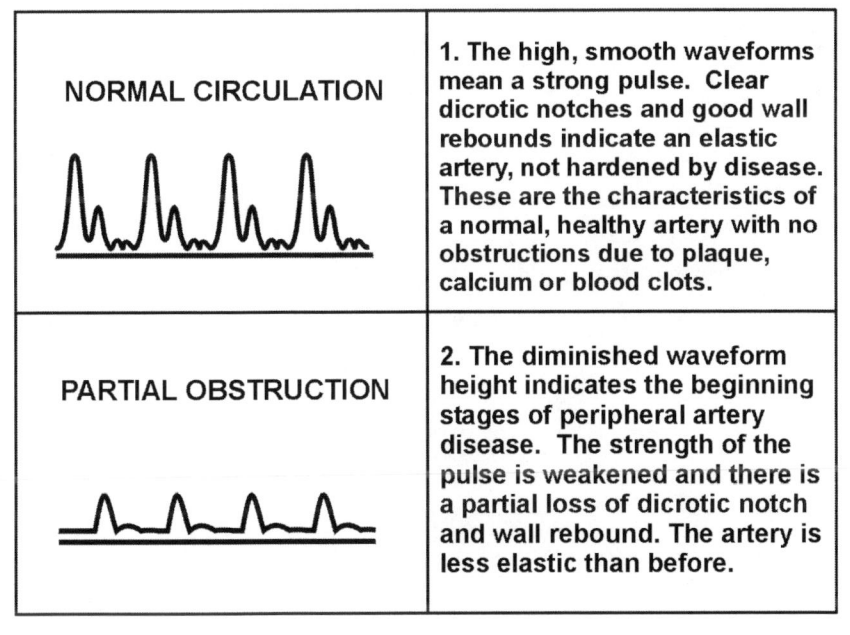

NORMAL CIRCULATION	1. The high, smooth waveforms mean a strong pulse. Clear dicrotic notches and good wall rebounds indicate an elastic artery, not hardened by disease. These are the characteristics of a normal, healthy artery with no obstructions due to plaque, calcium or blood clots.
PARTIAL OBSTRUCTION	2. The diminished waveform height indicates the beginning stages of peripheral artery disease. The strength of the pulse is weakened and there is a partial loss of dicrotic notch and wall rebound. The artery is less elastic than before.

DOPPLER ULTRASOUND TRACINGS OF DECLINING CIRCULATION IN A PERIPHERAL ARTERY

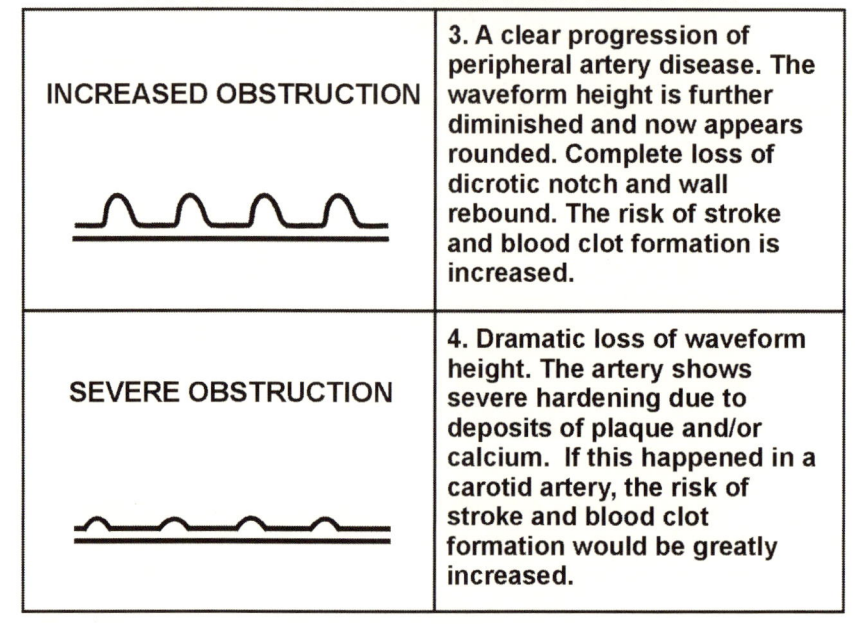

INCREASED OBSTRUCTION	3. A clear progression of peripheral artery disease. The waveform height is further diminished and now appears rounded. Complete loss of dicrotic notch and wall rebound. The risk of stroke and blood clot formation is increased.
SEVERE OBSTRUCTION	4. Dramatic loss of waveform height. The artery shows severe hardening due to deposits of plaque and/or calcium. If this happened in a carotid artery, the risk of stroke and blood clot formation would be greatly increased.

There's another way that Doppler ultrasound can also be used to determine the presence and severity of peripheral artery disease: the *Ankle/Brachial Index* or *ABI*.

The Ankle/Brachial Index is a number that compares the systolic blood pressure of the ankle to the systolic blood pressure of the arm. (The word *brachial* refers to the arm.)

Why would a pressure comparison of the ankles and the arms be important? Because, as a general rule, the arteries of the ankles have a higher blood pressure than the arteries in the arms. But people suffering from peripheral artery disease have just the opposite—the ankle blood pressure is lower than the arm.

So, if I find a typical blood pressure in your arm with an elevated pressure at the ankle, that's considered very good. But if the ankle blood pressure is lower than the pressure in your arm, that's considered a bad prognostic sign. Combine this with symptoms such as claudication, and it's a pretty sure bet that there is trouble with the circulation; something is blocking the free flow of blood to your lower limbs, and that something is probably peripheral artery disease.

The ABI test is similar to a standard blood pressure examination, using pressure cuffs around the arm and ankle. The Doppler ultrasound probe is used chiefly as an aid to detect the pulse during the procedure.

The ABI number is arrived at by dividing the ankle pressure by the arm pressure, for example, 130/120.

Since the ankle should have a higher number than the arm, an ABI number of 1 or higher is considered normal. If the number is *lower* than 1, it would indicate that your peripheral arteries are becoming clogged by cholesterol plaque.

As a rule of thumb, the severity of PAD is categorized by the following ABI numbers:

The Stages of Peripheral Artery Disease (PAD)

ABI Number	CARDIOVASCULAR ASSESSMENT
1 or above	Normal
.9—1	The beginning stages of PAD, often without symptoms present.
.5—.9	Symptomatic PAD, with leg pain when walking.
Less than .5	Severe PAD, with leg pain present during periods of rest.

Changing ABI numbers over the course of time are a good indication of the progression of atherosclerotic disease. It also allows me to note the effectiveness of treatment—if the number stays the same or decreases, I know whether additional steps will need to be taken.

Once again, Doppler and ABI examinations point to the need for establishing a baseline of cardiovascular health early in the patient's life. Many of the medical judgements I make depend on knowing what changes have taken place over the course of years. The four ultrasound tests I've outlined here are an immense help in diagnosing illness and tracking the results of treatment.

At the end of the physical examination, I'll have my nurse draw blood samples from the patient and send them to a diagnostic laboratory for analysis. This procedure begins the second step of WIN/WIN Therapy…

Step 2
In addition to a standard blood test and cholesterol screening, test for inflammatory risk factors—such as C-reactive protein and fibrinogen levels—and for infectious risk factors, such as Chlamydia pneumoniae and the other germs of cardiovascular disease.

Laboratory testing of blood samples is used to confirm or exclude a diagnosis, or to verify that a treatment is working—or, at the very least, doing no harm.

Blood testing measures various components of the blood to determine if they fall within normal values. It also detects the presence or absence of abnormal substances. In this way, a standard blood test can reveal organ malfunction long before the patient or his doctor suspects that anything is wrong.

For many years now, cholesterol levels have been added to the standard blood test as a predictor of cardiovascular disease. As we've seen, however, cholesterol by itself is an unpredictable predictor.

But thanks to the recent discoveries of infection and inflammation as a source of cardiovascular disease, new tests have been created that specifically target these twin evils, greatly enhancing your doctor's ability to predict stroke, heart attack and other cardiovascular troubles.

Along with the standard blood test and cholesterol testing, the new infection and inflammation tests I recommend are:

- High-Sensitivity C-Reactive Protein
- Fibrinogen Levels
- Cardiovascular Germs
  - *Chlamydia pneumoniae*
  - *Helicobacter pylori*
  - Cytomegalovirus
  - Herpes simplex

In my opinion, it should be standard practice for physicians to order these tests for every patient over the age of 40 who comes in for examination. Testing at age 40 not only confers the benefits of early detection but it also establishes a baseline for additional testing in later years.

If your doctor does not ordinarily include these tests in his examination, you can ask him to order these tests for you at a nearby clinic or testing facility.

It's important to note, however, that it is not necessary for a physician to order many of these tests. You can order your own blood testing at laboratories such as Health Check USA. You simply set up an appointment by telephone or over the Web and have your blood drawn at a local facility. At the moment, Health Check USA offers standard blood testing along with the new cardiovascular CRP test.

To give you a better understanding of the uses and benefits of laboratory testing, let's begin with a discussion of...

The Standard Blood Test

On the following pages are the results of a recent standard blood test performed on an 80-year-old male who has been a patient of mine ever since I started practice. Here's a brief summary of how I would evaluate his standard blood test, paying attention to topics that deal directly with cardiovascular disease.

PATIENT NAME	DATE	AGE	SEX	LAB NUMBER	LAB
XXXXXX, XXXXX	09/05/2000	80	M	XXXXXXXXXXX	REPORT

```
HEMOTOLOGY:
  RBC-----------------------------    4.81    M/CMM    ( 4.4-5.9  )
  HEMOGLOBIN ---------------------   15.8     CM/DL    (14.0-18.0 )
  HEMATOCRIT ---------------------   46.9     %        (40.0-52.0 )
  MCV-----------------------------   98       FL       (  80-100  )
  MCH-----------------------------   32.8     PG       (26.4-34.0 )
  MCHC----------------------------   33.6     G/DL     (31.0-36.0 )
  WBC-----------------------------    5.7     K/CMM    ( 3.9-11.3 )
  BANDS---------------------------    0       %        (  0-10    )
  NEUTROPHILS,   %----------------   59       %        ( 42-78    )
  LYMPHOCYTES,   %----------------   27       %        ( 15-45    )
  MONOCYTES,     %----------------   10       %        (  0-12    )
  EOSINOPHILS,   %----------------    3       %        (  0-7     )
  BASOPHILS,     %----------------    1       %        (  0-2     )
  ATYPICAL LYMPHOCYTES,  %--------    0       %        (  0-4     )
  COMMENT:
```

  Platelets appear adequate.

```
PLATELET COUNT--------------------   192      K/CMM    ( 140-440  )
MPV------------------------------      7.8    FL       ( 6.3-10.3 )

MONOCYTES, ABSOLUTE---------------   570      /CMM     (  60-900  )

LYMPHOCYTES, ABSOLUTE-------------  1539      /CMM     (1050-3600 )

BASOPHILS, ABSOLUTE---------------    57      /CMM     (  0-150   )

SEGMENTED NEUTROPHILS, ABSOLUTE---  3363      /CMM     (1650-8330 )

EOSINOPHILS, ABSOLUTE-------------   171      /CMM     (  0-550   )

RDW------------------------------     12.7    %        (11.5-14.5 )
```

PATIENT NAME	DATE	AGE	SEX	LAB NUMBER	LAB REPORT
XXXXXX, XXXXX	09/05/2000	80	M	XXXXXXXXXX	

CONTINUATION OF REPORT -- PAGE 2

```
CHEMISTRY:
*GLUCOSE--------------------------     121    MG/DL   (  65-115  )
 UREA NITROGEN--------------------      18    MG/DL   (   8-25   )
 CREATININE-----------------------     1.0    MG/DL   ( 0.5-1.6  )
 BUN/CREATININE RATIO-------------    18.0            (   5-25   )
 A/G RATIO------------------------     1.6            ( 0.9-2.6  )
 CALCIUM--------------------------     9.5    MG/DL   ( 8.6-10.6 )
 POTASSIUM------------------------     4.7    MEQ/L   ( 3.5-5.5  )
 GLOBULIN, CALCULATED-------------     2.9    G/DL    ( 1.4-4.5  )
 CARBON DIOXIDE-------------------      28    MEQ/L   (  18-30   )
 SODIUM---------------------------     143    MEQ/L   ( 134-146  )
 ALT------------------------------      20    IU/L    (   0-45   )
 CHLORIDE-------------------------     105    MEQ/L   (  95-110  )
 BILIRUBIN, TOTAL-----------------     1.0    MG/DL   ( 0.2-1.5  )
 AST------------------------------      21    IU/L    (   8-45   )
 ALBUMIN--------------------------     4.7    G/DL    ( 3.1-4.8  )
 ALKALINE PHOSPHATASE-------------      49    IU/L    (  30-130  )
 PROTEIN, TOTAL-------------------     7.6    G/DL    ( 6.1-8.3  )

*CHOLESTEROL---------------------     310    MG/DL   (   0-200  )
 TRIGLYCERIDE--------------------     149    MG/DL   (  20-200  )
 HDL CHOLESTEROL-----------------      47    MG/DL   (  35-100  )
*LDL CHOLESTEROL, CALCULATED------     233    MG/DL   (          )
 CHOLESTEROL/HDL RATIO-----------    6.60            (          )
```

(** Reference Values **)
(Chol Trig LDL)
(Desirable: <200 <200 <130 *)
(Borderline High: 200-239 200-399 130-159)
(High: >=240 400-999 >=160)
(Very High: >=1000)
(Note: LDL <=100 mg/dL optimal for coronary heart)
(disease patients)

First, a word on how to read this report.

The standard blood test report that comes back from the lab has two sections: *hematology*, which is the study of blood cells, and *chemistry*, which tests for various substances in the blood.

Each section is further divided into four columns. The first column names the type of cell or substance being examined. The second and third columns list a numerical quantity of the substance and the unit of measurement (or simply a percentage). The final column shows a range of "normal values" for the cell or substance. If the measured value falls outside the range—either too much or too little—the entire line is flagged with an asterisk to bring it to the attention of the physician.

The "normal" range of values is determined by the measurements that continually show up in healthy patients. Generally speaking, 95% of healthy patients will have values within this range. There are many reasons other than illness why a number may fall outside the "normal" range—age, race, sex, diet, drugs, physical activity, etc. So just because a number is higher or lower than normal does not necessarily indicate the presence of disease.

Hematology

Let's consider this patient's hematology section first, often refereed to as the ***Complete Blood Count (CBC)***.

The CBC tells us the number, shape, size and appearance of the red cells, white cells and platelets, those little particles that have a great influence on blood clotting. And analysis of the CBC can indicate anemia, leukemia, bleeding, inadequate nutrition, body toxicity and a host of other problems.

Hemoglobin is a substance in red blood cells that gives the blood its red color. Among its many jobs, hemoglobin transports oxygen and carbon dioxide to and from the tissues of the body. It also transports nitrogen oxide, which plays an important role in regulating blood pressure and the dilation or constriction of blood vessels.

Hematocrit is a measure of the relative volume of blood occupied by red blood cells. If the red blood count, hemoglobin and the hematocrit are all very high, the patient is more likely to create blood clots. If I'm dealing with a patient who has a blood clot disease, I might order a separate fibrinogen test. In interpreting these numbers, you have to take into account where the patient lives. People who live in higher elevations may have elevated numbers to compensate for the lack of oxygen, so their blood tends to be thicker.

Neutrophils, lymphocytes, monocytes, eosinophils and *basophils* are all types of white blood cells. Their numbers refer to the percentages of each type of cell compared to the total number of white blood cells. As you can see, the neutrophils are most prevalent. Changes in percentages are an indication that the body is undergoing some kind of stress, such as infection, allergy, trauma and so on.

The notation in the report that "platelets appear adequate" means that the lab technician, upon viewing a slide of the sample blood, determined that the platelets were normal in number and appearance. Abnormal platelets may indicate bleeding disorders.

Every tested item on this patient's hematology report falls within normal values. Since nothing stands out as an indication of ill cardiovascular health, we can move on and consider the patient's…

Blood Chemistry, Including Cholesterol Testing

Several organs in the body can have a direct bearing on cardiovascular disease. Blood chemistry lets me know how well these organs are functioning and whether they are affecting your cardiovascular health.

The first item tested in this report is *glucose*, which measures the sugar level in the blood. In this instance, the tested level of 121 is slightly higher than the normal upper range of 115. High levels of glucose in the blood are associated with diabetes, which is a risk factor for cardiovascular disease. At this stage, however, it's not possible to conclude very much from this one test. This patient's sugar levels may be high because the patient ate a meal close to the time when the blood was drawn—most blood tests require a fasting period of about eight hours prior to giving a sample. Because the number is only slightly high, it may be that the patient has a precursor to diabetes called *impaired fasting glucose.* At any rate, to make any kind of firm diagnosis, the patient would have to be tested again on a different day.

With everything I know about this patient, I suspect that this small elevation is simply an individual trait with no real significance. But if this patient had high blood pressure along with diabetes, then there is a possibility of great damage being done to his blood vessels and also his kidneys.

Which is why I want to check his *BUN* and *creatinine* levels, next.

BUN (Blood Urea Nitrogen) and creatinine are both waste products of body metabolism. The main job of the kidneys is to help cleanse the blood of waste products such as these. Abnormal numbers of the *BUN/Creatinine Ratio* tell me that the kidneys are not working properly and you are much more likely to have serious hypertension. Since healthy kidneys play a major role in determining normal blood pressure, I need to know if the kidneys are damaged.

Albumin and *globulin* are blood proteins that are bellwethers of your overall health and nutrition. Abnormal numbers in the *A/G Ratio (Albumin/Globulin Ratio)* are an indication of chronic liver disease. If the liver isn't working well, it limits the type of medicine that I might prescribe for cardiovascular disease, such as the statin drugs. Regular blood testing is necessary for statins, to keep a close eye on liver function.

The levels of *sodium, potassium, chloride* and *carbon dioxide* inform me about the salt balance of the bloodstream. These tests are very useful when prescribing *diuretics,* commonly known as *"water pills,"* for my patients. The main function of diuretics is to rid the body of excess salt. This type of medication may be prescribed for the treatment of high blood pressure. As diuretics remove the salt, the water follows (if there is an excess amount) and the blood pressure may be lowered.

Potassium is very important for the proper functioning of nerve and muscle. Since the heart is practically nothing *but* nerve and muscle, potassium has a big effect on the heart. Too much either way can cause problems, such as fibrillation. Potassium levels, which are controlled by the kidneys, play an important part in regulating blood pressure. Much of cardiovascular treatment has to do with changing potassium levels, either elevating or decreasing them.

So far, all of this patient's blood chemistry looks pretty good, but his cholesterol numbers at the bottom of the second page look a little shaky.

You already know why *cholesterol* and *LDL cholesterol* levels are important—elevated numbers are associated with increased cardiovascular risk. Just the opposite is true of the *HDL cholesterol* numbers—elevated levels here indicate a decrease in cardiovascular risk.

Like cholesterol, *triglycerides* are another type of lipid. Triglyceride levels rise in response to fat intake almost immediately after the consumption of a fatty meal. When triglycerides are elevated along with high cholesterol levels (called *combined hyperlipidemia*), there is a marked increase in the risk for atherosclerosis.

Many blood tests will include a *Cholesterol/HDL Ratio* in an attempt to interpret the cardiovascular risk of the patient. Typically, the risk breaks down this way:

Relative Risk	Cholesterol/HDL Ratio
Negative/Low	less than 3.43
Below Average	3.43 - 4.96
Average	4.97
Above Average	4.98 - 9.55
High/Major	greater than 9.55

What stands out most in this sample blood test are the patient's high cholesterol levels.

This patient has a significantly higher than normal cholesterol number of 310 and a high LDL cholesterol number of 233. Plus, his cholesterol/HDL ratio is 6.60, which puts him in the "above average" risk for cardiovascular disease.

I know this patient's history very well, and his cholesterol numbers have been very high for at least the past 30 years. And he comes from a family with a history of cardiovascular problems. Despite these risks, he's never suffered a stroke or heart attack or had diminished intellectual ability due to cerebrovascular disease. In fact, at the age of 80, he still worked at a very demanding job that he went to every day.

I'd like to think this patient owes some of his good health to the cardiovascular examinations and treatments I've given him for the past 50 years.

Especially since the patient is me.

Yep…I used my own recent blood test for the example in this book. I thought it was a good illustration of how cholesterol numbers are not the full story behind cardiovascular disease.

At my advanced age (now 83!), I can't guarantee that I won't eventually develop some type of cardiovascular problem. But the key phrase here is "advanced age." I made it much further than my family history or the conventional risk factors would indicate. By any measure, I've successfully held cardiovascular disease at bay for a good, long time.

And the reason for my success is WIN/WIN Therapy. Long ago I understood that cholesterol levels are only part of the story. More important are the twin factors of infection and inflammation which, thankfully, are now easily discovered with…

The New Cardiovascular Blood Tests for Infection and Inflammation

Hs-CRP

In Chapter Nine, we discussed the new inflammatory risk factors for cardiovascular disease. Thanks to our new understanding of chronic inflammation, a powerful tool has been created for diagnosing cardiovascular troubles, even in patients who feel well and have no outward signs of disease. The measurement of C-reactive protein (CRP) in the body is leaving the experimental world of research labs and medical journals and is becoming an essential predictive tool in doctors' offices and hospitals throughout the nation.

As you recall, CRP testing is a method for predicting a healthy person's risk of heart attack and other cardiovascular problems, especially when the CRP test is combined with other risk factors such as high cholesterol levels. And while standard CRP testing has been around for several years, only the new, highly sensitive CRP tests can detect the chronic, low-level inflammation that is associated with atherosclerosis, strokes and heart attacks.

These new tests are referred to as "*hs-CRP*" or "*high sensitivity-CRP.*" Until recently, these tests were only available at research laboratories. But now, the FDA has approved a number of hs-CRP tests that will cost between $10 and $20, making this test affordable and available to everyone.[336]

In March of 2002, the Centers for Disease Control and Prevention and the American Heart Association convened a meeting of 50 experts in Atlanta to study cardiovascular inflammation. From this meeting, new federal regulations will be written that, as the Associated Press reported, "will urge doctors to test millions of middle-aged Americans" for chronic levels of CRP.[337]

The reason is simple—chronic inflammation is the hidden factor behind all atherosclerotic cardiovascular disease. The hs-CRP test reveals this hidden inflammation, making elevated CRP levels an important risk factor. In fact, it may be that CRP levels are the single most important risk factor in the prediction of cardiovascular disease.

That's because conventional risk factors fail to identify nearly half of the people who end up with heart attacks. But, as an article about Dr. Paul Ridker—an associate professor at Harvard School of Medicine and one of the chief researchers into CRP—points out, measuring high sensitivity C-reactive protein allows your doctor "to detect cardiovascular risk even among healthy people with no symptoms or other risk factors—people who would otherwise be missed with a standard lipid test...." Dr. Ridker and his associates note that, "To date, ten prospective studies, six in the U.S. and four in Europe, have consistently shown that hs-CRP is a powerful predictor of future first coronary event in apparently healthy men and women."[338]

In one of the latest studies, it was *the* most powerful predictor. WebMD Medical News reports that researchers collected data from more than 20,000 postmenopausal women and compared 12 different risk factors for heart disease, including cholesterol, cigarette smoking, obesity, and diabetes. After examining the data, Dr. Ridker concluded that, "high-sensitivity CRP was the strongest single predictor" for a first time heart attack. The WebMD article explained that "the risk of heart attack was more than four times higher for women with the highest levels of hs-CRP, compared to those with the lowest levels."[339]

And in April of 2002, the Minnesota Health Technology Advisory Committee issued an Executive Summary that included this assessment of the predictive benefits of hs-CRP testing in healthy people who have no signs of cardiovascular disease:

> "Risks for Coronary Artery Disease or cardiovascular disease (CVD) are increased by 2-to 7-fold in individuals with the highest levels of CRP compared with those with the lowest level. Increased CRP levels can be detected several years before the clinical onset of Coronary Artery Disease."[340]

Clearly, hs-CRP testing is a great advancement in predicting future cardiovascular troubles. And because the hs-CRP test is only now being made widely available, a Center for Disease Control committee of physicians is creating guidelines for the use and interpretation of hs-CRP testing. Just about the time that this book goes to press, the guidelines should be in place. They're slated to be published in the November 2002 issue of *Circulation*, an official journal of the American Heart

Association, followed by a national campaign of education about the test, for both doctors and their patients.

But let me state my own recommendation right now: *everyone over the age of 40 should include hs-CRP testing as part of his cardiovascular examination.*

The detection of chronic inflammation in the body is one of the strongest early indicators of cardiovascular trouble. Despite the newness of the hs-CRP test, it immediately jumps to the head of the pack as an important predictive tool and a necessary step of WIN/WIN Therapy.

How necessary? Well, as the Associated Press reported, in 2001, the White House doctors who gave President George W. Bush his first annual physical checkup as Chief Executive included the new hs-CRP test as part of his examination.

The desirable range of CRP in the blood is different for men and women. In men, we like to see levels less than .55 mg/L and for women it should be less than 1.5 mg/L. If your test comes back with numbers higher than these, then you are considered to be at risk for future stroke, heart attack or peripheral artery disease. Generally speaking, the higher the number, the greater the risk. You should consult your own physician on the significance of your number.

It was good news for President Bush—his numbers were very low. But the advanced hs-CRP test is no longer limited to Chief Executives and Heads of State. It's now available to anyone who needs it—which is just about everyone.

Fibrinogen

As we discovered in Chapter Nine, fibrinogen is a protein that helps to create blood clots. Fibrinogen is closely associated with levels of inflammation in the blood and has been linked to the severity and extent of atherosclerosis in the heart and brain.

In adults, normal levels of fibrinogen are between 150–350 mg/dL. If your blood test comes back with levels higher than 350, you are considered to be at an increased risk for cardiovascular disease, heart attack and cerebrovascular disease.

Although as yet no drug has been designed specifically to lower fibrinogen levels, there are ways to naturally lessen the amount of fibrinogen in the body. Perhaps the most significant reduction can be achieved by quitting smoking, because smoking is greatly associated with high fibrinogen levels. Other steps to take include losing weight, lowering cholesterol and exercising regularly, all of which have been shown to reduce fibrinogen levels.

Infections have also been linked to increased amounts of fibrinogen in the body, which leads us to testing for…

Cardiovascular Germs

All the germs of cardiovascular disease can be detected through testing for antibodies in *serum*, the fluid portion of the blood. The germs stimulate the body to produce antibodies to each specific germ. A positive finding of antibodies indicates a current or past infection by the germ.

A positive finding of *Chlamydia pneumoniae*—the Heart Attack Germ—generally means you are at increased risk for stroke, heart attack and other cardiovascular troubles. Positive findings for the other germs—*Helicobacter pylori*, cytomegalovirus and Herpes simplex—also indicate an increased risk for cardiovascular disease. The total "infectious burden" also comes into play; if you have positive findings to two or more of the cardiovascular germs, your risk increases dramatically.

Because using antibiotics and antiviral drugs to treat cardiovascular disease is still in its infancy, some doctors may be reluctant to treat their patients with these drugs. But if you can demonstrate to your doctor that you have an active infection by a specific germ or bacteria, he is much more likely to prescribe these medicines. And by treating a particular infection, he is also treating you for cardiovascular disease.

To detect an active infection—as opposed to a chronic or past infection—a second blood test may be ordered after a few weeks to see if the level of antibodies has risen.

Other factors that might influence your doctor's choice to use antibiotics are your CRP and fibrinogen levels. Both proteins are indications of possible infection. Infection by one or more of the cardiovascular germs along with above-average levels of CRP and fibrinogen makes you a good candidate for antibiotic or antiviral therapy.

With blood testing completed, it's time to move on to...

Step 3
Use conventional therapy to treat the diseases and conditions that contribute to strokes and heart attacks.

Step 3 is likely to be the shortest section in this chapter, and with good reason.

When I sat down to write *The Heart Attack Germ*, I was determined not to simply repeat the same material that could be found in other health books. I wanted *The Heart Attack Germ* to be unique—filled with information that the reader couldn't find anywhere else, yet was vital to his understanding of cardiovascular disease.

That's why this chapter on conventional therapy will be a short one.

Modern medicine has many effective drugs and treatments to control the cardiovascular problems I find upon examination—such as angina and arrhythmias—as well as the various diseases and conditions that contribute to cardiovascular problems, such as diabetes and hypertension. I use these treatments every day in my office, which is why they are a part of WIN/WIN Therapy.

For example, arrhythmias can often be stabilized with medications such as **beta blockers**, which block certain actions of the sympathetic nervous system. High blood pressure can be controlled through simple weight loss and drugs such as beta blockers, **calcium channel blockers**, which widen blood vessels, and **ACE inhibitors**, which also work to reduce the constriction of blood vessels, thus reducing hypertension. Calcium channel blockers also reduce spasm in the arteries, which can help prevent the cracking of cholesterol plaque. Damaged heart valves can be surgically replaced with artificial valves. Even the symptoms of heart failure can be helped with the proper combination of treatments.

Conventional treatments are certainly a large part of my practice, and Step 3 is a critical part of WIN/WIN Therapy. But information on these and other conventional treatments can be found elsewhere, in literally thousands of health books, pamphlets and magazine articles.

So despite the importance of conventional treatments, there's no reason to spend time on this material in *The Heart Attack Germ*. You're certain to find all the information you need from other sources. It's better that we push forward and explore the advanced treatments that specifically target the infections and inflammation that are the source of most strokes and heart attacks. So, it's onward to…

Step 4
Use antibiotic, antiviral and anti-inflammatory drugs to control cardiovascular infection and inflammation.

If, during the course of examination, I detected the presence of atherosclerosis—even in the beginning stages—I would prescribe a course of antibiotic drugs. By the time a patient has reached middle age, it is nearly certain that he has been infected by one or more of the chronic germs of cardiovascular disease.

In my own practice, it seems beside the point to test patients for infection by *Chlamydia pneumoniae* or the other germs of cardiovascular disease. From my experience, the discovery of atherosclerosis is *in itself* a sign of infection, so antibiotics or antiviral drugs are called for. Since most cardiovascular infections such as *Chlamydia pneumoniae* are hidden, producing no visible symptoms, it isn't necessary for the patient to exhibit outward signs of infection—the presence of atherosclerosis is symptom enough.

Generally, I prescribe a ten-day course of the antibiotic azithromycin, which has been shown to be particularly effective against *Chlamydia pneumoniae* germs. But as we've learned in this book, *Chlamydia* is a very tough germ to eradicate completely. The body can't do it alone, and often the antibiotic can't completely eliminate the germ either.

Generally speaking, if the antibiotic can find the germ, it will kill it. The problem with the *Cp* germ is that it is often beyond the reach of the antibiotic. *Cp* bacteria can live inside cholesterol plaque, which has no blood supply. Therefore, the antibiotic may be unsuccessful in reaching all the germs, leaving a reservoir of infection. This may be why *Cp* infections are so often chronic in nature.

The most you can expect is to control the germ—to keep a lid on it and prevent it from doing serious damage, which the azithromycin is able to accomplish. Reinfection is a hallmark of *Chlamydia*, so I always advise my patients to return once a year for another examination to see how they're doing. If the atherosclerosis shows signs of progressing, another round of antibiotics is called for. This can be repeated indefinitely.

If I discover signs of viral infection in the patient, then I will prescribe antiviral drugs to treat both the acute infection and its influence on atherosclerosis. Whenever I see an outbreak of herpes zoster or herpes simplex on a patient, I'm always suspicious that's it's igniting something in the cardiovascular system, too. A typical drug to use would be Valtrex, 1000 mg three times a day for a week, then one a day for about a month.

If a person seems sickly, losing their strength or generally not progressing properly in their health, I'm likely to prescribe a course of antiviral drugs, especially if the patient is older, when hidden infections are likely. Such patients almost always respond very positively to this therapy—they feel better, think better and act better when chronic viral infections are brought under control.

In previous chapters, I made a point of presenting the many different ways that infection and inflammation combine to create cardiovascular troubles. Here at last we can put all of that knowledge to practical use with additional therapies aimed at reducing infection and inflammation.

For example, in Chapter 10 we discussed the link between heart disease and gum infections. So proper oral hygiene and visiting your dentist on a regular basis is an effective way to prevent infection and inflammation from contributing to cardiovascular troubles.

Also in Chapter 10, we discussed the link between respiratory infection and strokes and heart attacks. So I recommend that patients get their yearly flu shot as a way of reducing their cardiovascular risks.

In Chapter 9, we discussed how aspirin reduces the risk of death in patients with heart disease. So for patients who suffer from previous heart attacks or unstable angina, daily aspirin use is a standard part of anti-inflammatory and anti-clotting therapy.

And finally, in Chapter 14, we discussed the link between cardiovascular germs, stroke and the symptoms of Alzheimer's disease. So patients with Alzheimer's who have evidence of cerebrovascular disease should also be treated with antibiotic and antiviral drugs to prevent stroke and reduce the symptoms of Alzheimer's.

The final step of WIN/WIN Therapy is…

Step 5
Control personal risk factors that contribute to arterial injury and inflammation.

The combination of risk factors and cardiovascular infection does more damage than either element individually. "Reducing risk factors" is simply another way of saying "reducing artery injury and inflammation," so it makes sense to do what you can about risk factors.

Your physician can take care of risk factor diseases or medical conditions such as diabetes, hypertension and, to some extent, cholesterol levels. But personal risk factors such as smoking, obesity, diet and exercise depend on your own intervention.

There are many books that will guide you through personal risk reduction, but let me offer a few suggestions based on the experiences of my patients.

When people make the effort to set aside the time for regular, daily exercise, it seems to create a mindset for taking care of the body is other ways. People willing to exercise just naturally begin to take an interest in their health, motivating them to watch what they eat, quit smoking and so on.

Regular exercise reduces obesity and cholesterol levels, while toning the cardiovascular system, so it's an efficient way to tackle a number of factors at once. If you're exercising, you're not eating ice cream or candy, you're probably not stressing like you would at the office, you're not smoking—in short, you're doing a whole lot of other things that may be giving you more benefit than just the physical exercise.

It is important, however, not to overdo it, especially at first. Recently, three friends of mine began exercise programs to improve their cardiovascular fitness. All three of them had to give up after a few months because of foot and knee injuries. Instead of helping to make them healthier, their overly ambitious exercise programs had the exact opposite effect!

Moreover, there is no long-term cardiovascular benefit to strenuous exercise. Moderate exercise—such as brisk walking for 30 minutes to an hour—is all that's necessary to achieve results. As a general rule, the *amount of time* you spend exercising is more important than the intensity of the exercise.

Diets are notoriously difficult to stick with. Eating should not be a science project, but diets almost demand that you treat them as such. It's boring and bothersome to plan and prepare special meals, to spend time figuring out the caloric values of specific portions, and so on. Eventually, the diet becomes so difficult to maintain that it's abandoned.

So I give my patients this simple bit of advice that eliminates much of the anxiety and difficulty surrounding a healthy diet: *eat a colorful plate at every meal.*

Most people with poor diets eat plates of food that are basically one or two colors—gray or white. Pasta, meats, potatoes, breads—they're all variations on the same two colors. And they keep eating large portions of these same two colors, day in and day out.

In contrast, a plate with five or six different colors on it will always assure a varied diet that is generally much healthier. Almost all fruits and vegetables are colorful—orange carrots, green peas, different colored melons, radishes, etc. A colorful plate doesn't require keeping track of calories or special preparation or all of those other tasks that make dieting so onerous. Simply by making sure that each meal contains five or six different colors, you'll go a long way towards a healthier diet.

Perhaps you've noticed that I've barely mentioned dietary salt in this book. A few years ago, it would have been unthinkable that a book about cardiovascular disease wouldn't have emphasized the reduction of salt intake by the average person as necessary step for cardiovascular health.

For the past two decades, Americans have been told repeatedly that eating too much salt increases the average person's risk of heart disease and stroke by raising blood pressure. We've also been told that, to protect against the risk, we need to reduce our salt intake.

As a result, every aisle in the supermarket has dozens of low sodium products for "healthy eating" and many people with no cardiovascular problems have banned salt from their tables.

However, a number of studies beginning in the mid-1990s challenged the conventional wisdom of salt reduction by the average person. A 1996 study published in the Journal of the American Medical Association analyzed 56 previous studies and found that healthy people—and even some patients with high blood pressure—gained little from lowering the salt in their diet.[341] And a separate study found that hypertensive patients with the lowest salt in their diets were four times *more likely* to have a heart attack compared to the other participants.[342]

If you'll notice, restricting the intake of dietary salt is mentioned less and less in stories about reducing cardiovascular risk factors. It's all still a matter of controversy, and whether you should reduce salt in your diet is a matter between you and your physician. In my own practice, I don't advise my healthy patients to reduce their normal intake of salt. And if they suffer from hypertension, the medicines we have today are a far superior way of lowering blood pressure.

3

An Added Advantage of WIN/WIN Therapy

Not only does WIN/WIN Therapy reduce the risk of acute cardiovascular events, it provides an additional benefit by limiting the need for invasive surgery such as angioplasty and coronary bypass surgery.

This is an extremely significant advantage of WIN/WIN Therapy.

All surgery is inherently dangerous, expensive, time-consuming and painful. Some kinds of cardiovascular surgery, such as pacemaker implantation and valve replacement, have proven to be beneficial. But surgery rarely cures a metabolic disease, and atherosclerotic disease is no exception.

Many patients are not fully aware of what cardiovascular surgery will—and will not—accomplish. They assume that their doctors are suggesting the drastic step of surgery because a cardiac crisis is imminent and an operation is the only way to prevent the crisis.

In truth, angioplasties and bypass surgeries are often undertaken when there is no immediate danger for the patient, but simply because there is an indication of heart disease—perhaps pain in the chest, or an angiogram showing cholesterol plaque in one or more of the coronary arteries of the heart. These non-emergency operations are called *elective surgery*.

But, except for situations that meet certain, specific criteria, there is little evidence that either angioplasty or coronary artery bypass reduces the rate of heart attacks or increases the longevity of patients compared to non-surgical treatments using medications.

For example, a long-term study released in 1999 compared statistics for two groups of stable angina patients—those who initially received surgical treatment for their angina and those who received non-surgical medical treatment. The study found that initial bypass surgery neither improved the rate of survival for low-risk patients nor reduced the overall risk of heart attack, compared to the nonsurgical patients. The study also found that, for high-risk patients, the long term survival rates were essentially the same for both the surgical and nonsurgical groups.[343]

In fact, much of the cardiovascular surgery done today can *increase* your risk for a stroke or heart attack. As odd as it sounds, cardiovascular surgery itself is responsible for a significant percentage of all strokes and heart attacks.

During the trauma of cardiovascular surgery, particles of plaque and blood clots are introduced into the bloodstream where they travel as emboli, eventually becoming lodged in the arteries of brain. Either immediately or a few days after surgery, these emboli cause occlusions resulting in both mini-strokes and more serious strokes. The damage from these strokes can cause various kinds of neurologic damage such as confusion, memory loss and personality changes in the patient

How serious is this problem? A 2000 article in *Stroke*, a journal of the American Medical Association, put it this way:

> "Current estimates indicate that more than 50% of patients who undergo cardiopulmonary bypass have neurologic or neuropsychological deficits during the first week after surgery.... 10 to 30% have long-term or permanent deficits and 1 to 5% suffer severe disability or death."[344]

Elective angioplasty also has its risks. A 1997 article from *Family Practice News* reveals that, "Angina patients who have elective coronary angioplasty have a nearly two-fold higher risk of death or [heart attack] than similar patients who are managed medically." Dr. Chamberlain, a physician at the Royal Sussex County Hospital, England, who served as chair of the study, advised that, "You lose nothing by waiting to perform angioplasty, and there is no automatic prognostic benefit from angioplasty."[345]

Here's a similar example from 1997 concerning carotid endarterectomy, the surgical procedure to remove cholesterol plaque from inside carotid arteries. An article from the publication *Patient Care* had this to say:

> "The European Carotid Surgery Trial concluded that carotid endarterectomy is not beneficial and may even be harmful in patients who have a mild [narrowing of the artery from cholesterol plaque]....Interim results from the continuation of the trial have shown that endarterectomy is not indicated for most and possibly all patients who have moderate (30–69%) carotid [narrowing]. The trial investigators concluded that the time before any advantage in stroke-free life expectancy could be achieved would be four–five years in the 50–69% [narrowed] groups and six–seven years in that 30–49% [narrowed] group. The likelihood of the patient ever realizing that advantage is small...."[346]

As this article indicates, endarterectomies are not advised for patients who have a mild or even moderate narrowing of the carotid arteries.

The bottom line: most cardiovascular surgery is an admission of failure by your doctor. Surgery is a "do-or-die" tactic—a physician's way of saying, "I give up!" If surgery were truly effective, doctors would use it as their *first* option. But, of course, they don't. They always save it for last because they know just how poor an option it is.

A much better alternative is to limit the growth and consequences of atherosclerotic disease with safe, painless and inexpensive anti-infective and anti-inflammatory therapy—just what WIN/WIN Therapy provides.

4

The Future of WIN/WIN Therapy and the Heart Attack Germ

WIN/WIN Therapy is a work in progress.

Science has only just discovered the role of infection and inflammation as a source of cardiovascular illness. The medicines that we're using now to treat cardiovascular infection and inflammation are off-the-shelf remedies, created for other illnesses but pressed into service against strokes and heart attacks.

This will change in the future.

New antibiotic and antiviral drugs will be designed to target the specific germs of cardiovascular disease such as *Chlamydia pneumoniae*. Stronger anti-inflammatory agents will be perfected and directed against the particular inflammatory process found inside blood vessels.

And work has already begun on what may prove to be the decisive answer in the fight against the germs of cardiovascular disease: vaccination.

A *vaccine* is a substance containing a weakened or dead germ that is introduced to the body. The body responds to the vaccine by boosting the immune system's ability to recognize and destroy the germ. So if the real thing ever tries to infect the body, the immune system is fully prepared to quickly eliminate the threat. In this way, the body is inoculated against the germ and kept free of disease.

A vaccine against strokes and heart attacks would have been an absurd idea a few, short years ago. But the breakthrough discovery of cardiovascular germs has turned the unthinkable into a common sense proposal.

As it happens, the development of vaccines against the germs of cardiovascular disease, such as cytomegalovirus and *Chlamydia pneumoniae*, is already ongoing.[347, 348, 349, 350] And researchers are designing trial experiments to test the effectiveness of these vaccines.

Most likely, vaccination will not be of much help to patients already suffering from cardiovascular disease—antibiotics and antiviral drugs will still be the drugs of choice. But a preventive vaccine is the ultimate goal for researchers.

Perhaps the best way to explain why vaccination holds such promise for the future is to take a look at a triumph of vaccination from the past…

The Fight against Polio as a Model for the Fight against Strokes and Heart Attacks

There are many similarities between medicine's early treatments for polio and the current conventional treatments to prevent strokes and heart attacks.

Medicine has a history of treating the symptoms, rather than the causes, of infective disease—mostly because it is either unaware of, or unable to treat, the underlying infection. The struggle against polio is a classic example of the difference between treating the symptoms of infection and treating the infection itself.

First, a few facts about polio.

Poliomyelitis, or *polio*, is an infective disease that can lead to paralysis. Although polio has existed for many centuries, it was not until 1912 that the cause of this disease was firmly established to be a virus.

But even with this knowledge, there was no effective treatment for polio at the time of the nationwide epidemic that struck more than 50,000 Americans in the early 1950s. Treatment was limited to alleviating the paralytic *symptoms* of the disease; there was no treatment against the virus itself.

Perhaps the most famous treatment for polio victims of the 1950s was the "iron lung"—a large, metal respirator that encased a victim who, because of paralyzed breathing muscles, was unable to breathe for himself. The iron lung—complex, costly and labor-intensive—didn't cure the patient, but it helped him through critical moments until the acute stage of the illness passed. Heavy metal braces were also used to assist the paralyzed muscles of the legs. But both braces and the iron lung did nothing to prevent polio—they were only attempts to treat its symptoms.

It wasn't until 1954, when a vaccine against polio was finally available, that medicine had an effective way to prevent the disease. This change in therapy was revolutionary, sweeping away everything that had gone before. A vast segment of the medical profession collapsed into irrelevance—no more hospital polio wards, polio specialists or crude therapies like the iron lung. In the space of a decade they were all rendered obsolete by a few simple injections of polio vaccine.

The lesson of the polio story is clear: *treating the infection, instead of the mere symptoms of infection, makes all the difference.*

And it's a lesson that is finally being applied to strokes and heart attacks.

Right now, the usual treatments for atherosclerosis, strokes and heart attacks are in the "iron lung" stage. Angioplasty, bypass surgery, cardiac wards, stroke rehabilitation centers—these are "iron lung" treatments. We wait until the body is injured by infection, and then attempt to treat the symptoms of the injury.

But antibiotics and antiviral drugs—safe, painless and inexpensive—can significantly reduce the risk of a stroke or heart attack by treating the underlying infection. Already, these drugs are easing the need for dangerous and often ineffective cardiovascular therapies such as angioplasty and bypass surgery.

And the future holds the promise of a preventive vaccine. Vaccinating a child before he becomes infected will completely eliminate the atherosclerosis, strokes and heart attacks associated with the germs of cardiovascular disease. With a successful cardiovascular vaccine, many of the present-day cardiovascular treatments of rehabilitation and surgery may be rendered as obsolete as the iron lung.

And that will be medicine's ultimate victory over the Heart Attack Germ.

5

The Heart Attack Germ on the Web at www.theheartattackgerm.com

If this book has made you reconsider the cause and prevention of cardiovascular disease, it's understandable that you'd like to find additional sources of information on the topics we've covered.

But the discovery that infection and inflammation are the hidden players behind strokes, heart attacks and the symptoms of Alzheimer's is so new that—if you went to your local library or bookstore in search of more information—the only book you'd find on the subject is the very one you're now holding in your hands.

As a physician, I'm able to subscribe to many professional journals and medical newspapers that arrive at my house and office by the boatload. Most of these journals specialize in cardiovascular news, keeping me abreast of the latest developments in the link between infection, inflammation and cardiovascular disease.

But aside from the occasional newspaper or magazine article, the average reader had no place to turn to for the latest news about these topics. That's why I created…

theheartattackgerm.com

theheartattackgerm.com is a companion web site for this book, dedicated to informing my readers—and the public at large—of the continuing research into infection, inflammation and cardiovascular disease.

Every week, the site is updated with the latest research studies and medical journal articles from around the world, concerning topics such as cardiovascular germs, antibiotic therapy, inflammatory risk factors, vulnerable plaque, blood vessel spasm—in short, every key issue that I've covered in the book.

Also every week, I include my own personal commentary on the meaning and significance of these scientific studies, in language that the average reader can understand.

theheartattackgerm.com also features links to media web pages that run stories concerning these same issues. For example, when *Fox News* or *Good Morning America* airs a medical segment of interest, I'll link to their on-line site for a transcript or video rerun of the program. That way, you'll catch the important stories that you might otherwise miss.

In addition, theheartattackgerm.com contains text and animated movies that further explain the role of infection and inflammation in cardiovascular disease.

So come visit me on-line and get the latest. You will definitely be inside the loop, ahead of the curve and up to speed on the breakthrough discoveries of *The Heart Attack Germ*.

About the Authors

Dr. Louis A. Dvonch was a scholarship student at the Julliard School of Music in 1937–38. He attended Loyola University and graduated from the Loyola Medical School with a Doctor of Medicine degree in 1945. After serving in the U.S. Army Medical Corps, Dr. Dvonch went into private practice as a surgeon and general practitioner in 1947. He joined the staff of St. Anne's Hospital in Chicago, Illinois, where he held the posts of Chairman of the Emergency Room Department and Chairman of the Post Graduate Teaching Department. In 1976, he moved his practice to Naples, Florida and joined the staff of Naples Community Hospital, becoming Chairman of the Department of Family Practice.

Russell Dvonch is a writer living in North Hollywood, California.

Endnotes

1. Falck G, Heyman L, Gnarpe J, Gnarpe H: *Chlamydia pneumoniae* and chronic pharyngitis. Scand J Infect Dis1995; 27(2): 179–82

    "*Chlamydia pneumoniae* has been implicated as an etiological agent for both upper and lower respiratory tract infections. We describe 4 cases of chronic pharyngitis where *Chlamydia pneumoniae* appears to be the etiological agent."

2. Falck G, Heyman L, Gnarpe J, Gnarpe H: *Chlamydia pneumoniae* (TWAR): a common agent in acute bronchitis. Scand J Infect Dis 1994; 26(2): 179–87

    "We conclude that *C. pneumoniae* can be a major cause of acute bronchitis."

3. Saikku P: The epidemiology and significance of *Chlamydia pneumoniae*. J Infect 1992 Jul; 25 Suppl 1: 27–34

    "It is the commonest *Chlamydia* of mankind but fortunately the overwhelming majority of infections are mild, it has been estimated that 10% of all pneumonias are caused by this species."

4. Odeh M, Oliven A: Chlamydial infections of the heart. Eur J Clin Microbiol Infect Dis 1992 Oct; 11(10): 885–93

    "These organisms are documented to cause endocarditis, myocarditis and pericarditis."

5. Gnarpe H, Gnarpe J, Gastrin B, Hallander H: *Chlamydia pneumoniae* and myocarditis. Scand J Infect Dis Suppl 1997; 104: 50–2

"The findings were discussed and it was concluded that *C. pneumoniae* may be associated with inflammatory heart disease."

6. Saikku P, Wang SP, Kleemola M, Brander E, Rusanen E, Grayston JT: An epidemic of mild pneumonia due to an unusual strain of *Chlamydia psittaci*. J Infect Dis 1985 May, 151(5): 832–9
7. Grayston JT, Kuo CC, Wang SP, Altman J: A new *Chlamydia psittaci* strain, TWAR, isolated in acute respiratory tract infections. N Engl J Med 1986 Jul 17; 315(3): 161–8
8. Saikku P, Leinonen M, Tenkanen L, Linnanmaki E, Ekman MR, Manninen V, Manttari M, Frick MH, Huttunen JK: Chronic *Chlamydia pneumoniae* infection as a risk factor for coronary heart disease in the Helsinki Heart Study. Ann Intern Med 1992 Feb 15; 116(4): 273–8

    "The results suggest that chronic *C. pneumoniae* infection may be a significant risk factor for the development of coronary heart disease."

9. Falck G, Gnarpe J, Gnarpe H: Prevalence of *Chlamydia pneumoniae* in healthy children and in children with respiratory tract infections. Pediatr Infect Dis J 1997 Jun; 16(6): 549–54

    "The findings suggest that *C. pneumoniae* is common among children with respiratory tract infections."

10. Monno R, Di Bitonto G, Marcuccio L, Valenza M, Marcuccio C: Antibodies to *Chlamydia pneumoniae* in healthy children from Bari, south Italy. New Microbiol 1998 Jul; 21(3): 281–4
11. Heiskanen-Kosma T, Korppi M, Jokinen C, Kurki S, Heiskanen L, Juvonen H, Kallinen S, Sten M, Tarkiainen A, Ronnberg PR, Kleemola M, Makela PH, Leinonen M: Etiology of childhood pneumonia: serologic results of a prospective, population-based study. Pediatr Infect Dis J 1998 Nov; 17(11): 986–91

"*M. pneumoniae* and *Chlamydia pneumoniae* are important from the age of 5 years onwards."

12. Kuo CC, Shor A, Campbell LA, Fukushi H, Patton DL, Grayston JT: Demonstration of *Chlamydia pneumoniae* in atherosclerotic lesions of coronary arteries. J Infect Dis 1993 Apr; 167(4): 841–9

    "Antibody prevalence studies have shown that virtually everyone is infected with the *C. pneumoniae* organisms at some time and that reinfection is common."

13. Nalepa P: *Chlamydia pneumoniae* as an etiologic factor in disease of the respiratory tract. Pol Merkuriusz Lek 1997 Oct; 3(16): 208–9

    "The described recently species of *Chlamydia pneumoniae* is the subject of a large number of scientific reports. The majority of infections caused by this microorganism are asymptomatic."

14. Hyman CL, Roblin PM, Gaydos CA, Quinn TC, Schachter J, Hammerschlag MR: Prevalence of asymptomatic nasopharyngeal carriage of *Chlamydia pneumoniae* in subjectively healthy adults: assessment by polymerase chain reaction-enzyme immunoassay and culture. Clin Infect Dis 1995 May; 20(5): 1174–8

    "Although *Chlamydia pneumoniae* is a well-described and common respiratory tract pathogen, up to 90% of infections with this organism are thought to be asymptomatic."

15. Theunissen HJ, Lemmens-den Toom NA, Burggraaf A, Stolz E, Michel MF: Influence of temperature and relative humidity on the survival of *Chlamydia pneumoniae* in aerosols. Appl Environ Microbiol 1993 Aug; 59(8): 2589–93

    "It was concluded that transmission of *C. pneumoniae* via aerosols was possible. There is probably a direct transmission from person to person, taking into account the relatively short survival period of *C. pneumoniae* in aerosols."

16. Falsey AR, Walsh EE: Transmission of *Chlamydia pneumoniae*. J Infect Dis 1993 Aug; 168(2): 493–6

    "These observations suggest that several mechanisms of transmission of *C. pneumoniae* are possible, including the transfer of fomites from environmental surfaces with subsequent autoinoculation."

17. Normann E, Gnarpe J, Gnarpe H, Wettergren B: *Chlamydia pneumoniae* in children attending day-care centers in Gavle, Sweden. Pediatr Infect Dis J 1998 Jun; 17(6): 474–8

    "The organism seems to be easily communicable among individuals living in close proximity."

18. Normann E, Gnarpe J, Gnarpe H occurrence of *Chlamydia pneumoniae* infection. Ugeskr Laeger 1996 Feb 26; 158(9): 1228–9

    "The clinical courses of six patients involved in a family outbreak of *Chlamydia pneumoniae* respiratory tract infection are described."

19. Csango PA, Haraldstad S, Pedersen JE, Jagars G, Foreland I: Respiratory tract infection due to *Chlamydia pneumoniae* in military personnel. Scand J Infect Dis Suppl 1997; 104: 26–9

    "The objective of this investigation was to determine whether *Chlamydia pneumoniae* was involved in an outbreak of respiratory disease among military recruits...The combination of serological methods showed that 40 out of 52 (76.9%) had an acute infection with possible Chlamydial aetiology."

20. Normann E, Gnarpe J, Gnarpe H, Wettergren B: *Chlamydia pneumoniae* in children attending day-care centers in Gavle, Sweden. Pediatr Infect Dis J 1998 Jun; 17(6): 474–8

"*C. pneumoniae* can be commonly found in young children attending day care. Most of the youngest children did not develop specific antibodies. Children may have subclinical infections with *C. pneumoniae*."

21. Troy CJ, Peeling RW, Ellis AG, Hockin JC, Bennett DA, Murphy MR, Spika JS: *Chlamydia pneumoniae* as a new source of infectious outbreaks in nursing homes. JAMA 1997 Apr 16; 277(15): 1214–8

"*Chlamydia pneumoniae* caused serious morbidity and mortality among residents and morbidity among staff; *C. pneumoniae* is an important cause of respiratory disease outbreaks in nursing homes, and diagnostic tests must be readily available for early recognition of *C. pneumoniae* infections."

22. Magee, R: Arterial disease in antiquity. Medical Journal of Australia 1998; 169: 663–666.

"In 1975, Aidan Cockburn and co-workers published the findings of an autopsy on the mummy known as Pum II (Pennsylvania University Museum mummy number II). The wrappings, resins and tissues were all examined in great detail. The aorta was found to contain large and small atheromatous plaques, and other vessels in organs returned to the body cavity in visceral packages showed some intimal fibrous thickening consistent with arteriolar sclerosis."

23. AHA Medical/Scientific Statement: A Definition of Initial, Fatty Streak, and Intermediate Lesions of Atherosclerosis. Circulation. 1994; 89: 2462–2478

24. Muhlestein JB: The Link Between *Chlamydia pneumoniae* and Atherosclerosis. Infect Med 14(5): 380–382,392,426, 1997

25. Brown BG, Zhao XQ, Sacco DE, Albers JJ: Lipid lowering and plaque regression. New insights into prevention of plaque dis-

ruption and clinical events in coronary disease. Circulation 1993 Jun; 87(6): 1781–91

"Lesions with these characteristics constitute only 10–20% of the overall lesion population but account for 80–90% of the acute clinical events."

26. Davies MJ, Woolf N, Rowles P, Richardson PD: Lipid and cellular constituents of unstable human aortic plaques. Basic Res Cardiol 1994; 89 Suppl 1: 33–9

"It is therefore possible to define a vulnerable plaque as one in which the lipid core is disproportionately large, the cap thin, and in which monocytes preponderate over smooth muscle cells."

27. Davies MJ: Acute coronary thrombosis—the role of plaque disruption and its initiation and prevention. Eur Heart J 1995 Nov; 16 Suppl L: 3–7

"Studies comparing intact and disrupted plaques have been used to define the characteristics of vulnerable plaques i.e. those at risk of disruption. The characteristics are a lipid core occupying over 50% of overall plaque volume, a thin plaque cap, a large absolute number and density of macrophages, and a reduction in the smooth muscle content of the plaque."

28. Inflammation, Infection, and Coronary Artery Disease. Reinsuance Notes Vol.1, No.11, 1998

29. van der Wal AC, Becker AE, van der Loos CM, Tigges AJ, Das PK: Fibrous and lipid-rich atherosclerotic plaques are part of interchangeable morphologies related to inflammation: a concept. Coron Artery Dis 1994 Jun; 5(6): 463–9

"Our observations support the concept that inflammatory mechanisms modulate plaque morphology, by promoting either synthesis or lysis of the fibrous cap."

30. Richardson PD, Davis MJ, Born GVR: Influence of plaque configuration and stress distribution on fissuring of coronary atherosclerotic plaques. Lancet. 1989; 2: 941–944.

31. Davies, M: Remarks at Asian-Pacific Congress on Vascular Disease Prevention Vascular Disease Prevention.—Singapore. Report titled "Atherosclerotic Plaques-Why do they rupture?" at **http://www.medinfo.co.za/data/med_info/athero.htm**

32. Davies, MJ: The Composition of Coronary-Artery Plaques. The New England Journal of Medicine—May 1, 1997—Vol. 336, No. 18

33. Kornfeld, JL: Macrophages in Coronary Lesions Are Likely Contributors to Acute Ischemia. American College of Cardiology Conference Watch 1995

    "The macrophage product TF is known to instigate thrombosis in vitro. In autopsy studies, it is more abundant in ACS-associated lesions than in counterpart lesions from stable angina patients, and it tended to concentrate in the lipid-rich pool, a plaque region that appears to be highly thrombogenic when exposed by rupture (Basic Res Cardiol 1994; 89 [suppl 1]: 33.)."

34. Glim, M: Old at Heart. Physician's Weekly Dec. 13, 1999 Volume XVI, No. 47

35. Ihling, Christian: Pathomorphologic Classification of Coronary Atherosclerosis. Herz 23: 69–77, (1998)

    "Functionally, active plaques are characterized by a locally enhanced vasoreactivity with evidence coming from our own recent investigations that localised chronic inflammatory processes within the atherosclerotic plaque are responsible not only for the plaque rupture itself…"

36. Hademenos, George J: The Biophysics of Stroke. American Scientist May-June 1997

"Since the velocity of the blood is also higher, flow through the stenosed vessel has a greater tendency to become turbulent. Turbulent flow allows the blood's kinetic energy to be transferred into the cracks and crevices of plaque, potentially dislodging chunks of plaque into the bloodstream."

37. Willich SN, Klatt S, Arntz HR: Circadian variation and triggers of acute coronary syndromes. Eur Heart J 1998 Apr; 19 Suppl C: C12–23

38. Reuters Health Anger Expression Ups Stroke Risk. Mar 18, 1999 (SOURCE: Stroke 1999; 30: 523–528.)

39. Verrier RL, Mittleman MA: Life-threatening cardiovascular consequences of anger in patients with coronary heart disease. Cardiol Clin 1996 May; 14(2): 289–307

40. Cocco G, Iselin HU: Cardiac risk of speed traps. Clin Cardiol 1992 Jun; 15(6): 441–4

"Twenty-two patients with stable cardiac disease drove into a radar trap while having an ambulatory electrocardiogram. All patients reported cardiac symptoms, heart rate increases, and appearance of repetitive ventricular arrhythmias. Myoca dial ischemia was observed in some patients. Being caught while car speeding under the stresses of daily life may induce potentially dangerous cardiac effects. The data confirm the effects of stress and adrenergic tone on ventricular arrhythmias."

41. Leor J, Poole WK, Kloner RA: Sudden cardiac death triggered by an earthquake. N Engl J Med 1996 Feb 15; 334(7): 413–9

"The Northridge earthquake was a significant trigger of sudden death due to cardiac causes, independently of physical exerion. This finding, along with the unusually low incidence of such deaths in the week after the earthquake, suggests that emotional stress may precipitate cardiac events in peoplewho are predisposed to such events."

42. Auch-Schwelk W: Coronary spasm—a clinically relevant problem? Herz 1998 Mar; 23(2): 106–15

    "Pure coronary vasospasm does not lead to increased mortality."

43. Hellstrom HR: Evidence in favor of the vasospastic cause of coronary artery thrombosis. Am Heart J 1979 Apr; 97(4): 449–52

44. Thomas B. Graboys, MD and Charles M. Blatts, MD: Angina Pectoris: Management Strategies and Guide to Interventions. Professional Communications, Inc. (PCI) 1997

    "Vasospasm can injure the endothelial surface and result in intracoronary thrombus formation, and this may be an important factor in the rupture of endothelial plaque."

45. Lin CS, Penha PD, Zak FG, Lin JC: Morphodynamic interprtation of acute coronary thrombosis, with special reference to volcano-like eruption of atheromatous plaque caused by coronary artery spasm. Angiology 1988 Jun; 39(6): 535–47.

46. Kalsner S: Coronary artery spasm. Multiple causes and multiple roles in heart disease. Biochem Pharmacol 1995 Mar 30; 49(7): 859–71

    "Myocardial infarction and sudden cardiac death may be initiated by a sudden intense localized contraction of coronary artery smooth muscle. When this event occurs around a vulnerable eccentric lipid-filled plaque, rupture and extrusion of plaque contents and exposure of collagen occur. This may sometimes be a silent and self-limiting event; other times it leads to thrombus formation."

47. Yeung AC, Vekshtein VI, Krantz DS, Vita JA, Ryan TJ Jr, Ganz P, Selwyn AP: The effect of atherosclerosis on the vasomotor response of coronary arteries to mental stress. N Engl J Med 1991 Nov 28; 325(22): 1551–6

48. Heistad DD, Armstrong ML, Lopez JA: What causes spasm of atherosclerotic arteries. Trans Am Clin Climatol Assoc 1989; 101: 103–10

"...atherosclerosis produces a profound alteration of vascular responses, which may lead to spasm in several vascular beds."

49. Shimokawa H: Primary endothelial dysfunction: atherosclerosis. J Mol Cell Cardiol 1999 Jan; 31(1): 23–37

"Endothelial dysfunction by aging, menopause and hypercholesterolemia is involved in the development of atherosclerotic vascular lesions, and predisposes the blood vessel to several vascular disorders, such as vasospasm and thrombosis."

50. Sellke FW, Boyle EM Jr, Verrier ED: Endothelial cell injury in cardiovascular surgery: the pathophysiology of vasomotor dysfunction. Ann Thorac Surg 1997 Mar; 63(3): 885–94

51. Ihling C: Pathomorphologic Classification of Coronary Atherosclerosis. Herz 23: 69–77, (1998)

"Functionally, active plaques are characterized by a locally enhanced vasoreactivity with evidence coming from our own recent investigations that localised chronic inflammatory processes within the atherosclerotic plaque are responsible not only for the plaque rupture itself, but also for the hyperreactivity of these vessels to vasoconstrictor stimuli."

52. Ludmer PL, Selwyn AP, Shook TL, Wayne RR, Mudge GH, Alexander RW, Ganz P: Paradoxical vasoconstriction induced by acetylcholine in atherosclerotic coronary arteries. N Engl J Med 1986 Oct 23; 315(17): 1046–51

53. Maseri A, Sanna T: The role of plaque fissures in unstable angina: fact or fiction? Eur Heart J 1998 Sep; 19 Suppl K: K2–4

"Activated inflammatory cells produce cytokines which can activate the endothelium making it prothrombotic and vasoco strictive…"

54. Ganz P, Alexander RW: New insights into the cellular mechanisms of vasospasm. Am J Cardiol 1985 Sep 18; 56(9): 11E–15E

    "More recent evidence, however, suggests that the basic abnormality may be hypercontractility of the arterial wall associated with the atherosclerotic process itself."

55. Hoak JC: The endothelium, platelets, and coronary vasospasm. Adv Intern Med 1989; 34: 353–75.

56. Gottdiener JS, Krantz DS, Howell RH, Hecht GM, Klein J, Falconer JJ, Rozanski A: Induction of silent myocardial ischemia with mental stress testing: relation to the triggers of ischemia during daily life activities and to ischemic functional severity. J Am Coll Cardiol 1994 Dec; 24(7): 1645–51

57. Swint, S: Level of Mental Stress May Help Doctors Predict Heart Attack. WebMD Medical News Dec. 8, 1999

    "Gottdiener, who was a professor of medicine at Georgetown University Medical Center in Washington while participating in the study, says about half of the people who have restricted blood flow while exercising also will have restricted blood flow brought on by mental stress."

58. Gottdiener JS, Krantz DS, Howell RH, Hecht GM, Klein J, Falconer JJ, Rozanski A: Induction of silent myocardial ischemia with mental stress testing: relation to the triggers of ischemia during daily life activities and to ischemic functional severity. J Am Coll Cardiol 1994 Dec; 24(7): 1645–51

    "Patients with ischemia during mental stress testing also have increased ischemia during sedentary activities in daily life."

59. Legault SE, Langer A, Armstrong PW, Freeman MR: Usefulness of ischemic response to mental stress in predicting silent myocardial ischemia during ambulatory monitoring. Am J Cardiol 1995 May 15; 75(15): 1007–11

    "In conclusion, an ischemic response to mental stress is significantly associated with higher prevalence, longer duration, and more frequent episodes of ambulatory ischemia."

60. Gullette EC, Blumenthal JA, Babyak M, Jiang W, Waugh RA, Frid DJ, O'Connor CM, Morris JJ, Krantz DS: Effects of mental stress on myocardial ischemia during daily life. JAMA 1997 May 21; 277(19): 1521–6

    "Mental stress during daily life, including reported feelings of tension, frustration, and sadness, can more than double the risk of myocardial ischemia in the subsequent hour."

61. Rozanski A, Krantz DS, Bairey CN: Ventricular responses to mental stress testing in patients with coronary artery disease. Pathophysiological implications. Circulation 1991 Apr; 83(4 Suppl): II137–44

    "This research has consistently revealed that mental stress-induced myocardial ischemia occurs frequently during laboratory stress testing, particularly among patients with exercise-induced ischemia. This ischemia is usually silent…"

62. Vassiliadis IV, Fountos AI, Papadimitriou AG, Sbonias EC: Mental stress-induced silent myocardial ischemia detected during ambulatory ventricular function monitoring. Int J Card Imaging 1998 Jun; 14(3): 171–7

    "The results provide evidence that there is marked disparity in the incidence of chest pain and ST-segment changes, despite similar ischemic ejection fraction response between mental and physical stress. This is indicative of a major role of mental stress in provoking silent ischemia that potentially might provide additional clinical information compared to exercise test."

63. Singh N, Langer A: Current status of silent myocardial ischemia. Can J Cardiol 1995 Apr; 11(4): 286–9

 "Up to 75% of ischemic episodes in patients are silent."

64. Jiang W, Babyak M, Krantz DS, Waugh RA, Coleman RE, Hanson MM, Frid DJ, McNulty S, Morris JJ, O'Connor CM, Blumenthal JA: Mental stress-induced myocardial ischemia and cardiac events. JAMA 1996 Jun 5; 275(21): 1651–6

65. American Heart Association Press Release December 1, 1997

66. Doctor's Guide On-Line Edition Better Stress Management Could Help Reduce Women's Stroke Risk. PSL Consulting Group Inc. Aug. 6, 1998

 "Researchers report in this month's issue of the journal Stroke that women who exhibit large increases in blood pressure and heart rate during mental stress may develop accelerated atherosclerosis—the disease process that obstructs blood vessels and triggers a heart attack or stroke—in the carotid arteries, the vessels that carry blood to the brain."

67. Gutstein WH: Vasospasm, vascular injury, and atherogenesis: a perspective. Hum Pathol 1999 Apr; 30(4): 365–71

 "Based on early work by the author and a selective review of the literature, evidence is presented to show how a common cardiovascular event, vasospasm, may be one of the factors responsible for this tissue damage, because it produces a substantial arteriopathy in the very vessel in which it occurs."

68. American Heart Association Press Release December 1, 1997

 "Just like elevated cholesterol, mental stress over time may injure blood vessels and promote atherosclerosis in susceptible individuals, Kamarck says."

69. Giles TD Factors affecting circadian variability Blood Press Monit 2000; 5 Suppl 1: S3–7

    "Myocardial infarction and ischemia, sudden cardiac death and stroke occur with greater frequency in the morning hours after awakening. Multiple biologic functions such as blood pressure, heart rate, sympathetic neurotransmission, vascular tone, platelet aggregability, and coagulation parameters also show a diurnal variation and appear to contribute to adverse cardiac outcomes."

70. Yasue H, Kugiyama K Coronary spasm: clinical features and pathogenesis. Intern Med 1997 Nov; 36(11): 760–5

    "Coronary spasm occurs most often from midnight to early morning when the patient is at rest and it is usually not induced by exercise in the daytime."

71. Muller JE, Kaufmann PG, Luepker RV, Weisfeldt ML, Deedwania PC, Willerson JT: Mechanisms precipitating acute cardiac events: review and recommendations of an NHLBI workshop. National Heart, Lung, and Blood Institute. Mechanisms Precipitating Acute Cardiac Events Participants. Circulation 1997 Nov 4; 96(9): 3233–9

72. Lavery CE, Mittleman MA, Cohen MC, Muller JE, Verrier RL: Nonuniform nighttime distribution of acute cardiac events: a possible effect of sleep states. Circulation 1997 Nov 18; 96(10): 3321–7

73. Tuhrim S: Stroke Risk Factors CNS Spectrums 2000; 5(3): 70–74

74. Texas Heart Institute Heart Information Service: Heart Disease Risk Factors. May 2000

75. Chalmers J et al.: WHO-ISH Hypertension Guidelines Committee. 1999 World Health Organization-International Society of Hypertension Guidelines for the Management of Hypertension. J Hypertens, 1999, 17:151–185

76. Heart Information Network/Center for Cardiovascular Education, Inc.: Genetic Factors and Early Heart Disease.accessed at http://www.heartinfo.com
77. Reuters: Family Link Found in Artery Disease. January 29, 2001
78. Kiely DK, Wolf PA, Cupples LA, Beiser AS, Myers RH: Familial aggregation of stroke: the Framingham Study. Stroke. 1993; 24: 1366–1371.
79. Stewart JA, Dundas R, Howard RS, Rudd AG, Wolfe CD: Ethnic differences in incidence of stroke: prospective study with stroke register. BMJ 1999 Apr 10; 318(7189): 967–71
80. Gaines K: Regional and ethnic differences in stroke in the southeastern United States population. Ethn Dis 1997 Spring-Summer; 7(2): 150–64
81. Richards SB, Funk M, Milner KA: Differences between blacks and whites with coronary heart disease in initial symptoms and in delay in seeking care. Am J Crit Care 2000 Jul; 9(4): 237–44
82. Goff DC, Ramsey DJ, Labarthe DR, Nichaman MZ: Acute myocardial infarction and coronary heart disease mortality among Mexican Americans and non-Hispanic whites in Texas, 1980 through 1989. Ethn Dis 1993 Winter; 3(1): 64–9
83. Spencer C, Lip G: Hypertension. Pharmaceutical Journal August 21, 1999 Vol 263 No 7059 p280–283
84. American Heart Association: "Borderline" high systolic blood pressure raises risk of stroke, heart attack and death. News Release NR 97–4510 March 4, 1997
85. NIH: Publication No. 98–4080 The Sixth Report of the Joint National Committee On Prevention, Detection, Evaluation, and Treatment of High Blood Pressure. November 1997

86. Nathan D: Treating Type 2 Diabetes with Respect. Annals of Internal Medicine March 2, 1999 Volume 130 Number 5 Pages 440–441

87. Canadian Diabetes Association Diabetes Pamphlet #114001 June, 2000

88. WebMD Health Pages Publication: Understand Cholesterol. At Last. 1998. (Online)

89. The Picower Institute for Medical Research Press Release: New Molecular Research Explains Link Between Smoking and Strokes. May 3, 1996

    "Heart disease, not lung cancer, accounts for the majority of the estimated 419,000 deaths from smoking-related diseases each year in the United States. According to 1995 estimates, smoking-related heart disease kills 191,000 Americans each year—a figure 44% higher than death from smoking-related lung cancer."

90. 1964 Surgeon General Report: Reducing the Health Consequences of Smoking. p.322

91. Doyle JT, Dawber TR, Kannel WB, Heslin AS, Kahn HA: Cigarette smoking and coronary heart disease; combined experence of the Albany and Framingham studies. N. Engl. J. Med. 1962; 266: 796–801

92. Rubino F: Stroke Prevention. Jacksonville Medicine November 1998

93. Wolf PA, D'Agostino RB, Kannel WB, Bonita R, Belanger AJ: Cigarette smoking as a risk factor for stroke. The Framingham Study. JAMA 1988 Feb 19; 259(7): 1025–9

94. Gottlieb S, Fallavollita J, McDermott M, Brown M, Eberly S, Moss AJ: Cigarette smoking and the age at onset of a first non-

fatal myocardial infarction. Coron Artery Dis 1994 Aug; 5(8): 687–94

95. NIH: Publication No. 96–3795 Check Your Physical Activity & Heart Disease I.Q. Reprinted August 1996
96. Rippe JM, Ward A, Porcari JP, Freedson PS: Walking for health and fitness. JAMA. 1988; 259: 2720–2724.
97. Dr. JoAnn Manson, associate professor of medicine at Harvard Medical School: Findings were presented at the American Heart Association annual meeting in New Orleans November 12, 1996
98. Hubert HB, Feinleib M, McNamara PM, Castelli WP: Obesity as an independent risk factor for cardiovascular disease: a 26-year follow-up of participants in the Framingham Heart Study. Circulation 1983 May; 67(5): 968–77
99. Garrison RJ, Higgins MW, Kannel WB: Obesity and coronary heart disease. Curr Opin Lipidol 1996 Aug; 7(4): 199–202
100. Krauss R, Winston M, Fletcher B, Grundy S: Obesity: Impact on Cardiovascular Disease AHA Conference Proceedings. Circulation. 1998; 98: 000–000
101. Heart and Stroke Foundation of Canada: Heart Disease and Stroke in Canada. June, 1997
102. Nabel EG: Biology of the impaired endothelium. Am J Cardiol 1991 Nov 4; 68(12)6C–8C

    "The endothelium is a regulatory organ that mediates hemostsis, contractility, cellular proliferation, and inflammatory mechanisms in the vessel wall. Injury to the endothelium from hypertension, smoking, hyperlipidemia, and diabetes mellitus disrupts normal regulatory properties and results in abnormal endothelial cell function."

103. Vogel RA: Coronary risk factors, endothelial function, and atherosclerosis: a review. Clin Cardiol 1997 May; 20(5): 426–32

"The traditional risk factors for coronary heart disease, which includes hypercholesterolemia, hypertension, cigarette smoking, diabetes mellitus, and high-fat diet, have all been associated with impairments in endothelial function."

104. Vogel RA: Coronary risk factors, endothelial function, and atherosclerosis: a review. Clin Cardiol 1997 May; 20(5): 426–32

    "Impaired endothelial function may promote the development of atherosclerosis through its effect on vasoregulation, platelet and monocytes adhesion, vascular smooth muscle cells growth, and coagulation."

105. Vogel RA: Coronary risk factors, endothelial function, and atherosclerosis: a review. Clin Cardiol 1997 May; 20(5): 426–32

    "Risk factor modification, particularly lowering elevated concentrations of low-density lipoprotein cholesterol, improves endothelial function."

106. Merck Manual of Diagnosis and Therapy: Section 16. Cardiovascular Disorders Chapter 201. Atherosclerosis

107. Jialal I, Devaraj S: The role of oxidized low density lipoprotein in atherogenesis. J Nutr 1996 Apr; 126(4 Suppl): 1053S–7S

    "LDL can be oxidatively modified in cell-free systems by transition metals and by all the major cells of the arterial wall. Oxidatively modified LDL (Ox-LDL) is taken up by macrophage scavenger receptors, promoting cholesterol ester accumulation and foam cell formation. It also promotes atherosclerosis by recruitment and retention of monocytes in the intima, by its cytotoxicity toward endothelial cells and by stimulating monocyte adhesion to the endothelium."

108. Martinez-Gonzalez J, Llorente-Cortes V, Badimon L: Cellular and Molecular Biology of Atherosclerotic Lesions. Rev Esp Cardiol 2001 Feb; 54(2): 218–231

"In addition, macrophages and smooth muscle cells take up these LDL, through different receptors, and become foam cells. The accumulation of foam cells in the arterial wall contributes to lesion development. Therefore, lesion development involves the activation of endothelial cells, as well as smooth muscle cells and monocytes/macrophages."

109. Fialova L: New findings on the pathogenesis of atherosclerosis. Cesk Fysiol 1995 Jun; 44(2): 92–101

110. American Heart Association Press Release: Scientific Evidence Does Not Support Vitamin E or other Antioxidant Supplements. February 1, 1999

111. American Heart Association Press Release: White blood cell count a clue to CHD risk in elderly men. April 10, 1996

112. Baller D, Gleichmann U, Miche E, Mannebach H, Seggewiss H: Clinical significance of the cardiovascular risk factor fibrinogen in secondary prevention. Versicherungsmedizin 1995 Apr 1; 47(2): 55–60

    "Fibrinogen plays a central role in platelet aggregation and performs an essential substrate in the coagulation cascade. Thus, high fibrinogen levels may favor a hypercoagulable state resulting in final thrombotic events of cardiovascular disease."

113. Lee AJ, Lowe GD, Woodward M, Tunstall-Pedoe H: Fibrinogen in relation to personal history of prevalent hypertension, diabetes, stroke, intermittent claudication, coronary heart disease, and family history: the Scottish Heart Health Study. Br Heart J 1993 Apr; 69(4): 338–42

114. WebMD Medical News: Protein That Helps May Also Harm in High Amounts High Fibrinogen Levels Found to Be Heart Disease Risk Factor. Oct. 2, 2000

115. Kannel WB, D'Agostino RB, Belanger AJ: Update on fibrinogen as a cardiovascular risk factor. Ann Epidemiol 1992 Jul; 2(4): 457–66

    "Fibrinogen enhances the risk of cardiovascular disease in hypertensives, diabetics, and cigarette smokers. About half the cardiovascular risk of cigarette smoking appears due to the higher fibrinogen values."

116. Ernst E, Resch KL: Therapeutic interventions to lower plasma fibrinogen concentration. Eur Heart J 1995 Mar; 16 Suppl A: 47–52; discussion 52–3

117. Baller D, Gleichmann U, Miche E, Mannebach H, Seggewiss H: Clinical significance of the cardiovascular risk factor fibrinogen in secondary prevention. Versicherungsmedizin 1995 Apr 1; 47(2): 55–60

    "Fibrinogen is also involved in atherogenesis by stimulating proliferation and migration of smooth muscle cells."

118. Heinrich J, Assmann G: Fibrinogen and cardiovascular risk. J Cardiovasc Risk 1995 Jun; 2(3): 197–205

    "The plasma fibrinogen level is associated with both the severity and the extent of coronary, cerebral and peripheral atherosclerosis."

119. Reuters: Blood-clotting protein tied to heart risk. April 1, 1999

120. Stec JJ, Silbershatz H, Tofler GH, Matheney TH, Sutherland P, Lipinska I, Massaro JM, Wilson PF, Muller JE, D'Agostino RB: Association of fibrinogen with cardiovascular risk factors and cardiovascular disease in the Framingham offspring population. Circulation (Online) 2000 Oct 3; 102(14): 1634–8

121. Ridker PM, Cushman M, Stampfer MJ, Tracy RP, Hennekens CH: Inflammation, aspirin, and the risk of cardiovascular

disease in apparently healthy men. N Engl J Med 1997 Apr 3; 336(14): 973–9

"The men in the quartile with the highest levels of C-reactive protein values had three times the risk of myocardial infarction (relative risk, 2.9; P<0.001) and two times the risk of ischemic stroke (relative risk, 1.9; P=0.02) of the men in the lowest quartile."

122. PSL Group Doctor's Guide Web Site (**http://www.pslgroup.com/dg/ab49a.htm**): Blood Levels Of C-Reactive Protein May Predict Heart Attack, Stroke Aug. 24, 1998

"Overall, women with the highest levels of C-reactive protein had a five-fold increase in the risk of developing any cardiovascular disease and a seven-fold increase in risk of having a heart attack or a stroke, when compared to those with the lowest levels of C-reactive protein."

123. Anderson et al.: Inflammatory and Infectious Markers for MI. JACC Vol. 32, No. 1, July 1998: 35–41

"A multicenter group confirmed the predictive value of CRP for coronary events in both stable and unstable angina."

124. Mendall MA, Patel P, Ballam L, Strachan D, Northfield TC: C-reactive protein and its relation to cardiovascular risk factors: a population based cross sectional study. BMJ 1996 Apr 27; 312(7038): 1061–5

125. Paul M. Ridker, MD; Mary Cushman, MD; Meir J. Stampfer, MD; Russell P. Tracy, PhD; Charles H. Hennekens, MD: Plasma Concentration of C-Reactive Protein and Risk of Developing Peripheral Vascular Disease. Circulation. 1998; 97: 425–428.

"These prospective data indicate that among apparently healthy men, baseline levels of CRP predict future risk of developing symptomatic PAD and thus provide further support for the hypothesis that chronic inflammation is important in the pathogenesis of atherothrombosis."

126. Reuters Health: Blood Factors Help Predict Arterial Leg Disorder. May 28, 2001

    "A second marker, C-reactive protein (CRP), also strongly predicted the ailment. Those with the highest blood levels of CRP had more than double the risk of developing PAD as those with the lowest level."

127. Russell P. Tracy, PhD: Inflammation in Cardiovascular Disease. Circulation. 1998; 97: 2000–2002

    "In fact, there is some evidence that lipids and CRP are better predictors jointly than would be expected by adding up their individual predictive powers. CRP appeared to predict events in those at low risk on the basis of lipids, and CRP-lipid relationships to events were minimally altered by adjustment for other known CVD risk factors."

128. Torzewski M, Rist C, Mortensen RF, Zwaka TP, Bienek M, Waltenberger J, Koenig W, Schmitz G, Hombach V, Torzewski J: C-reactive protein in the arterial intima: role of C-reactive proteinreceptor-dependent monocyte recruitment in atherogenesis. Arterioscler Thromb Vasc Biol 2000 Sep; 20(9): 2094–9

    "In this study, we demonstrate that CRP deposition precedes the appearance of monocytes in early atherosclerotic lesions. CRP is chemotactic for freshly isolated human blood monocytes. A specific CRP receptor is demonstrated on monocytes in vitro as well as in vivo, and blockage of the receptor by use of a monoclonal anti-receptor antibody completely abolishes CRP-induced chemotaxis. CRP may play a major role in the recruitment of monocytes during atherogenesis."

129. Panichi V, Migliori M, De Pietro S, Taccola D, Andreini B, Metelli MR, Giovannini L, Palla R: The link of biocompatibility

to cytokine production. Kidney Int 2000 Aug; 58 Suppl 76: S96–103

"CRP may, in fact, directly interact with the atherosclerotic vessels or ischemic myocardium by activation of the complement system, thereby promoting inflammation and thrombosis."

130. Pasceri V, Willerson JT, Yeh ET: Direct proinflammatory effect of C-reactive protein on human endothelial cells. Circulation 2000 Oct 31; 102(18): 2165–8

"CRP induces adhesion molecule expression in human endothelial cells in the presence of serum. These findings support the hypothesis that CRP may play a direct role in promoting the inflammatory component of atherosclerosis and present a potential target for the treatment of atherosclerosis."

131. Bayer Aspirin: Heart Attack Fact Sheet. July 1999

"Aspirin reduces the risk of death by up to 23% if administered when a heart attack is suspected and for 30 days thereafter."

132. Cardiovascular Pharmacology: FDA approves new prescribed uses for aspirin. December 1998

"Ischemic stroke and TIA: In clinical trials of patients with TIAs due to fibrin platelet emboli or ischemic stroke, aspirin has been shown to significantly reduce the risk of the combined endpoint of stroke or death and the combined endpoint of TIA, stroke, or death by about 13% to 18%."

133. Bayer Aspirin: Landmark FDA Ruling on Aspirin Fact Sheet

"The FDA approved the use of aspirin to reduce the risk of stroke after TIA (transient ischemic attack or "ministroke"—the occurrence of stroke warning signs) in men. The ruling was based on two Canadian studies showing that aspirin reduced the risk of death or a major stroke by almost 50% by taking a 325mg aspirin tablet per day."

134. Bayer Aspirin: Landmark FDA Ruling on Aspirin Fact Sheet

    "In response to the volumes of supporting evidence, the FDA recognized the use of aspirin to prevent heart attack in patients who had suffered either a previous heart attack or who suffered from unstable angina. According to the FDA, daily doses of aspirin for people who already had a previous heart attack reduced the risk of a second heart attack by 20%. Adding patients suffering from unstable angina, the risk was reduced by fully 51%."

135. Guide to Clinical Preventive Services: Second Edition (1996) Government Printing Office (Stock No. 017–001–00525–8) Aspirin Prophylaxis for the Primary Prevention of Myocardial Infarction.

    "There is insufficient evidence to determine whether the proven benefits of routine aspirin prophylaxis given for the primary prevention of MI in asymptomatic men ages 40 to 84 years outweigh the proven harms, and thus the U.S. Preventive Services Task Force does not recommend for or against its use ("C" recommendation)."

136. The Michigan Daily Online: Study links heart disease, swelling Associated Press 04–03–97

137. Harvard Health Letter: The Search for New Culprits. May 1999; 24(8)

    "But in the 1997 investigation, the researchers found that aspirin was most protective in men with the highest blood levels of C-reactive protein, suggesting that part of its benefit may be its anti-inflammatory properties, not just its ability to inhibit platelet aggregation."

138. Scandinavian Simvastatin Survival Study Group: Randomized trial of cholesterol lowering in 4444 patients with coronary heart disease: the Scandinavian Simvastatin Survival Study (4S). Lancet 1994 Nov 19; 344(8934): 1383–9

139. Shepherd J, Cobbe SM, Ford I, Isles CG, Lorimer AR, MacFarlane PW, McKillop JH, Packard CJ: Prevention of coronary heart disease with pravastatin in men with hypercholesterolemia. West of Scotland Coronary Prevention Study Group. N Engl J Med 1995 Nov 16; 333(20): 1301–7

140. Byington RP, Davis BR, Plehn JF, White HD, Baker J, Cobbe SM, Shepherd J: Reduction of Stroke Events With Pravastatin : The Prospective Pravastatin Pooling (PPP) Project. Circulation 2001 Jan 23; 103(3): 387–392

"Pravastatin reduced the risk of stroke over a wide range of lipid values among patients with documented coronary disease."

141. Ridker PM, Rifai N, Pfeffer MA, Sacks FM, Moye LA, Goldman S, Flaker GC, Braunwald E: Inflammation, Pravastatin, and the Risk of Coronary Events After Myocardial Infarction in Patients With Average Cholesterol Levels. Circulation. 1998; 98: 839–844

142. Shah PK: Do Statins Change Plaque Composition in Humans? The 64th Annual Scientific Meeting of the Japanese Circulation Society Keynote Lecture April 1–3, 2000

143. Christensen D: Chronic Bronchitis May Increase Risk of MI, Mortality. Medical Tribune. September 26, 1996

"In the new study of 19,444 middle-aged men and women who were followed for up to 13 years, men with chronic bronchitis had a 52% higher risk of MI than other men, and a 74% increased coronary-mortality risk. Women with the chronic respiratory condition were 38% more likely than other women to suffer an MI and 49% more likely to suffer a coronary-related death, according to the study, published in The Lancet (1996; 348: 567–572)."

144. Penttinen J, Valonen P: The risk of myocardial infarction among Finnish farmers seeking medical care for an infection. Am J Public Health 1996 Oct; 86(10): 1440–2

"Men in this sample with recurrent or chronic infections of the upper respiratory tract exhibited a pronounced risk for myocardial infarction."

145. Reuters: Chronic Infections Hike Stroke Risk. September 9, 1997

"Those with frequent bouts of chronic bronchitis in the preceding two years had a 2.2 times greater risk for stroke or TIAs."

146. Modica P: Infections Linked To Onset Of Stroke. Medical Tribune News Service December 30, 1996

"In the first study, a team at the Tel Aviv University Medical Center in Tel Aviv, Israel found that among 182 patients who had been admitted to the hospital for stroke, about 24 percent of them had some type of short-term, severe infection, mostly in the urinary or respiratory tract. Almost all of the infections occurred one week before the stroke, said Dr. I.Y. Bova and colleagues of Tel Aviv's department of neurology."

147. Reuters: Bacteria Linked to Heart Attack. August 20, 1997

"In addition, approximately 20 percent of the patients reported respiratory symptoms during the three weeks prior to admission, consistent with the presence of an upper respiratory tract infection…"

148. Meier CR, Jick SS, Derby LE, Vasilakis C, Jick H: Acute respiratory-tract infections and risk of first-time acute myocardial infarction. Lancet 1998 May 16; 351(9114): 1467–71

"Our findings suggest that in people without a history of clinical risk factors for AMI, acute respiratory-tract infections are associated with an increased risk of AMI for a period of about 2 weeks."

149. Norton A: Flu Shot May Help Ward Off Heart Attack. Reuters Health December 18, 2000

    "In a study of 218 heart attack patients, the investigators linked flu vaccination to a 67% lower risk for a second heart attack."

150. Mattila KJ, Nieminen MS, Valtonen VV, Rasi VP, Kesaniemi YA, Syrjala SL, Jungell PS, Isoluoma M, Hietaniemi K, Jokinen MJ: Association between dental health and acute myocardial infarction. BMJ 1989 Mar 25; 298(6676): 779–81

151. Focus News from Harvard Medical, Dental, & Public Health Schools: Show Me Your Mouth, I'll Tell You About Your Heart. June 19, 1998

    "People with the most bone loss faced a 70% increased risk of developing symptoms of heart disease. Similar results applied to stroke."

152. DeStefano F, Anda RF, Kahn HS, Williamson DF, Russell CM: Dental disease and risk of coronary heart disease and mortality. BMJ 1993 Mar 13; 306(6879): 688–91

    "Among all 9760 subjects included in the analysis those with periodontitis had a 25% increased risk of coronary heart disease relative to those with minimal periodontal disease. Poor oral hygiene, determined by the extent of dental debris and calculus, was also associated with an increased incidence of coronary heart disease. In men younger than 50 years at baseline periodontal disease was a stronger risk factor for coronary heart disease; men with periodontitis had a relative risk of 1.72."

153. Reuters: Chronic Infections Hike Stroke Risk. September 8, 1997

"In addition, those with poor dental status (linked to gum disease) were at 2.6 times greater risk for stroke and TIAs."

154. Reuters Health: Gum disease linked to heart disease. Jan 26, 1998

"Men with extensive gum disease, with bleeding from essentially every tooth, were 4.5 times more likely to have coronary heart disease than men without gum disease.... 'Patients who saw a dentist at least once a year were four times less likely to have a history of cerebral vascular accident (stroke),' Loesche told Reuters Health."

155. Reuters Health: MI Patients More Likely to Have Periodontitis Than Healthy People. Nov 14, 2000

"The investigators found that 85% of patients with MI had periodontal disease compared with 29% of controls."

156. ABC (Australia) Online News: Another use for aspirin, by gum. March 2, 2000

"A study at Adelaide University's Dental School has found that men taking low-dose aspirin to prevent heart disease and stroke had inadvertently received another benefit: they had significantly less periodontitis."

157. Jousilahti P, Salomaa V, Rasi V, Vahtera E: Symptoms of chronic bronchitis, haemostatic factors, and coronary heart disease risk. Atherosclerosis 1999 Feb; 142(2): 403–7

"Plasma fibrinogen level was significantly higher, 3.70 versus 3.35 g/l ($P < 0.001$) in men and 3.64 versus 3.44 g/l ($P < 0.001$) in women, among subjects with symptoms of chronic bronchitis than among those without symptoms."

158. Mendall MA; Patel P; Ballam L; Strachan D; Northfield TC: C-reactive protein and its relation to cardiovascular risk factors: a population based cross sectional study. BMJ, 312(7038): 1061–5 1996 Apr 27

159. American Heart Association's Scientific Sessions 2000: Gum Disease Higher in Heart Attack Patients November 12, 2000

    "Deliargyris' team found that individuals with both periodontal disease and a first heart attack had higher blood levels of CRP than those without periodontal disease."

160. Reuters Health: Gum disease linked to blood clotting factors. Feb 23, 2000

    "People who have gum disease—indicated by red, swollen gums that bleed during tooth brushing—also tend to have higher blood levels of fibrinogen, a clotting factor, and C-reactive protein (CRP), an inflammatory molecule, according to a report in the February issue of the American Journal of Epidemiology. What's more, gum disease (known as periodontal disease) may also be linked with a higher cholesterol level..."

161. Loos BG, Craandijk J, Hoek FJ, Wertheim-van Dillen PM, van der Velden U: Elevation of systemic markers related to cardiovascular diseases in the peripheral blood of periodontitis patients. J Periodontol 2000 Oct; 71(10): 1528–34

    "Periodontitis results in higher systemic levels of CRP, IL-6, and neutrophils. These elevated inflammatory factors may increase inflammatory activity in atherosclerotic lesions, potentially increasing the risk for cardiac or cerebrovascular events."

162. Chiu B: Multiple infections in carotid atherosclerotic plaques. Am Heart J 1999 Nov; 138(5 Pt 2): S534–6

    "The current study is the first to report the detection of 2 major odontopathogens, *P gingivalis* and *S sanguis*, in atherosclerotic plaques. The immunolocalization of these micro-organisms within unstable plaque regions and their association with plaque ulceration, thrombosis, and apoptosis in vascular cells are intriguing."

163. Haraszthy VI, Zambon JJ, Trevisan M, Zeid M, Genco RJ: Identification of periodontal pathogens in atheromatous plaques. J Periodontol 2000 Oct; 71(10): 1554–60

    "Periodontal pathogens are present in atherosclerotic plaques where, like other infectious microorganisms such as *C. pneumoniae*, they may play a role in the development and progression of atherosclerosis leading to coronary vascular disease and other clinical sequelae."

164. Progulske-Fox A, Kozarov E, Dorn B, Dunn W Jr., Burks J, Wu Y: Porphyromonas gingivalis virulence factors and invasion of cells of the cardiovascular system. J Periodontal Res 1999 Oct; 34(7): 393

165. Danesh J: Epidemiological studies of infection and atherosclerosis. Submitted by the author to the International Symposium on Infections and Atherosclerosis Organized by Fondation Marcel Mérieux And the French National Institute of Health and Scientific Research (Inserm) With the support of Pasteur Mérieux Connaught Les Pensières, Veyrier-du-Lac 6–9 December 1998

    "More than 150 epidemiological or clinical studies have reported on associations of vascular disease and the presence of certain persistent bacterial and viral agents or of clinical conditions (e.g., periodontal disease) that are associated with persistent infection."

166. Haranaga S, Yamaguchi H, Friedman H, Izumi S, Yamamoto Y: *Chlamydia pneumoniae* infects and multiplies in lymphocytes in vitro. Infect Immun 2001 Dec; 69(12): 7753–9

"The results demonstrated that human peripheral blood lymphocytes as well as mouse spleen lymphocytes could be infected with *C. pneumoniae*. Furthermore, purified T lymphocytes as well as established T-lymphocyte cell line cells showed an obvious susceptibility to *C. pneumoniae* infection, indicating that T cells could be one of the host cells for this bacterial infection. These findings reveal a new infection site for *C. pneumoniae*, i.e., lymphocytes."

167. Airenne S, Surcel HM, Alakarppa H, Laitinen K, Paavonen J, Saikku P, Laurila A: *Chlamydia pneumoniae* infection in human monocytes. Infect Immun 1999 Mar; 67(3): 1445–9

"*Chlamydia pneumoniae* infection has been associated with cardiovascular diseases in seroepidemiological studies and by demonstration of the pathogen in atherosclerotic lesions. It has the capacity to infect several cell types, including monocyte-derived macrophages, which play an essential role in the development of atherosclerosis."

168. Godzik KL, O'Brien ER, Wang SK, Kuo CC: In vitro susceptibility of human vascular wall cells to infection with *Chlamydia pneumoniae*. J Clin Microbiol 1995 Sep; 33(9): 2411–4

"Endothelial cells, smooth muscle cells, and macrophages were capable of supporting *C. pneumoniae* growth in vitro."

169. Yang ZP, Kuo CC, Grayston JT: Systemic dissemination of *Chlamydia pneumoniae* following intranasal inoculation in mice. J Infect Dis 1995 Mar; 171(3): 736–8

170. Maass M, Bartels C, Engel PM, Mamat U, Sievers HH: Endovascular presence of viable *Chlamydia pneumoniae* is a common phenomenon in coronary artery disease. J Am Coll Cardiol 1998 Mar 15; 31(4): 827–32

"DNA sequencing of six different PCR products did not reveal differences between coronary isolates and respiratory reference strains, suggesting that common respiratory strains gain access to the systemic circulation."

171. Berger M, Schroder B, Daeschlein G, Schneider W, Busjahn A, Buchwalow I, Luft FC, Haller H: *Chlamydia pneumoniae* DNA in non-coronary atherosclerotic plaques and circulating leukocytes. J Lab Clin Med 2000 Sep; 136(3): 194–200

    "Earlier studies have associated atherosclerosis with *Chlamydia pneumoniae* infection. *C. pneumoniae* may circulate via monocytes and migrate into plaques by leukocyte infiltration…"

172. Kaul R, Wenman WM: *Chlamydia pneumoniae* facilitates monocyte adhesion to endothelial and smooth muscle cells. Microb Pathog 2001 Mar; 30(3): 149–55

    "Moreover, monocytes infected with viable *C. pneumoniae* adhered preferentially to HCAEC and HCSMC, as compared to uninfected monocytes or monocytes harbouring heat inactivated *Chlamydia*."

173. Gaydos CA: Growth in vascular cells and cytokine production by *Chlamydia pneumoniae*. J Infect Dis 2000 Jun; 181 Suppl 3: S473–8

    "U-937 macrophages infected with *C. pneumoniae* are capable of transmitting the infection to human coronary artery endothelial cells (CAEC) with direct cellular contact."

174. Knoebel E, Vijayagopal P, Figueroa JE 2nd, Martin DH: In vitro infection of smooth muscle cells by *Chlamydia pneumoniae*. Infect Immun 1997 Feb; 65(2): 503–6

    "The organism readily infected rabbit, bovine, and human aortic smooth muscle cells. Cholesterol-loaded smooth muscle cells were even more susceptible to *C. pneumoniae* infection."

175. Leinonen M: Interaction of *Chlamydia pneumoniae* Infection with Other Risk Factors of Atherosclerosis. Lecture during the International Symposium on Infections and Atherosclerosis Organized by Fondation Marcel Mérieux And the French National Institute of Health and Scientific Research (Inserm) With the support of Pasteur Mérieux Connaught Les Pensières, Veyrier-du-Lac 6–9 December 1998 Synthesis written by Dire La Science and validated by the lecturer

    "There are numerous risk factors affecting susceptibility to chronic infection with *C. pneumoniae*, including age, gender, smoking, heredity, physical activity, diet, stress, etc."

176. Medical Tribune News Service: Common Infection May Trigger High Blood Pressure. February 20, 1998

177. Movahed MR: Infection with *Chlamydia pneumoniae* and atherosclerosis: a review. J S C Med Assoc 1999 Aug; 95(8): 303–8

    "*C. pneumoniae* has been located in endothelium, smooth muscle cells and macrophages of arterial wall with atherosclerosis but not in normal arteries. Cellular models have shown that *C. pneumoniae* is able to replicate in endothelium, macrophages and smooth muscle cells."

178. Ngeh J, Gupta S: *C. pneumoniae* and Atherosclerosis: Causal or Coincidental. ASM News 2000; 66: 732

    "However, [Elementary Bodies] may unpredictably convert into a metabolically inactive form called [Persistent Body] within the cell, sometimes remaining dormant for extended periods. [Persistent Bodies] are not susceptible to the immune system or antibiotics."

179. DeLemos J: Emerging Role of *Chlamydia pneumoniae* in Inflammation and Coronary Artery Disease Chestpain Online In

Review(**http://www.chestpainonline.org/html/inrev0505.html**)

"This 'persistent body' appears to be larger than the RB, but metabolically inert."

180. Yamashita K, Ouchi K, Shirai M, Gondo T, Nakazawa T, Ito H: Distribution of *Chlamydia pneumoniae* infection in the atherosclerotic carotid artery. Stroke 1998 Apr; 29(4): 773–8

    "*C. pneumoniae* infection was observed in endothelial cells, macrophages and in smooth muscle cells that had migrated into the atheromatous plaque, as well as in smooth muscle cells and small arteries in the media underlying the atheromatous plaques. *C. pneumoniae* infection was most prominently observed in smooth muscle cells. The severity of the infection as demonstrated by immunohistochemistry was not significantly related to general risk factors for atherosclerosis. CONCLUSIONS: *C. pneumoniae* widely infects endothelial cells, macrophages, and smooth muscle cells in the atherosclerotic carotid artery."

181. Krull M, Klucken AC, Wuppermann FN, Fuhrmann O, Magerl C, Seybold J, Hippenstiel S, Hegemann JH, Jantos CA, Suttorp N: Signal transduction pathways activated in endothelial cells following infection with *Chlamydia pneumoniae*. J Immunol 1999 Apr 15; 162(8): 4834–41

    "In this study, we characterized *C. pneumoniae*-mediated activation of endothelial cells and demonstrated an enhanced expression of endothelial adhesion molecules followed by subsequent rolling, adhesion, and transmigration of leukocytes (monocytes, granulocytes)."

182. Kohara K, Tabara Y, Yamamoto Y, Igase M, Miki T: *Chlamydia pneumoniae* seropositivity is associated with increased plasma levels of soluble cellular adhesion molecules in community-

dwelling subjects: the Shimanami Health Promoting Program (J-SHIPP) study. Stroke 2002 Jun; 33(6): 1474–9

"These findings indicate that *C. pneumoniae* seropositivity is associated with higher plasma concentrations of soluble forms of adhesion molecules in the general population. The increase in circulating adhesion molecules may underlie the mechanisms linking *C. pneumoniae* infection and atherosclerosis in vivo."

183. Kalayoglu MV, Perkins BN, Byrne GI: *Chlamydia pneumoniae*-infected monocytes exhibit increased adherence to human aortic endothelial cells. Microbes Infect 2001 Oct; 3(12): 963–9

"These data show that *C. pneumoniae* can enhance the capacity of monocytes to adhere to primary human aortic endothelial cells. The enhanced adherence exhibited by infected monocytes may increase monocyte residence time in vascular sites with reduced wall shear stress and promote entry of infected cells into lesion-prone locations."

184. Inflammation caused by a bacterial infection may be involved in atherosclerosis. 97th General Meeting of the American Society for Microbiology May 4–8, 1997 Paper Number: D-017 Session Number: 027-D

"In a recent study, we found that *Chlamydia pneumoniae* is able to promote the movement of white blood cells such as neutrophilis and monocytes towards infected endothelial cells."

185. Molestina RE, Miller RD, Ramirez JA, Summersgill JT: Infection of human endothelial cells with *Chlamydia pneumoniae* stimulates transendothelial migration of neutrophils and monocytes. Infect Immun 1999 Mar; 67(3): 1323–30

"...levels of neutrophil and monocyte transendothelial migration were determined following 24 h of infection. Compared to mock-infected controls, significant increases in neutrophil migration were observed in response to most *C. pneumoniae* isolates examined (P < 0.001)."

186. Kalayoglu MV, Hoerneman B, LaVerda D, Morrison SG, Morrison RP, Byrne GI: Cellular oxidation of low-density lipoprotein by *Chlamydia pneumoniae*. J Infect Dis 1999 Sep; 180(3): 780–90

    "Although native LDL does not have atherogenic properties, cellular oxidation of LDL alters the lipoprotein into a highly atherogenic form. In this report, *C. pneumoniae* and chlamydial hsp60, an inflammatory antigen that was recently localized to atheromas, were found to induce cellular oxidation of LDL. These data provide initial evidence that an infectious agent can render LDL atherogenic and suggest a mechanism whereby *C. pneumoniae* may promote atheroma development."

187. Kalayoglu MV, Byrne GI: Induction of macrophage foam cell formation by *Chlamydia pneumoniae*. J Infect Dis 1998 Mar; 177(3): 725–9

    "It was found that the intracellular bacterium *Chlamydia pneumoniae* induces foam cell formation by human monocyte-derived macrophages."

188. Movahed MR: Infection with *Chlamydia pneumoniae* and atherosclerosis: a review. J S C Med Assoc 1999 Aug; 95(8): 303–8

    "A high *C. pneumoniae* antibody titer was found to correlate with high level of LDL and triglycerides and low level of HDL."

189. Tutuncu NB, Guvener N, Tutuncu T, Yilmaz M, Guvener M, Boke E, Pasaoglu I, Erbas T: *Chlamydia pneumonia* seropositivity correlates with serum fibrinogen and lipoprotein a levels: any role in atherosclerosis? Endocr J 2001 Apr; 48(2): 269–74

    "In the *C. pneumoniae* seropositive group, serum fibrinogen and lipoprotein a levels were found to be significantly higher than the seronegative group....The causal role of Chlamydial infections in atherosclerotic plaque formation might be due to their influence on the serum fibrinogen and lipoprotein a levels."

190. Coombes BK, Mahony JB: *Chlamydia pneumoniae* infection of human endothelial cells induces proliferation of smooth muscle cells via an endothelial cell-derived soluble factor(s). Infect Immun 1999 Jun; 67(6): 2909–15

"The ability of *C. pneumoniae* to elicit an endothelial cell-derived soluble factor(s) that stimulates SMC proliferation may be important in the pathogenesis of atherosclerosis."

191. Fryer RH, Schwobe EP, Woods ML, Rodgers GM: *Chlamydia* species infect human vascular endothelial cells and induce procoagulant activity. J Investig Med 1997 Apr; 45(4): 168–74

192. Liuba P, Karnani P, Pesonen E, Paakkari I, Forslid A, Johansson L, Persson K, Wadstrom T, Laurini R: Endothelial dysfunction after repeated *Chlamydia pneumoniae* infection in apolipoprotein E-knockout mice. Circulation (Online) 2000 Aug 29; 102(9): 1039–44

"*C. pneumoniae* impairs arterial endothelial function, and the NO pathway is principally involved. Cyclooxygenase-dependent vasoconstricting products may also account for the infection-induced impaired relaxation."

193. Mendall MA, Patel P, Ballam L, Strachan D, Northfield TC: C-reactive protein and its relation to cardiovascular risk factors: a population based cross sectional study. BMJ 1996 Apr 27; 312(7038): 1061–5

"Increasing age, smoking, symptoms of chronic bronchitis, *Helicobacter pylori* and *Chlamydia pneumoniae* infections, and body mass index were all associated with raised concentrations of C-reactive protein."

194. Roivainen M, Viik-Kajander M, Palosuo T, Toivanen P, Leinonen M, Saikku P, Tenkanen L, Manninen V, Hovi T: Manttari M: Infections, inflammation, and the risk of coronary heart disease. Circulation 2000 Jan 25; 101(3): 252–7

"Two chronic infections, HSV-1 and *Cpn*, increase the risk of coronary heart disease. The effect is emphasized in subjects with ongoing inflammation, denoted by increased CRP levels."

195. Toss H, Gnarpe J, Gnarpe H, Siegbahn A, Lindahl B, Wallentin L: Increased fibrinogen levels are associated with persistent *Chlamydia pneumoniae* infection in unstable coronary artery disease. Eur Heart J 1998 Apr; 19(4): 570–7

"Persistent *C. pneumoniae* infection is common in unstable coronary artery disease. The independent association between increased *C. pneumoniae* IgA antibody titres and fibrinogen levels indicates that chronic infection could be of importance for disease activity."

196. Tutuncu NB, Guvener N, Tutuncu T, *Yilmaz* M, Guvener M, Boke E, Pasaoglu I, Erbas T: *Chlamydia pneumonia* seropositivity correlates with serum fibrinogen and lipoprotein a levels: any role in atherosclerosis? Endocr J 2001 Apr; 48(2): 269–74

"In the C. pneumonia seropositive group, serum fibrinogen and lipoprotein a levels were found to be significantly higher than the seronegative group....The causal role of Chlamydial infections in atherosclerotic plaque formation might be due to their influence on the serum fibrinogen and lipoprotein a levels."

197. Shor A, Phillips J: Histological and ultrastructural findings suggesting an initiating role for *Chlamydia pneumoniae* in

the pathogenesis of atherosclerosis. Cardiovascular Journal of South Africa Volume 11 Supplement 1 February/March 2000

198. Kol A, Sukhova GK, Lichtman AH, Libby P: Chlamydial heat shock protein 60 localizes in human atheroma and regulates macrophage tumor necrosis factor-alpha and matrix metalloproteinase expression. Circulation 1998 Jul 28; 98(4): 300–7

"Chlamydial HSP 60 frequently colocalizes with human HSP 60 in plaque macrophages in human atherosclerotic lesions. Chlamydial and human HSP 60 induce TNF-alpha and MMP production by macrophages. Chlamydial HSP 60 might mediate the induction of these effects by *C. pneumoniae*. Induction of such macrophage functions provides potential mechanisms by which chlamydial infections may promote atherogenesis and precipitate acute ischemic events."

199. Song YG, Kwon HM, Kim JM, Hong BK, Kim DS, Huh AJ, Chang KH, Kim HY, Kang TS, Lee BK, Choi DH, Jang YS, Kim HS: Serologic and histopathologic study of *Chlamydia pneumoniae* infection in atherosclerosis: a possible pathogenetic mechanism of atherosclerosis induced by *Chlamydia pneumoniae*. Yonsei Med J 2000 Jun; 41(3): 319–27

200. Higuchi MD, Castelli JB, Aiello VD, Palomino S, Reis MM, Sambiase NV, Fukasawa S, Bezerra HG, Ramires JA: Great amount of *C. pneumoniae* in ruptured plaque vessel segments at autopsy. A comparative study with stable plaques. Arq Bras Cardiol 2000 Feb; 74(2): 149–51

201. Bauriedel G, Welsch U, Likungu JA, Welz A, Luderitz B: *Chlamydia pneumoniae* in coronary plaques: Increased detection with acute coronary syndrome. Dtsch Med Wochenschr 1999 Apr 1; 124(13): 375–80

"*Chlamydia pneumoniae* were detected in 32 of 51 (63%) coronary primary lesions of symptomatic patients. Most importantly, there was a highly significant prevalence of lesions associated with acute coronary syndrome. Predilection sites of *C. pneumoniae* were areas that revealed small healing activity and (or) propensity to plaque rupture. The present in situ findings indicate a pathogenic role of *Chlamydiae pneumoniae* in human (coronary) plaque rupture."

202. Bauriedel G, Andrie R, Likungu JA, Welz A, Braun P, Welsch U, Luderitz B: Persistence of *Chlamydia pneumoniae* in coronary plaque tissue. A contribution to infection and immune hypothesis in unstable angina pectoris. Dtsch Med Wochenschr 1999 Nov 26; 124(47): 1408–13

"It is most frequently found in macrophages/foam cells and is highly prevalent in the acute coronary syndrome."

203. Ashkenazi H, Rudensky B, Paz E, Raveh D, Balkin JA, Tzivoni D, Yinnon AM.: Incidence of immunoglobulin G antibodies to *Chlamydia pneumoniae* in acute myocardial infarction patients. Isr Med Assoc J 2001 Nov; 3(11): 818–21

204. Chandra HR, Choudhary N, O'Neill C, Boura J, Timmis GC, O'Neill WW: *Chlamydia pneumoniae* exposure and inflammatory markers in acute coronary syndrome (CIMACS).Am J Cardiol 2001 Aug 1; 88(3): 214–8

205. Shimada K, Daida H, Mokuno H, Watanabe Y, Sawano M, Iwama Y, Seki E, Kurata T, Sato H, Ohashi S, Suzuki H, Miyauchi K, Takaya J, Sakurai H, Yamaguchi H: Association of seropositivity for antibody to *Chlamydia*-specific lipopolysaccharide and coronary artery disease in Japanese men. Jpn Circ J 2001 Mar; 65(3): 182–7

206. Katsenis C, Kouskouni E, Kolokotronis L, Rizos D, Dimakakos P: The significance of *Chlamydia pneumoniae* in symptomatic carotid stenosis Angiology 2001 Sep; 52(9): 615–9

207. Virok D, Kis Z, Karai L, Intzedy L, Burian K, Szabo A, Ivanyi B, Gonczol E: *Chlamydia pneumoniae* in atherosclerotic middle cerebral artery. Stroke 2001 Sep; 32(9): 1973–6

208. Kawamoto R, Doi T, Tokunaga H, Konishi I: An association between an antibody against *Chlamydia pneumoniae* and common carotid atherosclerosis. Intern Med 2001 Mar; 40(3): 208–13

209. Linares-Palomino J, Gutierrez J, Lopez-Espada C, Ros E, Moreno J, Perez T, Rodriguez M, Maroto MC: Rev Neurol 2001 Feb 1–15; 32(3): 201–6 Comment in: Rev Neurol. 2001 Feb 1–15; 32(3): 232–3

210. Wolski A, Mazur E, Niedzwiadek J, Slepko J, Koziol-Montewka M, Michalak J: The relation between *Chlamydia pneumoniae* infection and abdominal aortic aneurysm. Pol Merkuriusz Lek 2001 Dec; 11(66): 491–4

    "Since all patients in this group were diagnosed as having symptomatic AAA, we suggest that active infection can exacerbate inflammation in the AAA wall and accelerate progresion of the disease. In our opinion patients with active *C. pnemoniae* infection may be candidates to the antimicrobial treatment."

211. Petersen E, Boman J, Wagberg F, Bergstrom S, Angquist KA: In vitro degradation of aortic elastin by *Chlamydia pneumoniae*. Eur J Vasc Endovasc Surg 2001 Nov; 22(5): 443–7

    "These results indicate that there is a relationship between the presence of *C. pneumoniae* and increased elastin degradation in the aortic wall in vitro. This suggests *C. pneumoniae* in the aortic wall directly or indirectly leads to the degradation of aortic elastin."

212. Reuters Health: Cold sores linked to heart attack risk. Nov 06, 2000

    "In a study of more than 600 people aged 65 and older, those who had HSV-1 antibodies in their blood were twice as likely to have had a heart attack or to have died from heart disease, researchers report in the November 7th issue of Circulation: Journal of the American Heart Association."

213. Reuters Health: Viruses may increase risk of heart disease. Feb 08, 2000

    "Chronic infection with the herpes simplex 1 or *Chlamydia* virus [sic] can increase the risk of developing heart disease, Finnish researchers suggest."

214. Roivainen M, et al.: Infections, Inflammation, and the Risk of Coronary Heart Disease Circulation. 2000; 101:252

    "Herpes simplex 1 (HSV-1) and HSV-2 viruses are found in atherosclerotic lesions."

215. Etingin OR, Silverstein RL, Hajjar DP: Identification of a monocyte receptor on herpesvirus-infected endothelial cells. Proc Natl Acad Sci U S A 1991 Aug 15; 88(16): 7200–3

    "We now demonstrate that HSV-infected endothelial cells express the adhesion molecule GMP140 and that this requires cell surface expression of HSV glycoprotein C and local thrombin generation."

216. Span AH, van Dam-Mieras MC, Mullers W, Endert J, Muller AD, Bruggeman CA: The effect of virus infection on the adherence of leukocytes or platelets to endothelial cells. Eur J Clin Invest 1991 Jun; 21(3): 331–8

    "In this study we show that early infection of endothelial cell monolayers with Herpes simplex virus type 1 (HSV-1) or cytomegalovirus (CMV) results in an increased monocyte (MC) and polymorphonuclear leukocyte (PMN) adherence…"

217. Key NS, Vercellotti GM, Winkelmann JC, Moldow CF, Goodman JL, Esmon NL, Esmon CT, Jacob HS: Infection of vascular endothelial cells with herpes simplex virus enhances tissue factor

activity and reduces thrombomodulin expression. Proc Natl Acad Sci U S A 1990 Sep; 87(18): 7095–9

"In a previous study, we found that cultured human umbilical vein endothelial cells (HUVECs) infected with herpes simplex virus 1 (HSV-1) became procoagulant, exemplified both by their enhanced assembly of the prothrombinase complex and by their inability to reduce adhesion of platelets. We now report two further procoagulant consequences of endothelial HSV infection: loss of surface thrombomodulin (TM) activity and induction of synthesis of tissue factor."

218. Saetta A, Fanourakis G, Agapitos E, Davaris PS Atherosclerosis of the carotid artery: absence of evidence for CMV involveme tin atheroma formation. Cardiovasc Pathol 2000 Ma Jun; 9(3): 181–3

"None of the specimens examined gave a positive result, indicating absence of CMV particles or CMV DNA sequences in the walls of carotid arteries. This finding suggests it is possible that CMV infection may not play a major role in the formation of atheroma. Therefore, further investigation is required in order to clarify the etiology of atherosclerosis."

219. al-Amro AA, al-Jafari AA, al-Fagih MR, Tajeldin M, Qavi HB: Frequency of occurrence of cytomegalovirus and *Chlamydia pneumoniae* in lymphocytes of atherosclerotic patients. Cent Eur J Public Health 2001 May; 9(2): 106–8

"These results demonstrate that atherosclerotic patients are more frequently infected with CMV or *C. pneumoniae* or both."

220. Reuters Health: Cytomegalovirus linked to heart disease. July 13, 2000

"In a study of more than 700 men and women, those with the highest levels of antibodies to CMV had a 76% greater chance of developing heart disease over 5 years, compared with adults who had few or no CMV antibodies. The presence of antibodies indicates that a previous infection has occurred."

221. Sorlie PD, Adam E, Melnick SL, Folsom A, Skelton T, Chambless LE, Barnes R, Melnick JL: Cytomegalovirus/herpesvirus and carotid atherosclerosis: the ARIC Study. J Med Virol 1994 Jan; 42(1): 33–7

    "These results suggest a modest association between CMV and asymptomatic carotid wall thickening consistent with early atherosclerosis."

222. Espinola-Klein C, Rupprecht HJ, Blankenberg S, Bickel C, Kopp H, Rippin G, Hafner G, Pfeifer U, Meyer J: Are morphological or functional changes in the carotid artery wall associated with *Chlamydia pneumoniae, Helicobacter pylori*, cytomegalovirus, or herpes simplex virus infection? Stroke 2000 Sep; 31(9): 2127–33

    "We found a significant association of IgG antibodies against *C. pneumoniae* and CMV with early and advanced carotid atherosclerosis."

223. Gattone M, Iacoviello L, Colombo M, Castelnuovo AD, Soffantino F, Gramoni A, Picco D, Benedetta M, Giannuzzi P *Chlamydia pneumoniae* and cytomegalovirus seropositivity, inflammatory markers, and the risk of myocardial infarction at a young age. Am Heart J 2001 Oct; 142(4): 633–40

    "After adjustment for confounders, seropositivity to both *Cp* and CMV infections is associated with the diagnosis of premature MI. The combination of both infections is associated with an enhanced inflammatory response and a markedly increased risk of premature MI."

224. Muhlestein JB, Horne BD, Carlquist JF, Madsen TE, Bair TL, Pearson RR, Anderson JL: Cytomegalovirus seropositivity and C-reactive protein have independent and combined predictive

value for mortality in patients with angiographically demostrated coronary artery disease. Circulation 2000 Oct 17; 102(16): 1917–23

"CMV seropositivity and elevated CRP, especially when in combination, are strong, independent predictors of mortality in patients with CAD. This suggests an interesting hypothesis that a chronic, smoldering infection (CMV) might have the capacity to accelerate the atherothrombotic process."

225. Hu W, Liu J, Niu S, Liu M, Shi H, Wei L: Prevalence of CMV in arterial walls and leukocytes in patients with atherosclerosis. Chin Med J (Engl) 2001 Nov; 114(11): 1208–10

"CMV plays an important role in the pathologic process of the atherosclerosis and the atherosclerotic cerebral infarction."

226. Associated Press: Viruses may cause heart disease, new study says. August 28, 1996

"A study published Thursday found that the risk of angioplasty failure is five times higher than usual if people are infected with CMV."

227. Blum A, Giladi M, Weinberg M, Kaplan G, Pasternack H, Laniado S, Miller H: High anti-cytomegalovirus (CMV) IgG antibody titer is associated with coronary artery disease and may predict post-coronary balloon angioplasty restenosis. Am J Cardiol 1998 Apr 1; 81(7): 866–8

"...patients with high antibody titer...had a higher restenosis rate than seropositive patients with a low antibody titer..."

228. Doctor's Guide (PSL Consulting Group Inc.): Routine Use of Cholesterol-Lowering Drug Improves Outcomes for Heart Transplant Recipients. September 6, 1995

"Half of all heart transplant patients have significant coronary blockages within five years of surgery and the problem is one of the leading causes of death among heart transplant recipients."

229. Koskinen P, Lemstrom K, Mattila S, Hayry P, Nieminen MS: Cytomegalovirus infection associated accelerated heart allograft arteriosclerosis may impair the late function of the graft. Clin Transplant 1996 Dec; 10(6 Pt 1): 487–93

    "Taken together, these results suggest that CMV infection is associated with intense cardiac allograft arteriosclerosis affecting the whole coronary tree soon after transplantation."

230. Loebe M, Schuler S, Zais O, Warnecke H, Fleck E, Hetzer R: Role of cytomegalovirus infection in the development of coronary artery disease in the transplanted heart. J Heart Transplant 1990 Nov–Dec; 9(6): 707–11

    "Cytomegalovirus infection seems to be an important factor in the development of accelerated graft arteriosclerosis in the transplanted heart."

231. Grattan MT, Moreno-Cabral CE, Starnes VA, Oyer PE, Stinson EB, Shumway NE: Cytomegalovirus infection is associated with cardiac allograft rejection and atherosclerosis. JAMA 1989 Jun 23–30; 261(24): 3561–6

232. Woods HR: Take Heart. Standford Medicine Winter 1999/2000

    "Analysis of many risk factors found that the most significant predictors of transplant coronary disease in CMV-infected patients were not receiving ganciclovir (almost triple the risk)…"

233. Pellicano R, Mazzarello MG, Morelloni S, Allegri M, Arena V, Ferrari M, Rizzetto M, Ponzetto A: Acute myocardial infarction and *Helicobacter pylori* seropositivity. Int J Clin Lab Res 1999; 29(4): 141–4

"In conclusion, patients with acute myocardial infarction had a significantly higher prevalence of *Helicobacter pylori* infection than the control population."

234. Danesh J, Youngman L, Clark S, Parish S, Peto R, Collins R: *Helicobacter pylori* infection and early onset myocardial infartion: case-control and sibling pairs study. BMJ 1999 Oct 30; 319(7218): 1157–62

    "In the context of results from other relevant studies, these two studies suggest a moderate association between coronary heart disease and *H. pylori* seropositivity that cannot be fully accounted for by other risk factors."

235. Pieniazek P, Karczewska E, Duda A, Tracz W, Pasowicz M, Konturek SJ: Association of *Helicobacter pylori* infection with coronary heart disease. J Physiol Pharmacol 1999 Dec; 50(5): 743–51

    "Present data show that there is significant link between CAD and *HP* infection."

236. Kahan T, Lundman P, Olsson G, Wendt M: Greater than normal prevalence of seropositivity for *Helicobacter pylori* among patients who have suffered myocardial infarction. Coron Artery Dis 2000 Oct; 11(7): 523–6

    "The positive association between seropositivity for *H. pylori* and having previously suffered acute myocardial infarction found in this study provides further support for the hypothesis that there is a causal association between chronic infection with *H. pylori* and the development of coronary heart disease."

237. Hara K, Morita Y, Kamihata H, Iwasaka T, Takahashi H: Evidence for infection with *Helicobacter pylori* in patients with acute myocardial infarction. Clin Chim Acta 2001 Nov; 313 (1–2): 87–94

"These results suggest that an increased IgA antibody titer, which is an index of the active phase of *HP* infection, should be an etiological marker for acute myocardial infarction."

238. Zhu J, Quyyumi AA, Muhlestein JB, Nieto FJ, Horne BD, Zalles-Ganley A, Anderson JL, Epstein SE: Lack of association of *Helicobacter pylori* infection with coronary artery disease and frequency of acute myocardial infarction or death. Am J Cardiol 2002 Jan 15; 89(2): 155–8

    "Our data suggest that prior infection with *H. pylori* is not a major factor determining either risk of CAD, AMI, or death in patients with CAD."

239. Gunn M, Stephens JC, Thompson JR, Rathbone BJ, Samani NJ: Significant association of cagA positive *Helicobacter pylori* strains with risk of premature myocardial infarction. Heart 2000 Sep; 84(3): 267–71

    "The association of chronic *H. pylori* infection with risk of myocardial infarction appears to be restricted to cagA bearing strains. The association is age dependent and stronger in younger subjects. Genetic heterogeneity of *H. pylori* may explain some of the discordant findings with regard to the association of *H. pylori* with coronary heart disease."

240. Pasceri V, Cammarota G, Patti g, Cuoco L, Gasbarrini A, Grillo R, Fedeli G, Gasbarrini G, Maseri A: Association of Virulent *Helicobacter pylori* Strains With Ischemic Heart Disease. Circulation. 1998; 97:1675–1679

    "To the best of our knowledge, this is the first study to have shown an association between ischemic heart disease and chronic infection by virulent strains of a micro-organism, supporting the hypothesis that the pathogenetic link between chronic infections and ischemic heart disease may be the chronic inflammatory response caused by these infections."

241. Figura N, Palazzuoli A, Faglia S, Lenzi C, Borrello F, Palazzuoli V, Nami R, Dal Canto N, De Regis F, Vaira D, Gennari L, Giordano N, Gennari C: Infection by CagA-positive *Helicbacter pylori* strains in patients with ischemic heart disease: prevalence and association with exercise-induced electrocardiographic abnormalities. Dig Dis Sci 2002 Apr; 47(4): 831–6

    "In conclusion, genetic heterogeneity of *H. pylori* could possibly explain some conflicting results concerning the association of *H. pylori* infection with IHD. Coronary vessels of IHD patients infected by CagA-positive *H. pylori* strains may be damaged more severely than those of uninfected patients."

242. Grau AJ, Buggle F, Lichy C, Brandt T, Becher H, Rudi J: *Helicobacter pylori* infection as an independent risk factor for cerebral ischemia of atherothrombotic origin. J Neurol Sci 2001 May 1; 186(1–2): 1–5

    "*H. pylori* seropositivity may be an independent risk factor for stroke of atherothrombotic origin."

243. Ponzetto A, Marchet A, Pellicano R, Lovera N, Chianale G, Nobili M, Rizzetto M, Cerrato P: Association of *Helicobacter pylori* infection with ischemic stroke of non-cardiac origin: the BAT.MA.N. project study. Hepatogastroenterology 2002 May–Jun; 49(45): 631–4

    "CONCLUSIONS: *H. pylori* infection appears to be signifcantly more frequent in middle-aged patients with acute ischemic stroke than in controls."

244. Ameriso SF, Fridman EA, Leiguarda RC, Sevlever GE: Detection of *Helicobacter pylori* in human carotid atherosclerotic plaques. Stroke 2001 Feb; 32(2): 385–91

    "CONCLUSIONS: *H. pylori* is present in a substantial number of carotid atherosclerotic lesions and is associated with features of inflammatory cell response. This study provides additional evidence of the relationship between *H. pylori* infection and atherosclerotic disease."

245. FDA Consumer magazine. Combination Drug Treatment Approved for Ulcers July–August 1996

    "The first antibiotic treatment for eradicating *Helicobacter pylori*, the bacteria associated with active duodenal ulcers, has been approved by FDA."

246. Armitage GC: Periodontal infections and cardiovascular diease—how strong is the association? Oral Dis 2000 Nov; 6(6): 335–50

247. Zhu J, Quyyumi AA, Norman JE, Csako G, Waclawiw MA, Shearer GM, Epstein SE: Effects of total pathogen burden on coronary artery disease risk and C-reactive protein levels. Am J Cardiol 2000 Jan 15; 85(2): 140–6

248. Zhu J, Nieto FJ, Horne BD, Anderson JL, Muhlestein JB, Epstein SE: Prospective study of pathogen burden and risk of myocardial infarction or death. Circulation 2001 Jan 2; 103(1): 45-51

    "The results suggest that infection plays an important role in *incident* MI or death and that the risk posed by infection is independently related to the pathogen burden."

249. Rupprecht HJ, Blankenberg S, Bickel C, Rippin G, Hafner G, Prellwitz W, Schlumberger W, Meyer J: Impact of viral and bacterial infectious burden on long-term prognosis in patients with coronary artery disease. 296: Circulation 2001 Jul 3; 104(1): 25–31

    "These results support the hypothesis that the number of infectious pathogens to which an individual has been exposed independently contributes to the long-term prognosis in patients with documented CAD."

250. Espinola-Klein C, Rupprecht HJ, Blankenberg S, Bickel C, Kopp H, Rippin G, Victor A, Hafner G, Schlumberger W, Meyer J: Impact of infectious burden on extent and long-term prognosis of atherosclerosis. Circulation 2002 Jan 1; 105(1): 15–21

251. Prasad A, Zhu J, Halcox JP, Waclawiw MA, Epstein SE, Quyyumi AA: Predisposition to atherosclerosis by infections: role of endothelial dysfunction. Circulation 2002 Jul 9; 106(2): 184–90

    "The immunoglobulin-G antibody response to multiple pathogens (pathogen burden) is an independent risk factor for endothelial dysfunction and the presence and severity of CAD. Endothelial dysfunction provides the crucial link by which pathogens may contribute to atherogenesis."

252. Jeffrey T. Kuvin, MD Carey D. Kimmelstiel MD: Infectious causes of atherosclerosis. American Heart Journal Volume 137 • Number 2 • February 1999

253. Hooper, J: A New Germ Theory. The Atlantic Monthly February 1999

254. Campbell LA, Kuo CC, Grayston JT: *Chlamydia pneumoniae* and cardiovascular disease. Emerg Infect Dis 1998 Oc Dec; 4(4): 571–9

    "Seroepidemiologic studies have associated *C. pneumoniae* antibody with coronary artery disease, myocardial infarction, carotid artery disease, and cerebrovascular disease."

255. Maass M: Persistence of *Chlamydia pneumoniae* in human arteriosclerotic plaque substance. Evidence and consequences. Herz 1998 May; 23(3): 178–84

    "Serological response to *Chlamydia pneumoniae* statistically indicates an increased risk of coronary artery disease and mycardial infarction."

256. Fagerberg B, Gnarpe J, Gnarpe H, Agewall S, Wikstrand J: *Chlamydia pneumoniae* but Not Cytomegalovirus Antibodies Are Associated With Future Risk of Stroke and Cardiovascular Disease : A Prospective Study in Middle-Aged to Elderly Men With Treated Hypertension. Stroke 1999 Feb; 30(2): 299–305

"Seropositivity for *C. pneumoniae*, but not for CMV, was associated with an increased risk for future cardiovascular disease and, in particular, stroke."

257. Cook PJ, Honeybourne D, Lip GY, Beevers DG, Wise R, Davies P: *Chlamydia pneumoniae* antibody titers are significantly associated with acute stroke and transient cerebral ischemia: the West Birmingham Stroke Project. Stroke 1998 Feb; 29(2): 404–10

"These data support the association of cerebral vascular disease with previous *C. pneumoniae* infection and the association of stroke and transient cerebral ischemia with recrudescence of infection."

258. Wimmer ML, Sandmann-Strupp R, Saikku P, Haberl RL: Association of chlamydial infection with cerebrovascular disease. Stroke 1996 Dec; 27(12): 2207–10

"We conclude that chronic infection with *C. pneumoniae* is associated with an increased risk of stroke and transient ischemic events."

259. Dake Y, Enomoto T, Shibano A, Sakoda T, Saito Y, Takahashi M: Epidemiologic study of *Chlamydia pneumoniae* with ELISA. Nippon Jibiinkoka Gakkai Kaiho 1998 Nov; 101(11): 1316–20

"It has been reported that infections from this bacterium are prevalent worldwide and that the proportion of the population having the antibody is high. It is, however, difficult to identify the pathogen by routine bacterial examination because it is an obligate cytozoic bacterium."

260. Lee Ann Campbell, Cho-Chou Kuo, and J. Thomas Grayston: *Chlamydia pneumoniae* and Cardiovascular Disease. Emerging Infectious Diseases Volume 4, Number 4 October–December 1998

    "The organism has been found in atherosclerotic lesions in 257 (52%) of 497 tissue specimens."

261. Qavi HB, Melnick JL, Adam E, Debakey ME: Frequency of coexistence of cytomegalovirus and *Chlamydia pneumoniae* in atherosclerotic plaques. Cent Eur J Public Health 2000 May; 8(2): 71–3

    "These results present evidence that CMV DNA and/or *C. pneumoniae* DNA can be detected in 71% of carotid atherosclerotic plaques and in some instances DNA of both agents in the same tissue."

262. Kuo CC, Grayston JT, Campbell LA, Goo YA, Wissler RW, Benditt EP: *Chlamydia pneumoniae* (TWAR) in coronary arteries of young adults (15–34 years old). Proc Natl Acad Sci U S A 1995 Jul 18; 92(15): 6911–4

    "…none of the 31 normal-appearing coronary samples were positive….Thus, *C. pneumoniae* is found in coronary lesions in young adults with atherosclerosis but is not found in normal-appearing coronary arteries of both persons with and without other evidence of atherosclerosis."

263. Taylor-Robinson D, Thomas BJ, Goldin R, Stanbridge R: *Chlamydia pneumoniae* in infrequently examined blood vessels. J Clin Pathol 2002 Mar; 55(3): 218–20

    "*Chlamydia pneumoniae* is often present in diseased areas of arteries, including the internal mammary arteries, and even in diseased areas of veins. It is not present in apparently healthy areas of either type of vessel."

264. Muhlestein JB, Hammond EH, Carlquist JF, Radicke E, Thomson MJ, Karagounis LA, Woods ML, Anderson JL: Increased incidence of *Chlamydia* species within the coronary arteries of patients with symptomatic atherosclerotic versus other forms of cardiovascular disease. J Am Coll Cardiol 1996 Jun; 27(7): 1555–61

"In contrast, only 1 (4%) of 24 nonatherosclerotic coronary specimens showed any evidence of *Chlamydia*...This high incidence of *Chlamydia* only in coronary arteries diseased by atherosclerosis suggests an etiologic role for *Chlamydia* infection in the development of coronary atherosclerosis that should be further studied."

265. Campbell LE, Cho-Chou Kuo, and J. Thomas Grayston: *Chlamydia pneumoniae* and Cardiovascular Disease. Emerging Infectious Diseases Volume 4, Number 4 October–December 1998

"In contrast, the organism has been found in only 5% of tissues that appear normal. Remarkably, the detection in diseased arterial tissue compared to normal arterial tissue represents an odds ratio of 10."

266. Muhlestein, JB: The Link Between *Chlamydia pneumoniae* and Atherosclerosis. Infect Med 14(5): 380–382,392,426, 1997

267. Ramirez JA: Isolation of *Chlamydia pneumoniae* from the coronary artery of a patient with coronary atherosclerosis. The *Chlamydia pneumoniae*/Atherosclerosis Study Group.Ann Intern Med 1996 Dec 15; 125(12): 979–82

"This study provides direct evidence of the presence of viable *C. pneumoniae* in atheromatous lesions. A chronic inflammatory response caused by a persistent infection of the coronary arteries may explain the link between *C. pneumoniae* and atherosclerosis."

268. Jackson LA, Campbell LA, Kuo CC, Rodriguez DI, Lee A, Grayston JT: Isolation of *Chlamydia pneumoniae* from a carotid endarterectomy specimen. J Infect Dis 1997 Jul; 176(1): 292–5

"*C. pneumoniae* was detected by PCR or ICC (or both) in 11 (69%) of 16 other endarterectomy specimens tested by both of these methods. These results provide further evidence for an association of *C. pneumoniae* and atherosclerosis by confiring the presence of viable bacteria within atherosclerotic plaque."

269. Melissa K. Conrad, MD, John T. Sinnott, IV, MD, FACP, and Michael Albrink, MD, FACS, and Pamela Sakalosky, BS: Infections in Oncology: Gastric Cancer: An Infectious Disease? Cancer Control Journal Vol 2, No. 6 November/December 1995

270. Saikku P, Laitinen K, Leinonen M: Animal models for *Chlamydia pneumoniae* infection. Atherosclerosis 1998 Oct; 140 Suppl 1:S17–9

271. Fong IW, Chiu B, Viira E, Fong MW, Jang D, Mahony J: Rabbit model for *Chlamydia pneumoniae* infection. J Clin Microbiol 1997 Jan; 35(1): 48–52

"Two study rabbits demonstrated, on histology, early and intermediate lesions of atherosclerosis: one animal (day 7) showed the accumulation of foamy macrophages (fatty streak) in the arch of the aorta, and the other animal (day 14) showed spindle-cell proliferation of smooth muscle cells (intermediate lesion)…"

272. Laitinen K, Laurila A, Pyhala L, Leinonen M, Saikku P: *Chlamydia pneumoniae* infection induces inflammatory changes in the aortas of rabbits. Infect Immun 1997 Nov; 65(11): 4832–5

273. Muhlestein JB, Anderson JL, Hammond EH, Zhao L, Trehan S, Schwobe EP, Carlquist JF: Infection with *Chlamydia pneumniae* accelerates the development of atherosclerosis and treament with azithromycin prevents it in a rabbit model. Circulation 1998 Feb 24; 97(7): 633–6

"Intranasal *C. pneumoniae* infection accelerates intimal thicke ing in rabbits given a modestly cholesterol-enhanced diet."

274. Muhlestein JB, Anderson JL, Hammond EH, Zhao L, Trehan S, Schwobe EP, Carlquist JF: Infection with *Chlamydia pneumoniae* accelerates the development of atherosclerosis and treatment with azithromycin prevents it in a rabbit model. Circulation 1998 Feb 24; 97(7): 633–6

"These findings are best explained by assigning a causative role to *C. pneumoniae* in the atherosclerotic process..."

275. Brown CJ: Catching a culprit in the act. Can Med Assoc J 1997; 156(3): 341

"Of 11 rabbits infected, one had a fatty streak and evidence of *C. pneumoniae* in the aorta and another had a grade III atherosclerotic lesion, from which *C. pneumoniae* was cultured."

276. Stille W, Dittmann R: Atherosclerosis as Consequence of Chronic Infection by *Chlamydia Pneumoniae*. Herz 23:185—192, (1998)

277. Stille W, Stephen C: Atherosclerosis—a chronic infectious disease caused by *Chlamydia pneumoniae*. Versicherungsmedizin 1999 Mar 1; 51(1): 12–7

"The reduction of incidence of atherosclerotic diseases since the 1960s, probably due to advanced antibiotic therapy."

278. Meier CR, Derby LE, Jick SS, Vasilakis C, Jick H: Antibiotics and risk of subsequent first-time acute myocardial infarction. JAMA 1999 Feb 3; 281(5): 427–3

279. Reuters Health: Antibiotics Tied To Reduced Heart Attack Risk. Feb 02, 1999 SOURCE: The Journal of the American Medical Association 1999; 281:427–431.

"The study findings fit well with the hypothesis that respiratory tract infections with *C. pneumoniae* may play a role in the etiology of ischemic heart disease, they conclude."

280. Lee Ann Campbell, Cho-Chou Kuo, and J. Thomas Grayston: *Chlamydia pneumoniae* and Cardiovascular Disease Emerging Infectious Disease. Volume 4 Number 4

"Three months after the final inoculation, the maximal intimal thickness (MIT) of the thoracic aortas increased in infected rabbits but not in controls. The MIT of azithromycin-treated rabbits was less than that of untreated infected rabbits and similar to that of controls."

281. Rizzato G, Montemurro L, Fraioli P, Montanari G, Fanti D, Pozzoli R, Magliano E: Efficacy of a three day course of azithrmycin in moderately severe community-acquired pneumonia. Eur Respir J. 1995; 8:398–402

282. Gupta S, Leatham EW, Carrington D, Mendall MA, Kaski JC, Camm AJ: Elevated *Chlamydia pneumoniae* antibodies, cardiovascular events, and azithromycin in male survivors of myocardial infarction. Circulation 1997 Jul 15; 96(2): 404–7

"The incidence of adverse cardiovascular events (over a mean follow-up period of 18+/-4 months) was recorded and shown to increase with increasing anti-*Cp* titre: *Cp*-ve, n=4 (7%); *Cp*-I, n=11 (15%); *Cp*+ve-NR, n=6 (30%); and *Cp*+ve-P, n=5 (25%). *Cp*+ve-NR and *Cp*+ve-P groups had a fourfold-increased risk for adverse cardiovascular events compared with the *Cp*-ve group (odds ratio [OR], 4.2; 95% confidence interval [CI], 1.2 to 15.5; P=.03)."

283. UK News Electronic Telegraph Wednesday 21 May 1997 Issue 726

"In the following 18 months, they had four times fewer admisions to hospital for cardiac problems, such as another heart attack or angina, than 20 other infected patients given a placebo dose, said Dr Sandeep Gupta, a British Heart Foundation research fellow at St George's."

284. Gupta S, Leatham EW, Carrington D, Mendall MA, Kaski JC, Camm AJ: Elevated *Chlamydia pneumoniae* antibodies, cardiovascular events, and azithromycin in male survivors of myocardial infarction. Circulation. 1997; 96:404–407.

285. Jackson LA, Wang S-P, Douglas K, Cooke DB, Grayston JT: Azithromycin treatment following percutaneous coronary revascularization procedures: a pilot study. Detection of *Chlamdia pneumoniae* bacteremia in patients with symptomatic coronary atherosclerosis. Abstracts of the 4th International Conference on the Macrolides, Azalides, Streptogramins and Ketolides; 1998; Barcelona, Spain. 1998; Abstract 4.16.

286. Melissano G, Blasi F, Esposito G, Tarsia P, Dordoni L, Arosio C, Tshomba Y, Fagetti L, Allegra L, Chiesa R: *Chlamydia pnemoniae* eradication from carotid plaques. Eur J Vasc Endovasc Surg 1999 Oct; 18(4): 355–9

"Roxithromycin seems effective in reducing the bacterial burden of *C. pneumoniae* within atherosclerotic plaques..."

287. Zoler, M: Macrolide Antibiotic Benefits Unstable Angina. Family Practice News November 1,1997

288. Henahan, Sean: Antibiotics for Heart Disease? Academic Excellence Science Updates August 28, 1997(**www.accessexcellence.org/WN/SUA11/roxis897.html**)

"It may be that we are seeing the beginning of a new era in the treatment of symptomatic atherosclerosis. Looking ahead, this approach might lead to new ways of intervening earlier in the process of artery hardening, possibly even a preventive vaccine."

289. Dr. Christopher O'Conner announced the results of the WIZARD trial on March 18, 2002 at the annual meeting of the American College of Cardiology. Johns Hopkins Division of Infectious Diseases Antibiotic Guide News March, 2002

290. Muhlestein JB, Anderson JL, Carlquist JF, Salunkhe K, Horne BD, Pearson RR, Bunch TJ, Allen A, Trehan S, Nielson C: Randomized secondary prevention trial of azithromycin in patients with coronary artery disease: primary clinical results of the ACADEMIC study. Circulation. 2000 Oct 10; 102(15): 1742-3.

"This study suggests that antibiotic therapy with azithromycin is not associated with marked early reductions (>/=50%) in ischemic events as suggested by an initial published report. However, a clinically worthwhile benefit (i.e., 20% to 30%) is still possible, although it may be delayed."

291. Parchure N, Zouridakis E, Kaski JC: Effect of Azithromycin Treatment on Endothelial Function in Patients With Coronary Artery Disease and Evidence of *Chlamydia Pneumoniae Infection*. Circulation 2002; 105:1298

"Our findings indicate that treatment with azithromycin has a favorable effect on endothelial function in patients with documented coronary artery disease and evidence of *CPn* infection irrespective of antibody titer levels."

292. Sinisalo J, Mattila K, Valtonen V, Anttonen O, Juvonen J, Melin J, Vuorinen-Markkola H, Nieminen MS,. Effect of 3 Months of Antimicrobial Treatment With Clarithromycin in Acute Non-Q-Wave Coronary Syndrome. Circulation. 2002; 105:1555

"Clarithromycin appears to reduce the risk of ischemic cardiovascular events in patients presenting with acute non-Q-wave infarction or unstable angina. No signs of this effect diminishing were observed during follow-up."

293. American Heart Association Press Release Three-Month Antibiotic Treatment Reduces Risk of Future Heart Attack Marcg 12, 2002

294. J. Gutiérrez, J. Linares-Palomino, C. Lopez-Espada, M. Rodríguez, E. Ros, G. Piédrola, M. del C. Maroto: *Chlamydia pneumoniae* DNA in the Arterial Wall of Patients with Periphral Vascular Disease. Infection 2001 Vol 29 No 4 pp 196–20

295. Wiesli P, Czerwenka W, Meniconi A, Maly FE, Hoffmann U, Vetter W, Schulthess G: Roxithromycin treatment prevents progression of peripheral arterial occlusive disease in *Chlamydia pneumoniae* seropositive men: a randomized, double-blind, placebo-controlled trial. Circulation 2002 Jun 4; 105(22): 2646–52

    "Carotid plaque areas monitored over 6 months decreased in the roxithromycin group (mean relative value, 94. 94.4%) but remained constant in the placebo group (100.2%). Regression of carotid plaque size observed in roxithromycin-treated patients was significant for soft plaques. CONCLUSIONS: This study indicates that macrolide treatment for 1 month is effective in preventing *C. pneumoniae* seropositive men from progression of lower limb atherosclerosis for several years."

296. Sousa JE, Costa MA, Abizaid AC, Rensing BJ, Abizaid AS, Tanajura LF, Kozuma K, Van Langenhove G, Sousa AG, Falotico R, Jaeger J, Popma JJ, Serruys PW: Sustained suppression of neointimal proliferation by sirolimus-eluting stents: one-year angiographic and intravascular ultrasound follow-up. Circulation 2001 Oct 23; 104(17): 2007–11

297. Associated Press: Coated Stents Seem to Keep Arteries Open. The New York Times March 18, 2002

298. WebMD: Doctors Excited by "Breakthrough" Heart Stent. Sept. 4, 2001

299. Foreman J: Coated Stents Show Huge Promise. **www.myhealthsense.com** May 7. 2002

300. Reuters News Agency: Antibiotics appear to cut heart risks. Washington Times August 20, 2002

301. Center for Cardiovascular Education Commentary for "How *Chlamydia* Bacteria Might Cause Heart Disease" May 25, 1999 (**www.heartinfo.com/news99/chlam052599.htm**)

"Rheumatic heart disease, once a common heart ailment following streptococcus infection, is caused by a similarity between the streptococcus organism and a heart muscle protein. The body mounts an immune response to the streptococcus and attacks the heart muscle in the process."

302. Steeg CN, Walsh CA, Glickstein JS: Rheumatic fever: No cause for complacence. Patient Care July 30, 2000 40–61

"Since no definitive diagnostic test for rheumatic fever exists, the precise incidence is uncertain."

303. US News and World Report On-Line Edition: Fight germs, fight heart disease? March 13, 2000

304. Itzhaki RF, Lin WR, Shang D, Wilcock GK, Faragher B, Jamieson GA: Herpes simplex virus type 1 in brain and risk of Alzheimer's disease. Lancet 1997 Jan 25; 349(9047): 241–4

305. Arvanitakis Z: Dementia And Vascular Disease. Jacksonville Medicine Volume 51, Number 2 February, 2000

306. Kalaria RN: The role of cerebral ischemia in Alzheimer's disease. Neurobiol Aging 2000 Mar–Apr; 21(2): 321–30

307. Skoog I: Vascular aspects in Alzheimer's disease. Neural Transm Suppl 2000; 59:37–43

308. Breteler MM: Vascular risk factors for Alzheimer's disease: an epidemiologic perspective. Neurobiol Aging 2000 Mar Apr; 21(2): 153–60

309. PBS NEWSHOUR: New Hope. airing March 12, 1997

310. TIME Magazine: A Gift of Love. March 24, 1997 VOL. 149 NO. 12

311. Alzheimers.com: Clean Arteries Help Preserve a Clear Mind. March 29, 1997

312. Reuters: Strokes Aggravate Alzheimer's. March 11, 1997

313. American Heart Association Journal Report: What you do know (quitting smoking, lowering blood pressure) can help prevent what you don't know (silent strokes). May 7, 1998

314. AScribe Newswire: Anti-inflammatory drug holds promise of sharply reducing risk for Alzheimer's disease researcher discover. August 7, 2000

315. McGeer EG: Brain inflammation in Alzheimer disease and the therapeutic implications. Alzheimer Dis Assoc Disord 2000; 14 Suppl 1:S54–61

"This hypothesis is supported by a number of epidemiological studies suggesting that the prevalence of AD in persons is reduced by 40–50% in persons using antiinflammatory drugs."

316. McGeer EG, McGeer PL: The importance of inflammatory mechanisms in Alzheimer disease. Exp Gerontol 1998 Aug; 33(5): 371–8

317. Akiyama H, Barger S, Barnum S, Bradt B, Bauer J, Cole GM, Cooper NR, Eikelenboom P, Emmerling M, Fiebich BL, Finch CE, Frautschy S, Griffin WS, Hampel H, Hull M, Landreth G, Lue L, Mrak R, Mackenzie IR, McGeer PL, O'Banion MK,

Pachter J, Pasinetti G, Plata-Salaman C, Rogers J, Rydel R, Shen Y, Streit W, Strohmeyer R, Tooyoma I, Van Muiswinkel FL, Veerhuis R, Walker D, Webster S, Wegrzyniak B, Wenk G, Wyss-Coray T: Inflammation and Alzheimer's disease. Neurobiol Aging 2000 May Jun; 21(3): 383–421

318. McGeer PL, McGeer EG, Yasojima K: Alzheimer disease and neuroinflammation. J Neural Transm Suppl 2000; 59:53–7

319. Lin WR, Shang D, Itzhaki RF: Neurotropic viruses and Alzheimer disease. Interaction of Herpes simplex type 1 virus and apolipoprotein E in the etiology of the disease. Mol Chem Neuropathol 1996 May–Aug; 28(1–3): 135–41

320. Leissring MA, Sugarman MC, LaFerla FM: Herpes simplex virus infections and Alzheimer's disease. Implications for drugtreatment and immunotherapy. Drugs Aging 1998 Sep; 13(3): 193–8

321. Reuters Health: Cold Sore Virus Mimics Alzheimer's Protein. Tuesday, January 30, 2001

322. Espinola-Klein C, Rupprecht H, Blankenberg S, Bickel C, Kopp H, Rippin G, Hafner G, Pfeifer U, Meyer J: Are Morphological or Functional Changes in the Carotid Artery Wall Associated With *Chlamydia pneumoniae, Helicobacter pylori*, Cytomegalovirus, or Herpes simplex Virus Infection? Stroke. 2000; 31:1521

323. Elkind MSV, Lin I, Grayston JT, Sacco RL: *Chlamydia pneumoniae* and the Risk of First Ischemic Stroke. Stroke 1999; 30: 299–305

324. Cook PJ, Honeybourne D, Lip GYH, Beevers DG, Wise R, Davies P: *Chlamydia pneumoniae* Antibody Titers Are Significantly Associated With Acute Stroke and Transient Cerebral Ischemia. Stroke 2000 Jul; 31(7): 1521–5

325. Balin BJ, Gerard HC, Arking EJ, Appelt DM, Branigan PJ, Abrams JT, Whittum-Hudson JA, Hudson AP: Identification

and localization of *Chlamydia pneumoniae* in the Alzheimer's brain. Med Microbiol Immunol (Berl) 1998 Jun; 187(1): 23–42

326. Reuters New Service: Common microbe may have role in Alzheimer's—study. August 11, 1998

327. Science News November 21, 1998 Vol. 154, No. 21, p. 325

328. Ring RH, Lyons JM: Failure to detect *Chlamydia pneumoniae* in the late-onset Alzheimer's brain. J Clin Microbiol 2000 Jul; 38(7): 2591–4

329. Mahony J, Woulfe J, Munoz D, Chong S, Browning D, Smieja M: *Chlamydia pneumoniae* in the brain of Alzheimer's disease patients. CACMID meeting in Ottawa: Nov. 4—7, 2000

330. Maugh T: Spreading a New Idea on Disease. Los Angeles Times April 22, 1999

331. Reuters Health: Gene linked to hormone replacement's heart effects. February 21, 2001

"In a recent study of women with heart disease—the HERS trial—hormone replacement therapy did not reduce the risk of heart attack. In fact, the risk increased during the first year of the study, although it declined later."

332. cbsnews.com: Red Flag On Hormone Replacement. July 9, 2002

333. Associated Press: Do your heart a favor: Skip the mental stress. June 5, 1996

334. Reuters Health: Imaging test predicts heart attack, stroke risk. January 6, 1999

335. Weitz JI: Diagnosis and Treatment of Chronic Arterial Insufficiency of the Lower Extremities: A Critical Review. AHA Medical/Scientific Statement Circulation. 1996; 94:3026–3049

"Because patients with either asymptomatic or symptomatic lower extremity arterial disease have widespread arterial disease, they have a significantly increased risk of stroke, myocardial infarction, and cardiovascular death."

336. Health Week Online: Beyond Cholesterol Washington Post Co. Program No. 411

337. Haney, DQ: Finding alters notion on heart attacks. Associated Press Aug 4, 2002

338. Great Smokies Connection Newsletter: Acute Phase Protein Offers Acute Insight Into Cardiovascular Disease May 16, 2001, Volume 12, Number 10

339. Peck, P: Blood Test Helps Identify Women at Risk for Heart Attack—Elevated Levels of a Specific Protein Predict Risk. WebMD Medical News March 22, 2000

340. Minnesota Health Technology Advisory Committee: C-Reactive Protein Screening of Coronary Artery Disease April 2002

341. Associated Press: Study questions need for low-salt diets. May 21, 1996

"Challenging the conventional wisdom among doctors and government experts, a study found that healthy people and even some patients with high blood pressure gain little from lowering the salt in their diet."

342. Dranov P: The Surprising Salt Shake-Up. Good Housekeeping August 1995

"The report, published in the June issue of Hypertension, found that patients with the lowest salt intake were actually four times more likely to have heart attacks than other participants."

343. Peduzzi P, Kamina A, Detre K: Twenty-two-year follow-up in the VA Cooperative Study of Coronary Artery Bypass Surgery for Stable Angina. Am J Cardiol 1998 Jun15; 81(12): 1393–9

"This trial provides strong evidence that initial bypass surgery did not improve survival for low-risk patients, and that it did not reduce the overall risk of myocardial infarction. Although there was an early survival benefit with surgery in high-risk patients (up to a decade), long-term survival rates became comparable in both treatment groups. In total, there were twice as many bypass procedures performed in the group assigned to surgery without any long-term survival or symptomatic benefit."

344. Heart Disease Weekly: Fat Particles Released During Heart Surgery Can Damage Brain. March 15, 2000
345. Family Practice News: October 15, 1997
346. Patient Care: November 30, 1997
347. Murdin AD, Gellin B, Brunham RC, et al.: Collaborative multidisciplinary workshop report: progress toward a *Chlamydia pneumoniae* vaccine. J Infect Dis 2000; 181 Suppl 3: S552–7.
348. Christiansen G, Pedersen AS, Hjerno K, Vandahl B, Birkelund S: Potential relevance of *Chlamydia pneumoniae* surface proteins to an effective vaccine. J Infect Dis 2000 Jun; 181 Suppl 3: S528–37
349. Makela PH: Is cardiovascular disease preventable by vaccination? Ann Med 1999 Feb; 31(1): 61–5
350. Plotkin SA: Vaccination against cytomegalovirus. Submitted by the author to the International Symposium on Infections and Atherosclerosis Organized by Fondation Marcel Mérieux And the French National Institute of Health and Scientific Research (Inserm) With the support of Pasteur Mérieux Connaught Les Pensières, Veyrier-du-Lac 6–9 December 1998

0-595-26220-1

Made in the USA
Columbia, SC
10 January 2020